CW01213253

Medical Robots and Devices:
New Developments and Advances

BIOMEDICAL ROBOTS AND DEVICES IN HEALTHCARE

Opportunities and Challenges for Future Applications

Edited by

FAIZ IQBAL

School of Engineering, University of Lincoln,
Lincoln, United Kingdom

PUSHPENDRA GUPTA

Department of Mechanical Engineering, Indian Institute of Technology Kharagpur, Kharagpur, West Bengal, India

VIDYAPATI KUMAR

Department of Mechanical Engineering, Indian Institute of Technology Kharagpur, Kharagpur, West Bengal, India

DILIP KUMAR PRATIHAR

Department of Mechanical Engineering, Indian Institute of Technology Kharagpur, Kharagpur, West Bengal, India

Series Editor

OLFA BOUBAKER

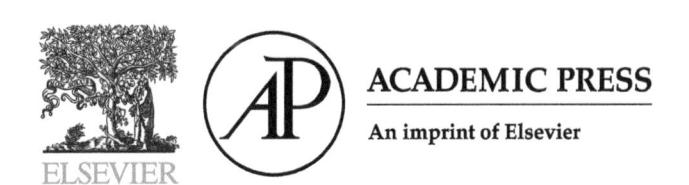

ACADEMIC PRESS

An imprint of Elsevier

ELSEVIER

Academic Press is an imprint of Elsevier
125 London Wall, London EC2Y 5AS, United Kingdom
525 B Street, Suite 1650, San Diego, CA 92101, United States
50 Hampshire Street, 5th Floor, Cambridge, MA 02139, United States

Copyright © 2025 Elsevier Inc. All rights are reserved, including those for text and data mining, AI training, and similar technologies.

Publisher's note: Elsevier takes a neutral position with respect to territorial disputes or jurisdictional claims in its published content, including in maps and institutional affiliations.

For accessibility purposes, images in this book are accompanied by alt text descriptions provided by Elsevier.

No part of this publication may be reproduced or transmitted in any form or by any means, electronic or mechanical, including photocopying, recording, or any information storage and retrieval system, without permission in writing from the publisher. Details on how to seek permission, further information about the Publisher's permissions policies and our arrangements with organizations such as the Copyright Clearance Center and the Copyright Licensing Agency, can be found at our website: www.elsevier.com/permissions.

This book and the individual contributions contained in it are protected under copyright by the Publisher (other than as may be noted herein).

Notices
Knowledge and best practice in this field are constantly changing. As new research and experience broaden our understanding, changes in research methods, professional practices, or medical treatment may become necessary.

Practitioners and researchers must always rely on their own experience and knowledge in evaluating and using any information, methods, compounds, or experiments described herein. In using such information or methods they should be mindful of their own safety and the safety of others, including parties for whom they have a professional responsibility.

To the fullest extent of the law, neither the Publisher nor the authors, contributors, or editors, assume any liability for any injury and/or damage to persons or property as a matter of products liability, negligence or otherwise, or from any use or operation of any methods, products, instructions, or ideas contained in the material herein.

ISBN 978-0-443-22206-1

For information on all Academic Press publications
visit our website at https://www.elsevier.com/books-and-journals

Publisher: Mara Conner
Acquisitions Editor: Sonnini Yura
Editorial Project Manager: Isabella Silva
Production Project Manager: Prem Kumar Kaliamoorthi
Cover Designer: Christian Bilbow

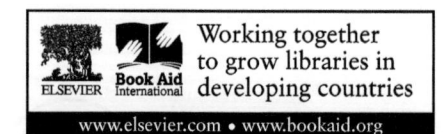

Typeset by STRAIVE, India
Transferred to Digital Printing 2024

Contents

Contributors ix

1. Soft robotics and computational intelligence: Transformative technologies reshaping biomedical engineering 1
Thomas Gaskins, Pushpendra Gupta, Vidyapati Kumar, Dilip Kumar Pratihar, and Faiz Iqbal

1.1 Introduction	1
1.2 Soft robotics: Brief introduction	5
1.3 Potential and ongoing applications of soft robots	6
1.4 Limitations in soft robotics	11
1.5 Summary	11
References	12

2. Advancements in biomedical devices: A comprehensive review 15
Mohammed Ubaid, Shadab Ahmad, Shanay Rab, Faiz Iqbal, and Yebing Tian

2.1 Introduction	15
2.2 Automation in biomedical devices	16
2.3 Technological advancements in automation—Cyber physical systems, robots, and integration with digital platforms, and their advantages	20
2.4 Case studies and applications	27
2.5 Regulatory and safety considerations	27
2.6 Drawbacks and challenges	30
2.7 Conclusion	35
References	35

3. Mathematics in biomedical robotics and devices and its role in healthcare delivery 41
Mo Sadique, Sapna Ratan Shah, and Sardar M.N. Islam

3.1 Introduction	41
3.2 Mathematical foundations of robotics and biomedical robotics	45
3.3 Applications of mathematics in biomedical robotics and devices	52
3.4 Future perspectives and limitations	58
3.5 Conclusion	59
References	60

4. Advancing ankle–foot orthosis design through biomechanics, robotics, and additive manufacturing: A review   65
Vidyapati Kumar, Pushpendra Gupta, and Dilip Kumar Pratihar

4.1 Introduction	65
4.2 Biomechanics of biological ankle and foot	67
4.3 Design of Orthoses for lower limb	69
4.4 Advances in orthotic manufacturing	74
4.5 Technical challenges	78
4.6 Summary	80
4.7 Future directions	81
References	82

5. Application of multibistatic frequency-domain measurements for enhanced medical sensing and imaging   85
Behnaz Sohani, Amir Rahmani, and Aliyu Aliyu

5.1 Introduction	85
5.2 Advantages of integrating multibistatic antennas in the development of detecting hemorrhagic brain strokes using a scanner	87
5.3 Experimental validation	101
5.4 Discussion	104
References	105

6. Sleep posture analysis: state-of-the-art and opportunities of wearable technologies from clinical, sensing and intelligent perception perspectives   109
Omar Elnaggar, Paolo Paoletti, Andrew Hopkinson, and Frans Coenen

6.1 Introduction	109
6.2 Health complications: A sleep behavior perspective	109
6.3 Sleep posture analysis: Current state of research	116
6.4 Monitoring sleep postures using wearable sensors	122
6.5 Temporal analysis of in-bed postural activity using wearable sensors	125
6.6 Conclusion	126
References	127

7. Comparative evaluation of deep learning techniques for multistage Alzheimer's prediction from magnetic resonance images   135
Pushpendra Gupta, Pradeep Nahak, Vidyapati Kumar, Dilip Kumar Pratihar, and Kalyanmoy Deb

7.1 Introduction	135
7.2 Methodology	137

7.3	Results and discussion	146
7.4	Conclusion	150
	References	150

8. Machine learning brain activation topography for individual skill classification: Need for leave-one-subject-out (LOSO) cross-validation — 153

Takahiro Manabe and Anirban Dutta

8.1	Background	153
8.2	Methods	155
8.3	Results	159
8.4	Discussion	162
	References	163

9. Transfer learning-based disease prognosis in Biomedicine 4.0: Challenges and opportunities — 165

Senthil Kumar Jagatheesaperumal and Sivasankar Ganesan

9.1	Introduction	165
9.2	Challenges in disease prognosis	166
9.3	AI/ML in disease prognosis	168
9.4	Transfer learning for disease prognosis	171
9.5	Enhancing disease prognosis models	174
9.6	Conclusion	177
	References	177

10. Voice and chatbot: A hybrid framework using XAI for improving mental health — 179

Debmitra Ghosh, Sayani Ghatak, and Hrithik Paul

10.1	Introduction	179
10.2	Problem statement	181
10.3	Literature survey	181
10.4	Preliminaries	184
10.5	Dataset description	187
10.6	Proposed method	188
10.7	Result and analysis	194
10.8	Limitation and conclusion	203
	Declaration of data availability	204
	Declaration of conflicts of interest statement	204
	References	204
	Further reading	205

11. Wearable sensors: The pathway to applications of on-body electronics — 207
Viktorija Makarovaite and Robert Horne

11.1	RFID wearables: Design consideration	208
11.2	RFID wearable sensor fabrication and applications	212
11.3	Wearable sensor mass fabrication	219
11.4	Conclusion	223
	References	224

Index — *227*

Contributors

Shadab Ahmad
School of Mechanical Engineering, Shandong University of Technology, Zibo, Shandong, People's Republic of China

Aliyu Aliyu
School of Engineering, University of Lincoln, Lincoln, United Kingdom

Frans Coenen
School of Electrical Engineering, Electronics and Computer Science, University of Liverpool, Liverpool, United Kingdom

Kalyanmoy Deb
Electrical and Computer Engineering, Michigan State University, East Lansing, MI, United States

Anirban Dutta
University of Lincoln, United Kingdom

Omar Elnaggar
School of Engineering, University of Liverpool, Liverpool, United Kingdom

Sivasankar Ganesan
Department of Mechanical Engineering, Amrita School of Engineering, Amrita Vishwa Vidyapeetham, Coimbatore, Tamil Nadu, India

Thomas Gaskins
School of Engineering, University of Lincoln, Lincoln, United Kingdom

Sayani Ghatak
CSE Department, JIS University, Kolkata, India

Debmitra Ghosh
CSE Department, JIS University, Kolkata, India

Pushpendra Gupta
Department of Mechanical Engineering, Indian Institute of Technology Kharagpur, Kharagpur, West Bengal, India

Andrew Hopkinson
School of Psychology, University of Liverpool, Liverpool, United Kingdom

Robert Horne
School of Engineering, University of Kent, Canterbury, United Kingdom

Faiz Iqbal
School of Engineering, University of Lincoln, Lincoln, United Kingdom

Sardar M.N. Islam
ISILC, Victoria University, Melbourne, VIC, Australia

Senthil Kumar Jagatheesaperumal
Department of Electronics and Communication Engineering, Mepco Schlenk Engineering College, Sivakasi, Tamil Nadu, India

Vidyapati Kumar
Department of Mechanical Engineering, Indian Institute of Technology Kharagpur, Kharagpur, West Bengal, India

Viktorija Makarovaite
School of Engineering, University of Kent, Canterbury, United Kingdom

Takahiro Manabe
University at Buffalo, Amherst, NY, United States

Pradeep Nahak
Department of Mechanical Engineering, Indian Institute of Technology Kharagpur, Kharagpur, West Bengal, India

Paolo Paoletti
School of Engineering, University of Liverpool, Liverpool, United Kingdom

Hrithik Paul
CSE Department, JIS University, Kolkata, India

Dilip Kumar Pratihar
Department of Mechanical Engineering, Indian Institute of Technology Kharagpur, Kharagpur, West Bengal, India

Shanay Rab
School of Architecture, Technology, and Engineering, University of Brighton, Brighton, United Kingdom

Amir Rahmani
School of Engineering, University of Lincoln, Lincoln, United Kingdom

Mo Sadique
School of Computational & Integrative Sciences, Jawaharlal Nehru University, New Delhi, India

Sapna Ratan Shah
School of Computational & Integrative Sciences, Jawaharlal Nehru University, New Delhi, India

Behnaz Sohani
Wolfson School of Mechanical, Electrical & Manufacturing Engineering, Loughborough University, Loughborough, United Kingdom

Yebing Tian
School of Mechanical Engineering, Shandong University of Technology, Zibo, Shandong, People's Republic of China

Mohammed Ubaid
Technische Fakultät, Friedrich Alexander Universität Erlangen-Nürnberg, Erlangen, Germany

CHAPTER 1

Soft robotics and computational intelligence: Transformative technologies reshaping biomedical engineering

Thomas Gaskins[a], Pushpendra Gupta[b], Vidyapati Kumar[b], Dilip Kumar Pratihar[b], and Faiz Iqbal[a]

[a]School of Engineering, University of Lincoln, Lincoln, United Kingdom
[b]Department of Mechanical Engineering, Indian Institute of Technology Kharagpur, Kharagpur, West Bengal, India

1.1 Introduction

The medical sector is undergoing a major transformation catalyzed by the integration of cutting-edge technologies like the Internet of Things (IoT), Software as Medical Devices (SaMD), and artificial intelligence (AI) [1]. The IoT has enabled interconnected devices for real-time diagnostics and treatment through remote care, while SaMD plays a pivotal role through software capabilities for monitoring and therapeutic interventions. Stringent guidelines ensure that SaMD solutions meet rigorous efficacy and safety standards. Meanwhile, AI is pioneering a shift toward advanced diagnostic support and data analytics, prompting regulatory endorsement of AI-driven devices like in diabetic retinopathy detection. However, ethical and cybersecurity concerns remain for AI-driven devices. Additionally, 3D printing [2] and additive manufacturing [3] are revolutionizing personalized, patient-tailored medical devices and procedures, also showing the potential to reduce costs and improve quality [4]. The combination of 3D printing with AI and the Internet of Medical Things can further optimize manufacturing. In essence, this book brings out how the seamless integration of these exponentially growing technologies can catalyze the medical sector toward remote care, improved diagnostics and treatments, and patient-centric solutions—charting the course for the future of healthcare. However, data security and ethical and interoperability challenges persist, demanding nuanced governance.

Expanding upon this technological evolution, computational intelligence, which includes deep learning (DL), machine learning (ML), and AI, is transforming the medical sector by improving healthcare system performance, quality, equity, and responsiveness. AI enables disease diagnosis, treatment personalization, and resource optimization [5].

It supports healthcare professionals in making data-driven decisions and providing tailored recommendations. The integration of biomedical robots and devices with computational intelligence creates new opportunities in healthcare, such as enhancing medical imaging analysis, disease diagnosis, and predictive modeling using DL [6]. DL uses convolutional neural networks (CNNs) to extract and classify complex features from various imaging modalities, such as CT, MRI, ultrasound, and X-ray, leading to more accurate detection and diagnosis of medical conditions. DL also analyzes large-scale healthcare datasets to facilitate early epidemic detection, disease spread modeling, and adverse event identification. However, DL faces challenges such as the need for large-labeled datasets, the interpretability of "black box" models, the standardization of medical images, and the requirement for domain-specific expertise. These challenges need to be addressed for the successful and ethical application of DL in medical image analysis and public health. Computational intelligence, especially DL, is essential for advancing healthcare delivery and outcomes.

Transitioning from computational intelligence, sleep analysis takes center stage in the pursuit of human well-being, which includes physical health and cognitive function. Leveraging DL and ML, especially convolutional neural networks, is instrumental in achieving precise recognition and analysis of sleep positions. The accuracy of sleep position recognition is paramount, and ML algorithms, especially CNNs, are instrumental in analyzing data from sleep monitoring devices [7]. These algorithms optimize feature extraction and classification, enabling the development of intelligent systems that can monitor sleep stages, posture, and duration. The integration of ML in sleep medicine exemplifies the broader impact of computational intelligence in healthcare, paving the way for advancements in medical diagnostics and personalized treatment, ultimately contributing to better health outcomes. The ongoing evolution of computational intelligence holds the promise of transforming healthcare by improving the accuracy and efficiency of sleep analysis and other medical applications.

Building upon the advancements in medical image analysis, transfer learning (TL) emerges as a pivotal technique, addressing challenges related to limited data and domain-specific expertise, thereby driving innovation in healthcare. The review in Ref. [8] underscores TL's ability to produce high-accuracy classification models with limited data, addressing the scarcity of labeled datasets and the need for domain-specific expertise. TL's success in transferring knowledge across domains is evident in its wide application in medical image analysis, where it has significantly improved disease diagnosis and treatment planning. Despite the need for further research to overcome current limitations, such as the lack of benchmarking comparisons and studies on specific disorders, TL continues to be a driving force in healthcare innovation, offering agile and efficient models for complex medical imaging data, thereby enhancing patient care and outcomes. The importance of TL in medical image analysis cannot be overstated, as it holds the potential for continued advancements in the field. Advanced signal processing techniques can further exploit the data from multiple transmitters and receivers to improve the sensitivity and resolution of medical imaging modalities. This approach aims to enable earlier and more accurate detection of pathologies such as breast cancer, brain abnormalities, and tissue characterization.

Robot-assisted rehabilitation is more effective than conventional therapy in enhancing upper limb motor function recovery in stroke patients, particularly those with chronic conditions [9]. While it may not significantly reduce muscle tone or improve daily living activities, the use of robotic devices in rehabilitation offers high-intensity, repetitive, and task-specific treatments that can positively impact arm function recovery. The integration of robot-assisted therapy with traditional methods may lead to higher-quality rehabilitation, allowing for more intensive and independent practice. This systematic review with meta-analysis underscores the potential of human–robot interaction (HRI) in providing a more efficient and effective approach to stroke rehabilitation. HRI is a burgeoning field that is instrumental in enhancing rehabilitation efforts and providing support to those in need, such as the elderly or disabled [10]. HRI enables close and safe interaction, leveraging cognitive computing and natural communication methods like gestures and speech to offer personalized support. Despite its potential, HRI faces challenges such as accommodating complex interactions, ensuring operational presence amid communication limitations, and understanding the human role in unexpected scenarios. The development of humanoid robots with human-like movements and expressions, coupled with advanced speech recognition and language understanding, is essential for effective HRI [11]. Addressing these challenges requires an interdisciplinary approach, drawing expertise from cognitive science, engineering, psychology, and human factors engineering, to advance the field and improve healthcare outcomes through innovative biomedical robots and devices.

Biomedical robots and computational intelligence are also making strides in mental healthcare by providing innovative solutions for monitoring and treating brain disorders. The cognitive smart healthcare system proposed by Ref. [12] utilizes a network of IoT sensors, including an electroencephalography (EEG) headband, to gather vital signs and neural data continuously. This data is analyzed in real-time by AI systems, which, coupled with DL models, can distinguish between pathological and normal brain patterns. Such analysis enables healthcare professionals to remotely evaluate a patient's mental state and intervene promptly. These advancements in robotics and AI not only enhance the accessibility and quality of mental healthcare but also make it more affordable. As technology progresses, the integration of edge robotics with human-like responsiveness could further aid in the recovery of mental faculties through cognitive and physical therapy, offering a beacon of hope for patients with mental health conditions. Biomedical robots have the potential to revolutionize mental healthcare by offering novel ways of diagnosis, intervention, and support for various mental health conditions. The study in Ref. [13] reviews some of the emerging applications of robots in this domain, such as aiding autistic children in social skills development, motivating stroke survivors to exercise, alleviating loneliness through companionship, and enhancing clinician training on disability awareness. One of the key benefits of robots is their ability to provide cognitive assistance without physical contact, which can be especially helpful for dementia patients who need stimulation and socialization. Another advantage is their effectiveness in promoting behavioral change, such as weight loss and healthy lifestyle, through personalized coaching and feedback. Furthermore, robots can enable objective and quantitative assessment of mental health status, such as using motion tracking to measure the social interactions of schizophrenic patients. However, the clinical impact of these robotic solutions still requires rigorous evaluation through randomized control trials and long-term studies that consider both patient outcomes and provider perspectives. As technology advances, robots can become more intelligent, responsive, and empathetic, and play a vital role in improving the mental health and well-being of people. However, the adoption of robots in mental healthcare also needs to be carefully paced and regulated to ensure ethical and safe use. Computational intelligence in biomedical engineering is also expanding its areas in extracting valuable information using brain activation topography. This area employs ML models, particularly CNNs, to analyze brain activation patterns from techniques such as EEG. However, rigorous evaluation methods, such as leave one subject out (LOSO) cross-validation, are crucial to ensure the generalizability of these models across individuals, enabling reliable classification of skill levels.

The healthcare industry is undergoing a paradigm shift as discussed earlier with the adoption of IoT devices [14] and assistive technologies [15] that enable remote patient monitoring, smart hospitals, mobile e-health platforms, and interactive patient aids. Among these technologies, wearable sensors [16] are particularly promising for improving health monitoring and personalized healthcare. They can collect and transmit vital signs, movement disorders, rehabilitation progress, and environmental exposure data continuously and noninvasively, while patients carry on with their normal activities. This can lead to better diagnosis, treatment, and prevention of various health conditions, such as Parkinson's disease, stroke, head injuries, and spine mobility issues. Wearable sensors are also part of the broader spectrum of assistive technologies that aim to enhance the health, healthcare, and quality of life of people, especially the aging population and those with impairments. These technologies provide functions such as emergency detection, disease management, health feedback, and advice, and allow patients to live more independently and receive quality care remotely. However, there are still challenges and opportunities for improving the privacy, scalability, reliability, integration, interoperability, reimbursement, and efficacy of these technologies. IoT devices and assistive technologies have the potential to transform healthcare delivery and relieve the burden on the healthcare system if these challenges can be effectively addressed.

This introduction chapter to the book as highlighted in the previous section introduces the book and then aims to introduce the first technology that makes an intriguing entrance into the world of biomedical engineering. The technology helps in both biomedical robots as well as biomedical devices which makes it ideally suited to kick-start this book. This technology is **Soft Robotics**, which is characterized by its pliable and adaptable materials and thus, holds immense promise in the realm of medicine. Their compatibility with biological tissues allows for a gentle distribution of forces, minimizing the risk of injury. The field of soft robotics is flourishing with applications that leverage this inherent flexibility for safe human interaction. These include surgical soft robotics, Exosuits, artificial organs, prosthetics, assistive devices, etc. Additionally, soft robotic gloves are emerging as valuable tools in rehabilitation therapy. Despite challenges in miniaturization, power supply, and modeling soft material behavior, soft robotics continues to advance, offering significant potential for biomedical applications due to its harmonious interaction with living tissues and resistance to wear and fatigue. The following sections discuss it in detail.

1.2 Soft robotics: Brief introduction

Soft robotics is a recent and emerging field of study. Soft robots are autonomous machines made from soft materials. These materials have similar moduli to those of soft biological materials and tissue found in nature. Utilizing these materials has the benefit of considerably reducing the potential, inadvertent harm of traditional robotic systems working in close proximity to humans and animals. Robots made from soft materials also exhibit superior adaptability to various objects and environments as well as improved maneuverability over soft substrates [17] without causing damage [18]. These properties of soft robots make them well-suited and highly promising for biomedical applications with further development. Fig. 1.1 shows a representation of a soft robot in a fruit-picking application; similar movements can assist in biomedical environments.

Soft robots are manufactured in a variety of ways, with the most common way being the curing of soft elastomers inside a mold with PDMS. PDMS is the most used material traditionally owing to its good properties for prototypes as well as commercial products and ease of use [20]. In recent years, PDMS has become economically tougher to get. This has led to an increased use of the EcoFlex range of soft elastomers [21–22] as well as some other soft elastomers [23,24]. Additive manufacturing is also commonly used in the fabrication of soft robots, mostly being utilized to fabricate the molds for curing elastomers with FDM and SLA technologies [25]. It is also utilized to construct soft robots directly and of particular interest is 4D printing, which has an outstanding potential for use in biomedical engineering. It has potential in soft robotics as well due to its energy source-specific transformation, volume reduction, biocompatibility, and the ability to be powered by biologically harmless energy sources. 4D printing is also able to produce robots at the submicroscale powered by external stimuli [26]. Soft robots are typically actuated by a pressurized fluid, often air, but can also be actuated by pulleys or tensile

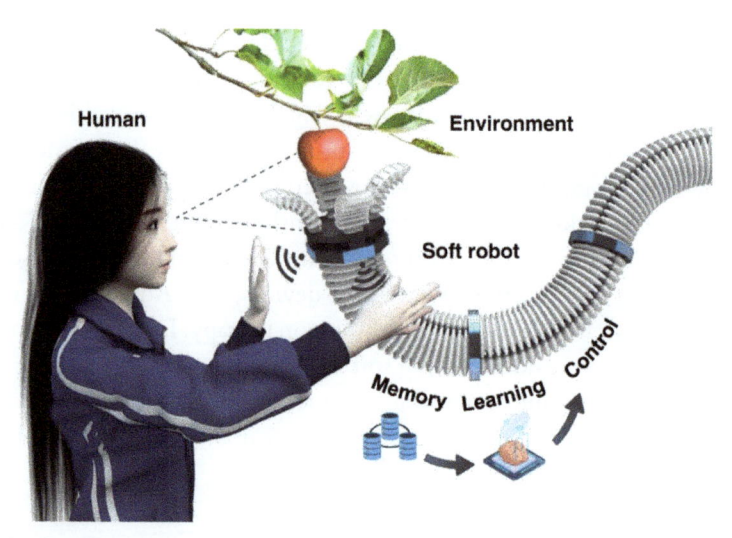

Fig. 1.1 A soft robot for a fruit-picking application [19].

or shape-memory actuators upon heating [17]. Recent research archives have reported experiments with hydrogels, which have the property to change their volume and shape when heated above a temperature known as the lower critical solution temperature. This is useful for building actuators in soft robots and drug delivery systems [27].

1.3 Potential and ongoing applications of soft robots

This section provides an overview of the various applications soft robots have and how they assist in biomedical research.

1.3.1 Surgical applications for soft robots

One of the most obvious uses for soft robots is robotic surgery. Minimally invasive surgery has some issues due to limited triangulation and instrument clashing because of the lack of motion of rigid surgical instruments. They also have the disadvantages of constrained workspace and impossible navigation around organs due to the rigidity [28]. Owing to their various advantages, soft robots provide a promising prospect for surgical systems as they can maneuver around organs without causing damage. Additionally, they can be made MRI-compatible with relative ease due to their elastomer construction [24].

Interest in soft robotic surgery research is given to retraction which is necessary when the surgical target is located below an organ or collapsed tissue and needs to be moved out of the way to get to the surgical site. This action can be quite invasive and often requires the use of considerable force. Retraction requires a compliant and safe interaction with the organs or tissue where soft robots offer a promising solution [24].

Traditional surgical robots require a large footprint in the operating theater and utilize rigid instruments with an articulating tip. These robots aid minimally invasive surgery, however, because of the lack of flexibility a more invasive open approach is required for areas that require a more delicate access. Continuum soft robots have the promise to solve these shortcomings with traditional surgical robots. Most medical continuum robots are single backbone continuum robots which means they have a central elastic structure that supports the passage of actuation or transmission elements and tools down the body of the manipulator. The development of single-backbone continuum robots is multibackbone robots. These consist of multiple parallel elastic elements constrained together. Some multibackbone robots utilize one primary central backbone with other secondary backbones that are offset from the central backbone. There are also concentric-tube continuum robots which are constructed from multiple precurved tubes nested inside of each other made from an elastomer. The base of each tube can be moved axially and rotated to control the overall shape of the robot structure. These tubes are typically made from a shape memory alloy in a super elastic phase so heat treatment can be used to shape each tube before being assembled [29].

Continuum robots have the potential to positively impact several fields of surgery listed as follows:

1.3.1.1 Brain surgery
Existing instruments for brain surgery are rigid and straight, limiting areas of the brain that are accessible. Continuum robots have the potential to introduce new surgical procedures where previously unreachable areas of the brain can be operated on via a nonlinear path [29].

1.3.1.2 Otolaryngology
Due to existing instruments being made from rigid materials, some regions cannot be accessed through the nostril, mouth, or ear canal and diseases in those regions require open surgery. Continuum robots may have the potential to reach these areas because of their flexibility [29].

1.3.1.3 Cardiac surgery
Some cardiac surgeries can be completed by minimally invasive procedures by stabilizing the region of the heart that is being operated on. However, there are some difficulties involving the limited ability to apply and control the necessary forces and the difficulties of positioning the instrument inside the beating heart. Soft continuum robots may be able to overcome these difficulties with enough research [29].

1.3.1.4 Vascular surgery
Catheters and guidewires are used to perform injections, drain fluids, and insert additional instruments in a minimally invasive way. However, steering the catheters can be difficult due to friction between the catheter and vascular walls. Steerable soft robotic catheters may be able to overcome this issue [29].

1.3.1.5 Abdominal interventions
Navigation of the ablator through the tissue to the surgical site for treating tumors and controlling the size of the necrosis zone is challenging. Small-scale continuum robots have the potential to solve these issues due to their highly flexible nature [29].

1.3.1.6 Urology
Continuum robots are promising to be deployed transurethral to treat prostate or bladder pathologies as they can be miniaturized to the scale required as well as provide good dexterity and flexible access [29].

1.3.2 Exosuits
Another potential use of soft robots in biomedical applications is in exosuit. Both to rehabilitate patients and to augment the strength of able-bodied people. Challenges are encountered in assisting able-bodied people or people with partial impairments as the exosuits must apply appropriate forces without increasing their metabolic expenditure to see the benefits. This is difficult for rigid exoskeletons because of two main reasons, weight and if the rigid joints are not perfectly aligned, they can work against the user's movement rather than assisting. Soft robots have the potential to solve these issues through the soft form of exoskeletons called exosuits which should be able to move with the user and flex with their movements as well as apply force. The properties of soft robots and soft actuators lend themselves well to this purpose as they are lighter than hard robots and can flex with the user but still be able to exert considerable force. Fig. 1.2 shows an exosuit being used in practice.

Soft robots do have a drawback compared to rigid exoskeletons though as they can deform while actuating which decreases the amount of force being transferred to the user which means careful design considerations must be made to how the user interfaces with the soft exosuit as well as the stiffness properties of the suit itself [31]. Perhaps a more practical use of soft robots is to rehabilitate certain parts of the body. Like the Exo-Glove which utilizes a soft tendon routing system inspired by the natural tendons of the human body. These are connected to a pulley system and the fingers by a thimble-like strap made from an inextensible fabric. This device was successful in restoring the grasping function to a disabled subject [32].

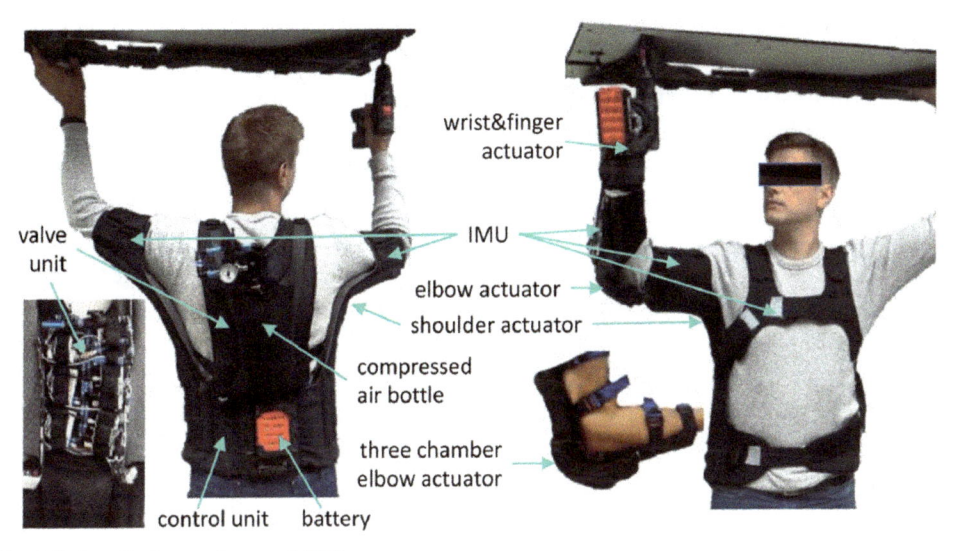

Fig. 1.2 Practical use of exosuit [30].

1.3.3 Prosthetics

The current state-of-the-art myoelectric hand prosthetic technology consists of prostheses made from rigid constructions. As a result of this construction, additional mechanisms are required to make interaction with humans and other objects safe. These additional mechanisms contribute to the high cost of prosthetic devices and increase the weight of the hand. The additional complexity also means higher standards of maintenance are needed and durability is potentially lowered. These factors significantly contribute to the high rates of prosthetic hand abandonment. Soft robotic prosthetic hands have the potential to solve these issues because of the inherent compliance of the materials used in the construction and the ability to utilize monolithic construction to fabricate the hand. This means that the overall weight of the prosthetic is lower than that of traditional rigid construction hands and the simplicity and quick production reduces the cost and maintenance of the prosthetic [33]. Currently, soft robotic hands have a low payload capacity (RBO Hand 2 has a payload of 0.5 kg) but a higher payload is achievable, if necessary, by utilizing stiffer rubbers and thicker hulls in the construction as well as potentially using hydraulic actuation instead of pneumatic actuation [34].

1.3.4 Artificial organs

There are two main uses for soft robots with artificial organs. Both develop artificial organs to implant and utilize soft robots to replicate human organs to study the mechanics of the organ. The mouth and swallowing system are of particular interest to replicate with soft robotic technology. Measuring the tongue movement and the interaction with its surroundings is difficult due to the structure of the oral cavity. Thus, it is desirable to construct a robotic replica to validate medical hypotheses about the oral cavity. The tongue is an entirely soft structure which makes soft robots well-suited to replicate it. Utilizing inextensible layers and pneumatic actuators embedded in the extensible layer, researchers were able to replicate the human tongue and they achieved roll-up, roll-down, elongation, groove, and twist as replicas of the movement of the natural tongue [22]. It is also desirable to replicate the esophagus since dysphagia (swallowing difficulty) affects a large proportion of the population and one approach to treatment is to modify the viscosity of the food. One way to experiment with food viscosity is to utilize a soft robotic esophagus which can mimic the human swallowing process to explore the mechanics of swallowing [35].

The heart is also of particular interest to replicate with a soft robot, this is because artificial hearts have several problems. Ventricle assist devices (VADs) are known for causing hemolysis, thrombosis, and infections following implantation. In addition to this, right ventricular failure following the implantation of a left ventricular assist device is common. All current VADs and total artificial hearts (TAH) are made of many mechanical components which increases the cost and risk of failure. Blood clots are also a problem associated with artificial hearts. Soft robots have the potential to solve some of these issues as they can replicate the motion of the human heart yielding a pulsing blood flow. A soft total artificial heart was designed from the CAD file of a healthy human heart and was then made from a soft elastomer and pneumatically driven. This approach shows promise from the low complexity of the heart and the ability to replicate the natural action of the human heart. However, further progress is needed as the prototypes had very limited durability [23]. Some research has also been done to mimic the ventricles of the heart too, primarily for studying the motion of the human heart to assist in the development of FE simulations of soft robotic hearts and the development of artificial hearts [36].

1.3.5 Assistive technologies

A potential use of soft robots is in assistive technology as assistive robots need to be safe for use at home which makes it an ideal field for soft robots. This combined with the aging population in most developed countries makes assistive soft robotics desirable. One assistive technology example that Soft Robotics is well-suited for is assisting elderly people in taking a shower, this is of particular focus of the EU-funded I-SUPPORT project which is pursuing a soft robot arm that mounts on the shower wall to softly wipe the person and pouring water and soap. It consists of three fluidic chambers and three longitudinal chambers. The fluidic chambers produce elongation and bending in all directions and the cables increase the force exerted [37]. Fig. 1.3 shows a soft robotic assistive robot in use.

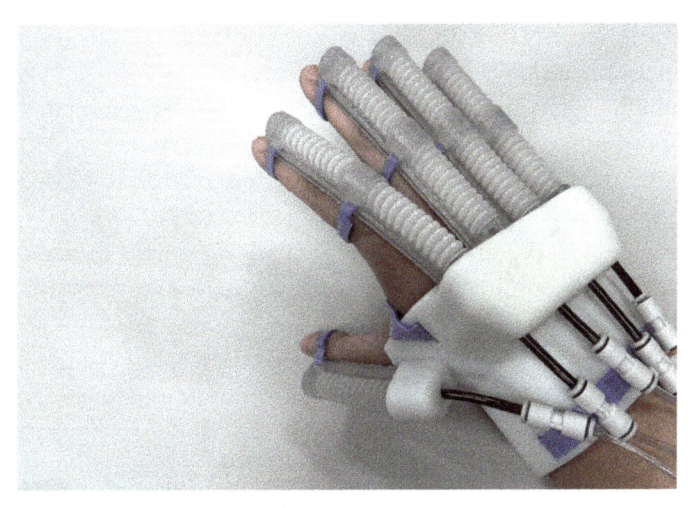

Fig. 1.3 Soft Robotic application for rehab [38].

1.4 Limitations in soft robotics

Despite the numerous benefits of soft robots, some limitations prevent their widespread adoption. They are currently unable to cope with heavy loads and survive many actuations. They also have issues with controls because of the near-infinite degrees of freedom which also makes modeling difficult. The flexibility is also a challenge as the robot can deform in undesirable and unpredictable ways from the weight of the robot or the environment and thus more work is required to model and control soft robots [35]. However, work is being done to create soft sensors utilizing mesh networks of conductive structures which could aid with the control of soft robots [39].

1.5 Summary

Soft Robotics has immense potential in biomedical engineering ranging from revolutionizing surgery through superior maneuverability in various surgical procedures to promising enhanced precision and accessibility. Other potentials include continuum soft robots which open avenues for diverse applications in brain surgery, otolaryngology, cardiac surgery, vascular surgery, abdominal interventions, and urology. Rehabilitation using exosuits is another well-suited benefit of soft robotics along with prosthetics and artificial organs. Assistive technologies, particularly in tasks like shower assistance for the elderly, showcasing their safety and adaptability in home environments is another benefit that arises from Soft Robotics. They do however have some limitations in load bearing and control complexities which with proper ongoing research can be mitigated; thus, Soft Robotics emerges as a transformative force in biomedical applications, paving the way for safer, more adaptable, and cost-effective solutions in surgery, rehabilitation, prosthetics, artificial organs, and assistive technologies.

The succeeding chapters in this book provide an in-depth exploration of the latest innovations, opportunities, and challenges across various domains of biomedical robots and devices. Beginning with Chapter 2 and continuing through to Chapter 11, the key topics covered are:

- Chapter 2 provides a comprehensive review of advancements in biomedical devices and the potential of automation, AI, and other technologies to revolutionize healthcare.
- Chapter 3 covers the role of mathematics in biomedical robotics and devices, including modeling, simulation, control algorithms, and optimization techniques. It explores the potential impact on healthcare delivery.
- Chapter 4 examines advancing ankle-foot orthosis design through integrating biomechanics, robotics, and additive manufacturing to improve mobility and quality of life.
- Chapter 5 deals with multibistatic frequency-domain measurements for enhanced medical sensing and imaging, with a focus on microwave imaging for applications like breast cancer detection.
- Chapter 6 reviews sleep posture analysis using wearable sensors from clinical, sensing, and intelligent perception perspectives. It discusses opportunities and challenges.
- Chapter 7 evaluates various DL techniques for multistage Alzheimer's disease prediction from magnetic resonance images. Findings validate complex deep CNNs can reliably distinguish early pathological changes.
- Chapter 8 presents a novel LOSO cross-validation-based ML application for individual skill classification using brain activation topography.
- Chapter 9 reviews machine learning for disease prognosis in Biomedicine 4.0, emphasizing transfer learning to improve accuracy and speed.
- Chapter 10 proposes a voice and chatbot framework using explainable AI to care for mental health and recommend doctors/hospitals.
- Chapter 11 explores wearable sensors as the pathway to diverse applications of on-body electronics, reviewing design aspects and considerations.

References

[1] F. Tettey, S.K. Parupelli, S. Desai, A review of biomedical devices: classification, regulatory guidelines, human factors, software as a medical device, and cybersecurity, Biomed. Mater. Devices (2023) 1–26.

[2] V. Kumar, A. Babbar, A. Sharma, R. Kumar, A. Tyagi, Polymer 3D bioprinting for bionics and tissue engineering applications, in: Additive Manufacturing of Polymers for Tissue Engineering, CRC Press, Boca Raton, 2022, pp. 17–39.

[3] V. Kumar, C. Prakash, A. Babbar, S. Choudhary, A. Sharma, A.S. Uppal, Additive manufacturing in biomedical engineering, Addit. Manuf. Process. Biomed. Eng. (2022) 143–164.

[4] H.B. Mamo, M. Adamiak, A. Kunwar, 3D printed biomedical devices and their applications: a review on state-of-the-art technologies, existing challenges, and future perspectives, J. Mech. Behav. Biomed. Mater. (2023) 105930.
[5] T. Panch, P. Szolovits, R. Atun, Artificial intelligence, machine learning and health systems, J. Glob. Health 8 (2) (2018).
[6] D. Ravì, C. Wong, F. Deligianni, M. Berthelot, J. Andreu-Perez, B. Lo, G.Z. Yang, Deep learning for health informatics, IEEE J. Biomed. Health Inform. 21 (1) (2016) 4–21.
[7] X. Li, Y. Gong, X. Jin, P. Shang, Sleep posture recognition based on machine learning: a systematic review, Pervasive Mob. Comput. (2023) 101752.
[8] P. Kora, C.P. Ooi, O. Faust, U. Raghavendra, A. Gudigar, W.Y. Chan, K. Meenakshi, K. Swaraja, P. Plawiak, U.R. Acharya, Transfer learning techniques for medical image analysis: a review, Biocybern. Biomed. Eng. 42 (1) (2022) 79–107.
[9] R. Bertani, C. Melegari, M.C. De Cola, A. Bramanti, P. Bramanti, R.S. Calabrò, Effects of robot-assisted upper limb rehabilitation in stroke patients: a systematic review with meta-analysis, Neurol. Sci. 38 (2017) 1561–1569.
[10] M.A. Goodrich, A.C. Schultz, Human–robot interaction: a survey. Foundations and trends®, Hum-Comput. Interact. 1 (3) (2008) 203–275.
[11] T.B. Sheridan, Human–robot interaction: status and challenges, Hum. Factors 58 (4) (2016) 525–532.
[12] S.U. Amin, M.S. Hossain, G. Muhammad, M. Alhussein, M.A. Rahman, Cognitive smart healthcare for pathology detection and monitoring, IEEE Access 7 (2019) 10745–10753.
[13] L.D. Riek, Robotics technology in mental health care, in: Artificial Intelligence in Behavioral and Mental Health Care, Academic Press, 2016, pp. 185–203.
[14] M.J. Baucas, P. Spachos, S. Gregori, Internet-of-things devices and assistive technologies for health care: applications, challenges, and opportunities, IEEE Signal Process. Mag. 38 (4) (2021) 65–77.
[15] R. Haux, S. Koch, N.H. Lovell, M. Marschollek, N. Nakashima, K.H. Wolf, Health-enabling and ambient assistive technologies: past, present, future, Yearb. Med. Inform. 25 (S 01) (2016) S76–S91.
[16] M.M. Rodgers, V.M. Pai, R.S. Conroy, Recent advances in wearable sensors for health monitoring, IEEE Sensors J. 15 (6) (2014) 3119–3126.
[17] D. Rus, M.T. Tolley, Design, fabrication and control of soft robots, Nature 521 (7553) (2015), https://doi.org/10.1038/nature14543. Art. no. 7553.
[18] T. Ashuri, A. Armani, R. Jalilzadeh Hamidi, T. Reasnor, S. Ahmadi, K. Iqbal, Biomedical soft robots: current status and perspective, Biomed. Eng. Lett. 10 (3) (2020), https://doi.org/10.1007/s13534-020-00157-6. Art. no. 3.
[19] W. Liu, Y. Duo, J. Liu, F. Yuan, L. Li, L. Li, L. Wen, Touchless interactive teaching of soft robots through flexible bimodal sensory interfaces, Nat. Commun. 13 (1) (2022) 5030.
[20] G.M. Whitesides, Soft robotics, Angew. Chem. Int. Ed. 57 (16) (2018) 4258–4273, https://doi.org/10.1002/anie.201800907.
[21] C. Majidi, R.F. Shepherd, R.K. Kramer, G.M. Whitesides, R.J. Wood, Influence of surface traction on soft robot undulation, Int. J. Robot. Res. 32 (13) (2013) 1577–1584, https://doi.org/10.1177/0278364913498432.
[22] X. Lu, W. Xu, X. Li, A soft robotic tongue—mechatronic design and surface reconstruction, IEEEASME Trans. Mechatron. 22 (5) (2017) 2102–2110, https://doi.org/10.1109/TMECH.2017.2748606.
[23] N.H. Cohrs, et al., A soft Total artificial heart—first concept evaluation on a hybrid mock circulation, Artif. Organs 41 (10) (2017) 948–958, https://doi.org/10.1111/aor.12956.
[24] T. Ranzani, M. Cianchetti, G. Gerboni, I.D. Falco, A. Menciassi, A soft modular manipulator for minimally invasive surgery: design and characterization of a single module, IEEE Trans. Robot. 32 (1) (2016) 187–200, https://doi.org/10.1109/TRO.2015.2507160.
[25] B. Venzac, et al., PDMS curing inhibition on 3D-printed molds: why? Also, how to avoid it? Anal. Chem. 93 (19) (2021) 7180–7187, https://doi.org/10.1021/acs.analchem.0c04944.
[26] S.Y. Hann, H. Cui, M. Nowicki, L.G. Zhang, 4D printing soft robotics for biomedical applications, Addit. Manuf. 36 (2020) 101567, https://doi.org/10.1016/j.addma.2020.101567.

[27] H. Banerjee, M. Suhail, H. Ren, Hydrogel actuators and sensors for biomedical soft robots: brief overview with impending challenges, Biomimetics 3 (3) (2018), https://doi.org/10.3390/biomimetics3030015. Art. no. 3.
[28] A. Diodato, et al., Soft robotic manipulator for improving dexterity in minimally invasive surgery, Surg. Innov. 25 (1) (2018) 69–76, https://doi.org/10.1177/1553350617745953.
[29] J. Burgner-Kahrs, D.C. Rucker, H. Choset, Continuum robots for medical applications: a survey, IEEE Trans. Robot. 31 (6) (2015) 1261–1280, https://doi.org/10.1109/TRO.2015.2489500.
[30] J. Kuschan, J. Krüger, Fatigue recognition in overhead assembly based on a soft robotic exosuit for worker assistance, CIRP Ann. 70 (1) (2021) 9–12.
[31] A.T. Asbeck, S.M.M. De Rossi, K.G. Holt, C.J. Walsh, A biologically inspired soft exosuit for walking assistance, Int. J. Robot. Res. 34 (6) (2015) 744–762, https://doi.org/10.1177/0278364914562476.
[32] H. In, B.B. Kang, M. Sin, K.-J. Cho, Exo-glove: a wearable robot for the hand with a soft tendon routing system, IEEE Robot. Autom. Mag. 22 (1) (2015) 97–105, https://doi.org/10.1109/MRA.2014.2362863.
[33] A. Mohammadi, et al., A practical 3D-printed soft robotic prosthetic hand with multi-articulating capabilities, PLoS One 15 (5) (2020) e0232766, https://doi.org/10.1371/journal.pone.0232766.
[34] R. Deimel, O. Brock, A novel type of compliant and underactuated robotic hand for dexterous grasping, Int. J. Robot. Res. 35 (1–3) (2016) 161–185, https://doi.org/10.1177/0278364915592961.
[35] M. Zhu, W. Xu, L.K. Cheng, Esophageal peristaltic control of a soft-bodied swallowing robot by the central pattern generator, IEEEASME Trans. Mechatron. 22 (1) (2017) 91–98, https://doi.org/10.1109/TMECH.2016.2609465.
[36] E.T. Roche, et al., A bioinspired soft actuated material, Adv. Mater. 26 (8) (2014) 1200–1206, https://doi.org/10.1002/adma.201304018.
[37] M. Cianchetti, C. Laschi, Pleasant to the touch: by emulating nature, scientists Hope to find innovative new uses for soft robotics in health-care technology, IEEE Pulse 7 (3) (2016) 34–37, https://doi.org/10.1109/MPUL.2016.2539799.
[38] H. Su, X. Hou, X. Zhang, W. Qi, S. Cai, X. Xiong, J. Guo, Pneumatic soft robots: Challenges and benefits, in: Actuators, vol. 11, No. 3, MDPI, 2022, p. 92.
[39] J.C. Yeo, H.K. Yap, W. Xi, Z. Wang, C.-H. Yeow, C.T. Lim, Flexible and stretchable strain sensing actuator for wearable soft robotic applications, Adv. Mater. Technol. 1 (3) (2016) 1600018, https://doi.org/10.1002/admt.201600018.

CHAPTER 2

Advancements in biomedical devices: A comprehensive review

Mohammed Ubaid[a], Shadab Ahmad[b], Shanay Rab[c], Faiz Iqbal[d], and Yebing Tian[b]

[a]Technische Fakultät, Friedrich Alexander Universität Erlangen-Nürnberg, Erlangen, Germany
[b]School of Mechanical Engineering, Shandong University of Technology, Zibo, Shandong, People's Republic of China
[c]School of Architecture, Technology, and Engineering, University of Brighton, Brighton, United Kingdom
[d]School of Engineering, University of Lincoln, Lincoln, United Kingdom

2.1 Introduction

2.1.1 Background

The idea toward complete automation/computerization of the manufacturing processes started with Industry 4.0 in West Europe (Germany) [1]. The goal was to upgrade to advanced manufacturing techniques, such as automated production and cyber physical system (CPS), which leverage Internet of Things (IoT), Machine Learning (ML), Artificial Intelligence (AI), and real-time data processing, to enhance capabilities of existing systems and practices. These techniques enable humans to make intelligent decisions across all domains, especially in the field of manufacturing. These techniques have not been limited for use in upgrading the efficiency of goods and services; however, they are gaining a lot of attention for their application in biomedical devices. These intelligent systems minimize human intervention for diagnosis, decision-making, and even support in surgeries by real-time data recording and processing [2]. The use of CPS in biomedical devices is transforming the healthcare sector and is aimed at providing a convergent approach for automation, biomedical engineering, and health informatics [3].

2.1.2 Objective

Significant research has been conducted highlighting the benefits of this alliance; however, articles covering all major attributes from manufacturing to implantation and successful working of biomedical devices are scarce in the literature. Studies have been performed on the role of AI and ML algorithms [2], the use of additive manufacturing for manufacturing of implants [4], cybersecurity of IoT enabled biomedical devices [5], and regulations and safety of biomedical devices [6]; however, all factors in a single article are merely addressed. This chapter aims to provide a comprehensive overview of the above parameters as a single window of information covering advantages and disadvantages considering a few case studies.

2.2 Automation in biomedical devices

2.2.1 Definition and scope

Automation refers to the idea of making a process self-sustaining and functioning with or without very little human intervention. To understand automation in scope of biomedical devices, let us divide them into three main categories:

1. Implantable devices
2. Wearable devices
3. Equipment for diagnosis and treatment

The combination of these devices is shown in Fig. 2.1. The idea of automation in biomedical devices is not only limited to advancements in manufacturing technologies but also emerging and developing to monitor their functioning as well as patients' health in

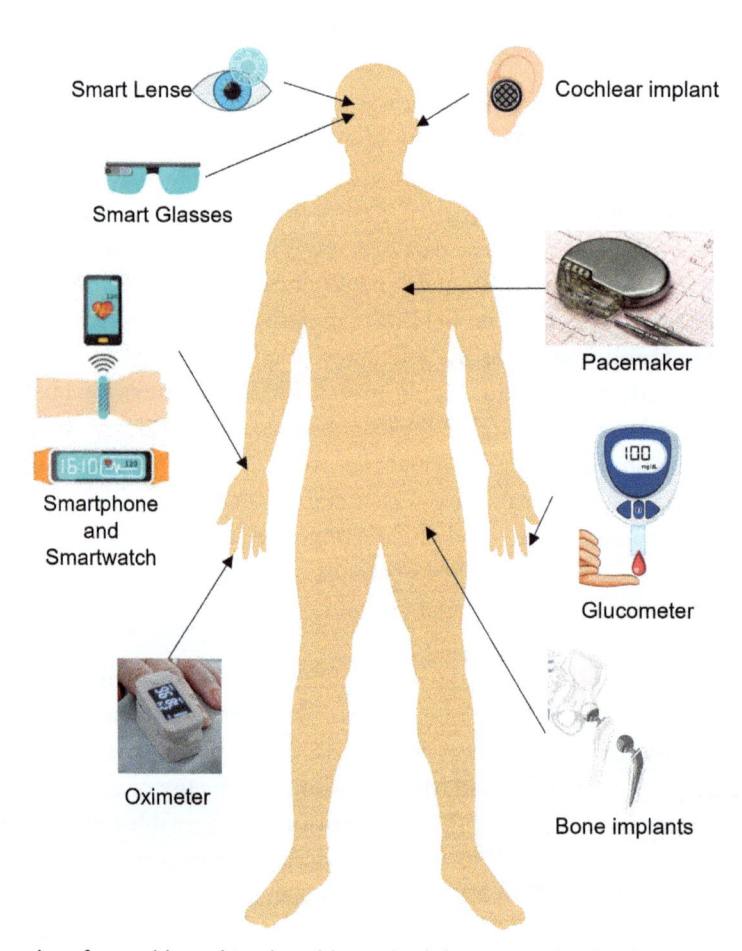

Fig. 2.1 Examples of wearable and implantable medical devices used in healthcare.

real time. This allows us to make intelligent and informed decisions for the diagnosis and treatment of the patients and to take appropriate steps in advance with suggestions from CPS to treat symptoms. Biomedical devices should not be short of the following characteristics: accuracy, reliability, repeatability, portability, and calibration [7].

2.2.2 Overview and emergence of automation

Biomedical devices are available in several types and are widely in use. They range from wearable, implants, andequipment. Combined with suitable automation techniques, biomedical devices have aided right from the beginning of diagnosis to finally performing surgeries by using CPS [7].

2.2.2.1 Implantable devices
The implantable devices can be further divided into two categories. Fig. 2.2 depicts their classification.

Biomedical devices interacting with tissues—For example, bone implants, etc.
The challenge for this category of biomedical devices is their requirement to be unique because their shape, size, form, and features vary from patient to patient. On top of it, the need for extremely high surface finish and low tolerance is an additional artifact faced in the manufacturing of these materials. Such characteristics of this category of biomedical devices make it a challenge to be produced using conventional methods of manufacturing that require high infrastructural investment and multiple steps for producing a single part having complex geometries [8]. AM has evolved to be a preferred method that not only overcomes the problems of conventional manufacturing but also provides ease in manufacturing such complex geometries with higher mechanical and surface features. Few AM techniques used are Stereolithography (SLA), Digital Light Processing (DLP), Selective Laser Sintering (SLS), Electron Beam Melting (EBM), Fused Deposition Modeling (FDM), Multijet/Polyjet 3D printing, Selective Laser Melting (SLM),

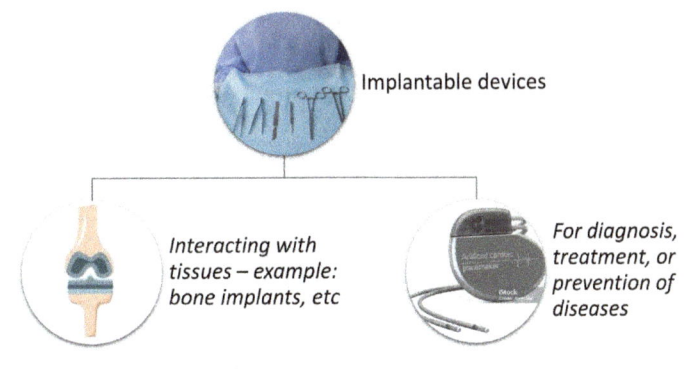

Fig. 2.2 Classification of implantable devices.

Laminated Object Manufacturing (LOM), and Friction Stir Additive Manufacturing, etc. These techniques use a variety of materials such as alloys, ceramics, polymers, composites, and biomaterials for a variety of applications [9], i.e., as per the part to be produced.

Biomedical devices for diagnosis, treatment, or prevention of diseases—For example, pacemakers, contact lenses, etc.

These biomedical devices are introduced inside the human body, do not interact with the tissues, and perform either of the following functions:

- Diagnosis—using cardioverter defibrillators that are implanted in the chest or abdomen. They monitor hearts rhythm and deliver a shock if an abnormal heart rhythm is noticed
- Treatment—using pacemakers and implantable drug pumps. Pacemakers are also implanted in the chest or abdomen and regulate heart rhythm by sending electrical impulses to the heart. Implantable drug pumps are implanted in the abdomen and are used to deliver medication directly into the body to treat various diseases
- Prevention—using implantable glucose monitoring devices that monitor the blood glucose level continuously and are useful for diabetic patients to maintain their blood sugar at normal levels

These examples are not exclusive but show how implantable devices are being used to soften the requirements of continuous monitoring without human intervention. The automation of these biomedical devices is the future of the healthcare industry. These technologies are now linked using AI with cloud computing and can collect and evaluate live patients' data using ML algorithms and big data analytics, resulting in errorless diagnosis, prevention, and treatment of any disease.

2.2.2.2 Wearable devices

The biomedical devices that can be worn by humans and removed from time to time, without the need for surgery for their introduction and/or removal, are called as wearable device. These are our daily interactive items like smart and sports watches, fitness trackers, smartphone-integrated devices, and electronic textiles, and garments [10] as shown in Fig. 2.3. These devices are connected via the Internet of Medical Things (IoMT), which is a subset of the IoT. IoMT allows digitization of traditional healthcare devices by connecting them to cloud computing, providing live tracking and analysis of patients' health without the need of any trained medical practitioner. It can transform how we perceive the present healthcare system for a better and integrated future.

2.2.2.3 Equipment for diagnosis and treatment

Diagnosis and treatment are the two major attributes of biomedical devices belonging to this category. It is important to understand that in view of the present study, this aspect of biomedical devices deals with large-scale machines, or say biomedical equipment like

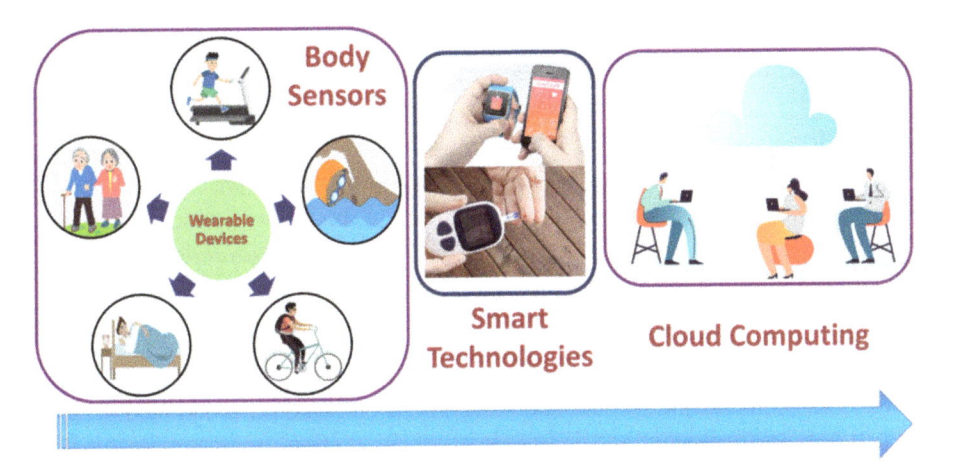

Fig. 2.3 Wearable devices used via IoMT [2].

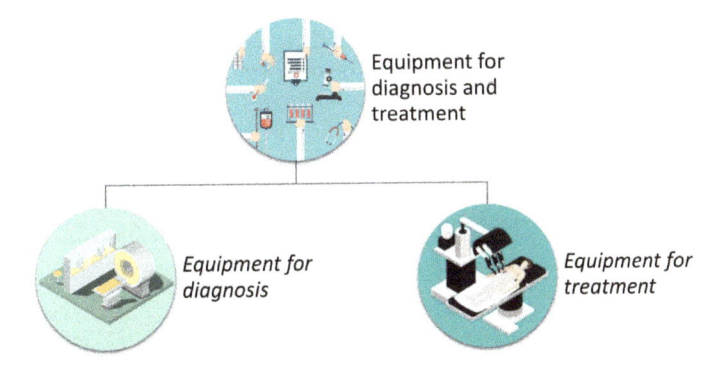

Fig. 2.4 Classification of equipment for diagnosis and treatment.

X-rays, ultrasound, magnetic resonance imaging (MRI), CT scan, Positron Emission Tomography (PET), ventilators, dialysis, surgical robots, catheter robots, etc. [11–16]. It will be easier to understand these devices by classifying them into the following broad categories as shown in Fig. 2.4.

Equipment for diagnosis

These are imaging techniques used to capture the inside of the human body to identify diseases for their treatment and/or prevention. Some examples include X-rays, ultrasound, MRI, CT scan, and PET. The automated analysis or diagnosis using these techniques assists in providing high-resolution images of the inside of the human body, allowing 3D reconstruction of the infected part and providing real-time dimensions of the infection. With the introduction of automation, these equipment for diagnosis can now be termed "smart diagnostics," as they identify potential infections and diseases, perform analysis, and helps in treating/eliminating infections and diseases.

Equipment for treatment

The shift from medical practitioners performing complicated procedures to robotic surgeries by implementing technological innovations in this branch of biomedical devices is no less than a boon for humanity. Automation in the field of surgeries has shaped the future of healthcare over the past decade. Its growing popularity among medical practitioners and patients is the proof of its success. Surgical robots, with their increasing precision day by day, can provide surgeons with very high-precision control for medical procedures along with high-resolution images, allowing them to perform minimally invasive surgeries that result in fast healing. Equipped with diagnostic devices, surgical robots can identify the position, location, and size of the infection/abnormality to be removed from the body [17].

2.3 Technological advancements in automation—Cyber physical systems, robots, and integration with digital platforms, and their advantages

2.3.1 Implantable devices

The need for patient-specific implants has been a major decelerating factor for implementation of automation in implantable biomedical devices. With few exceptions, all the implantable devices are required to be manufactured as per patients' requirements, i.e., their unique size, shape, and application-specific features.

2.3.1.1 Biomedical devices interacting with tissues

AM has provided us with the opportunity to produce patient-specific parts and set up the facilities for mass production. Compared to the time-consuming conventional methods, which require a multistep approach, AM has made it easier like never before to produce implants possessing the required biological characteristics and mechanical features. The literature has suggested that design and manufacturing of these complex and customized structures are moving toward customization, and the production of implants can be carried out very easily using the following steps [18,19]. These steps are specific to a bone replacement and can be easily repeated for other parts of the body. Fig. 2.5 depicts the steps with the help of a flow diagram.
- Use of imaging techniques (like MRI and CT scan) to mimic the implant on the computer through scanning
- Providing the surgeon with virtual 3D reconstruction to analyze the requirement for a specific implant, its shape, size, and the process to be followed for its replacement
- Digital reconstruction of the part to be replaced using computer-aided software

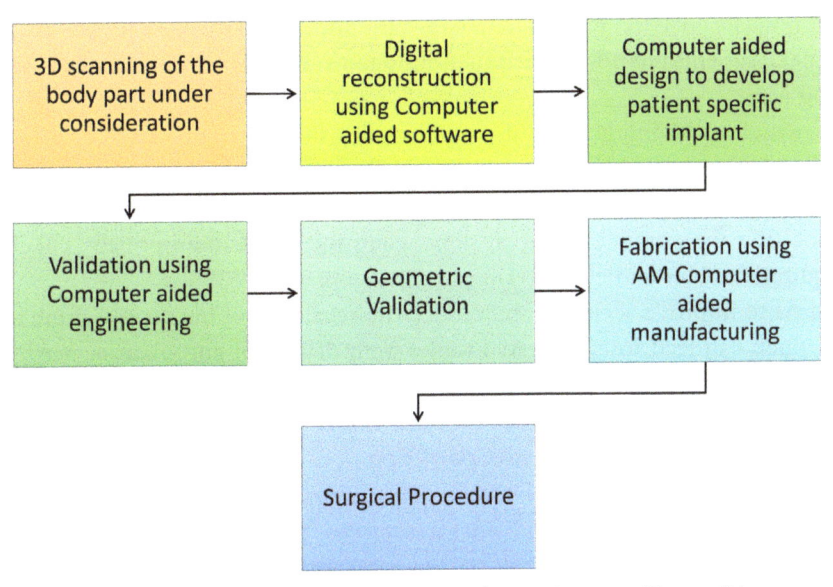

Fig. 2.5 Steps for replacement of an implant customized to patient-specific conditions.

- Computer-aided design to develop patient-specific biocompatible implants. Validation of mechanical properties using computer-aided engineering
- Geometrical validation
- Fabrication of implant using AM computer-aided manufacturing
- Surgical procedure

The combination of AM with living cells and bioactive materials to develop biocompatible materials is called bioprinting. Bioprinting is an extension of AM which is used to produce scaffolds or other biomaterials [20–22]. Few popular techniques for bioprinting include laser/light-based, inkjet-based, and extrusion-based bioprinting technologies [23].

The advancements in manufacturing and processing of these biomaterials/biomedical devices lie in their congregation with the computational field, which is referred to as "cyber CPS" [24], i.e., integration of AI, ML algorithms, cloud computing, big data analytics, and IoMT, which allows the systems to work on feedback thereby providing them with real-time inputs for better predictions, maintenance, and improved Product Lifecycle Management of the AM devices.

The above drawn steps are individual fields of studies and operations, each requiring input from the previous activity to start the next process. CPS have centralized the execution of these steps by networking them and thereby construing smart manufacturing facilities. The smart manufacturing facilities have the following advantages:

- Use of AM for the production of mass customized parts without time loss [25]

- Use of big data analytics to analyze a large amount of data from manufacturing units, customers, patients record, and production systems, which helps in real-time decision-making [26]
- IoMT which is the integration of manufacturing facilities with sensors enables us to monitor the equipment performance as well as the part being produced simultaneously, allowing us to make corrections at the initial stage of problem detection and not after the completion of all steps when the part is being finally checked for its required features and characteristics [27]
- Use of AI to improve accuracy and reduce the reliability of human-machine interaction, which can lead to errors. AI enables high degree of automation, performance enhancement, improved efficiency, and easy control over the processes [28,29]
- Use of ML with AI to allow better decision-making and improved predictability for machine performance and part manufacturing
- Use of AI for quality checks – AI-based quality inspection systems can check the product being formed in real time allowing for improved product quality, productivity [30] or corrective actions in real time or reproducing the product without further wastage of raw materials and resources
- Use of CPS for maintenance activities –machines and equipment are monitored during their usual operations and detection or projection of any problem/fault, which might occur in the future and provide suggestions for corrections

2.3.1.2 Biomedical devices for diagnosis, treatment, or prevention of diseases

The major advantage of these kinds of medical devices is that there is no need for mass customization. These are standard products available with various features to suit the requirements from patient to patient. The only requirement is correct detection of the problem and wherever required efficient function. As the manufacturing of these devices is standardized, there is not much requirement for the implementation of AM techniques. These devices are improving with advancements in the field of technology. With increased computing efficiency, the devices are becoming, smaller, faster, and reliable [31]. This section will particularly deal with the influence of advancements in data acquisition and processing with the use of CPS. We will look at how the CPS is influencing and shaping the healthcare sector for these biomedical devices.

The devices are implanted inside the human body and are equipped with internet connectivity and cloud storage facilities recording the patients' activities, blood levels, sugar levels, heart rate, and temperature. They allow users to track their vitals which helps in keeping a check on their health [2,32]. This also creates a large database for patients and doctors to evaluate the credentials of the patients and to predict the possibility of infections, diseases, or chronic problems.

Such aspects can only be realized through the integration of these devices with CPS. Each computing facility of CPS offers a characteristic advantage. Their integration with

biomedical devices is nothing less than a miraculous outcome in the field of diagnosis, treatment, and prevention. It offers doctors to remotely keep a check on the patients' health and their vitals and provide with consultation and steps to treat a particular condition. The benefits are many but not limited to the following:
- Early prediction and diagnosis of the disease
- Remote diagnosis without the presence of the patient in front of the doctor and to avoid utilization of dedicated hospital facilities
- Reduces burden on infrastructure of hospitals
- Data evaluation and processing in real time against the historical data for reliable predictions
- Alerts can be provided to both doctors and patients
- Reminders against increased/decreased levels of vitals in the body
- Treatment in real time without waiting for the in-person availability of the doctors
- Drug delivery at controlled level and at designated times without the patient's intervention

2.3.2 Wearable devices

These devices can track body movements from a variety of subsystems in the body [33]. Juxtaposing to the implantable devices, they do not require any dedicated surgery and/or a medical practitioner to implant them in the body. They can be worn easily and start to function as soon as they are setup by the user. This section deals with attributes of data collected from wearable biomedical devices and its analysis and informed decision-making by using CPS. The depiction of how human-worn sensors are connected is shown in Fig. 2.6.

These devices can connect with the patient's smartphone/or other available devices and provide vital information directly to the patient. Moreover, the devices are also connected to the cloud and are accessible to doctors for regular monitoring and controlling. The data from these devices are sent to the cloud and stored for computing using ML algorithms. The data are analyzed against available standards and using IoMT interfaced with patients for support via virtual assistants or to raise alarms for any foreseeable problems. They can also provide feedback to doctors for preventive measures, early detection, diagnosis, and for clinical procedures for treatment [3,34]. Applications for implementation of this smart healthcare technology have enabled medical practitioners to access patients' health remotely resulting in reduced visits to the hospitals. The added advantage is the reduced risk of catching another chronic disease from another patient or transferring the patient's disease to another hospital staff or visitors. Remote access to the data and the hospitals is the key feature of these wearable devices [3]. Allowing for monitoring the patients' vitals remotely thereby minimizing hospital visits and allowing doctors to patient's connections across the globe opens new avenues for improved healthcare

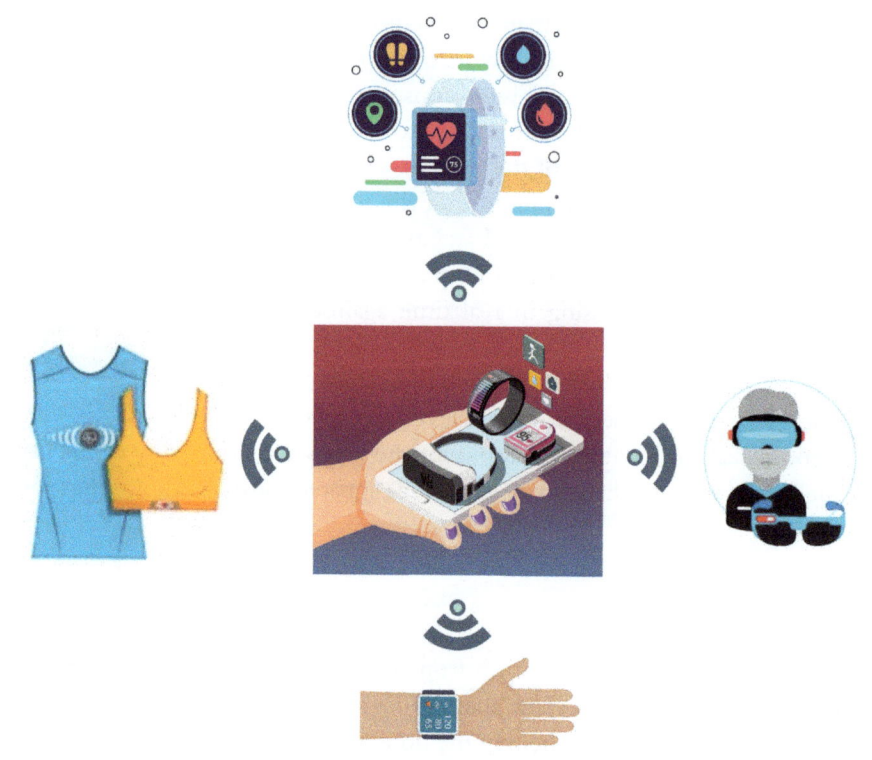

Fig. 2.6 Connection of wearable devices using IoT.

and reduced costs of medical diagnosis and treatment. The positive aspects of this technological leap in wearable biomedical devices are the following:
- No need for medical procedures
- Real-time prediction, prevention, and diagnosis
- Worldwide connectivity among doctors and patients through cloud-based systems
- Remote diagnosis and treatment by data evaluation against standard medical records or historical data
- Reduced need for hospitalization and its facilities making it cost effective
- Warning and/or alerts can be provided in real time to both doctors and patients against increased/decreased levels of vitals in the body

2.3.3 Equipment for diagnosis and treatment
2.3.3.1 Equipment for diagnosis
Initial prediction or diagnosis of certain diseases can be done via implantable, or wearable biomedical devices; however, detailed diagnosis and analysis can only be done by using sophisticated machines and/or equipment specifically designed to identify the presence of

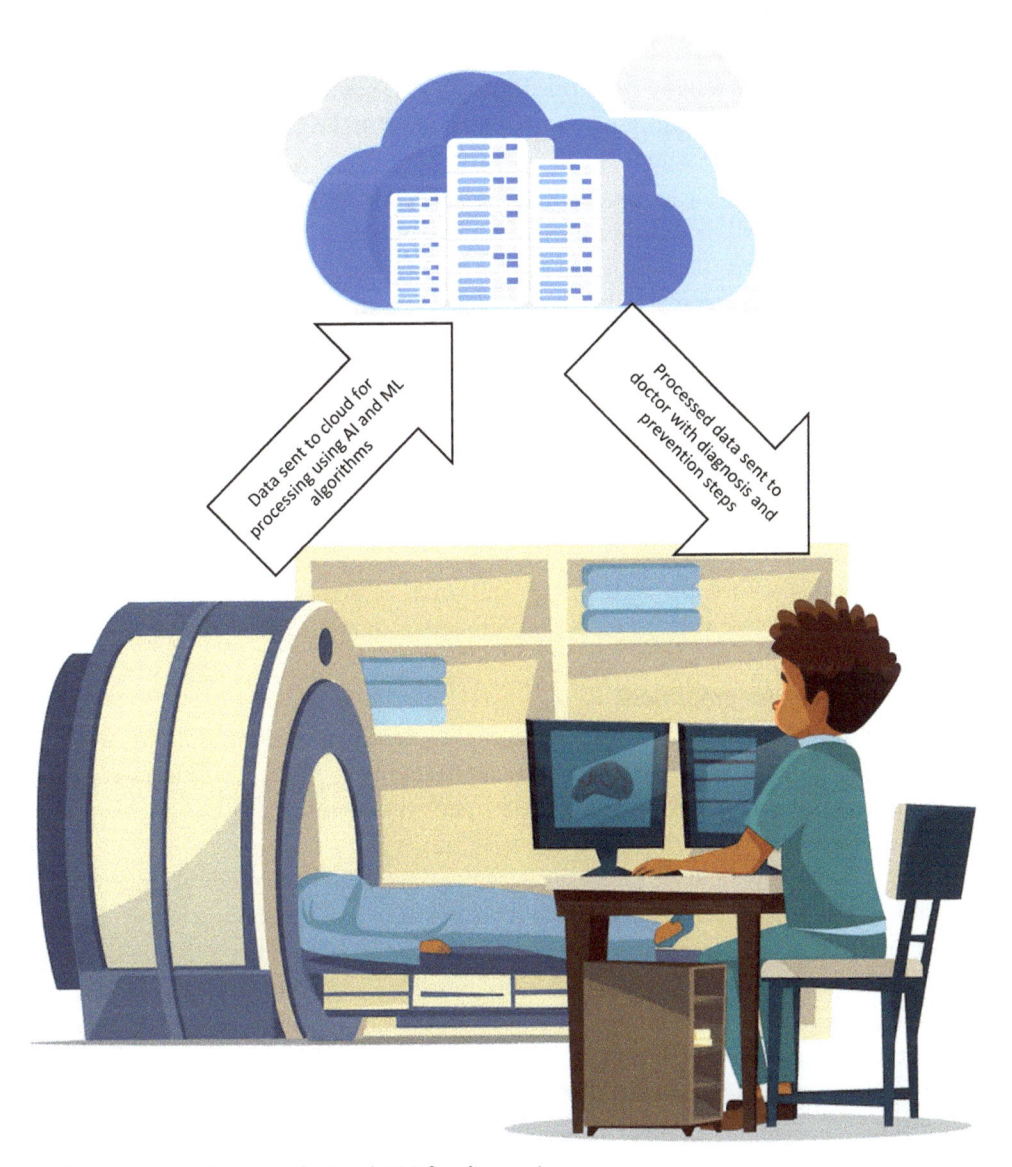

Fig. 2.7 Depicting the use of AI and CPS for diagnosis.

characteristic abnormalities or signals for a certain disease (Fig. 2.7). The integration of these machines and equipment with CPS allows them to evolve into Smart Diagnostic.

Smart diagnostics refers to the use of cloud-based software along with AI and ML algorithms for faster and more accurate identification of disease [35,36]. The imaging platforms are connected to the internet via IoMT and can be used to automate the diagnosis process allowing reduced human interaction, higher accuracy and precision, and reduced time due to faster diagnosis, thereby increasing the patient handling capacity. They are very useful for remote diagnosis allowing easy setting up of facilities at suitable places without the requirement of operators, and doctors to be physically present in front of the machines to operate them.

The live images are sent to the cloud where they are stored and analyzed instantaneously using AI and ML based algorithms against standard images or parameters, therefore providing erroneous detection and diagnosis. Moreover, they can also facilitate to provide information about any unheeded or unknown infection that might be present in the patients' body. The need is to equip these biomedical devices with internet and interfaces for remote operation and diagnosis. The pros of smart diagnostics explicitly include the following:
- Remote operation and diagnosis
- Detection of unnoticed or unknown infection and/or diseases
- Cloud-based software providing cloud storage and time-sensitive analysis
- High accuracy, precision, and reliability
- Reduced human efforts through self-identification of potential problems
- Increased transparency with patients allowing access to cloud computing based results

2.3.3.2 Equipment for treatment

Connecting the equipment of diagnosis with the cloud has yielded nothing short of self-sustained robotic surgical facilities. The feedback from smart diagnostics is fed to the equipment for treatment and is used to perform medical procedures like heart surgery, prostate surgery, or minimally invasive surgery.

Automation in this field of biomedical devices has equipped medical practitioners with tools of higher accuracy, precision, and erroneous features allowing highly delicate surgical procedures to be performed without much complexity. They offer higher flexibility, better reach inside the body which is not possible in conventional procedures, and enable surgeons to carry out minimally invasive surgeries, resulting in smaller incisions and faster healing and reduced hospitalization [11–13]. There is also a reduction of human error because the robotics arms are guided with very high accuracy allowing controlled movement.

Remote surgeries can also be performed without the presence of surgeons in the same room. A schematic of the same is shown in Fig. 2.8. Patients can be operated from across the globe without the need for availability of surgeons in front of the patient and/or machine [37]. As equipped with smart diagnostics, AI and ML algorithms can guide surgeons on how to perform the procedures and keep a live track of the removal of infections. The next step shall be to completely automate the surgical procedures requiring only the supervision of a medical practitioner, thereby reducing the workforce which in turn will be cost effective for patients and thereby reducing the burden on pockets of the marginalized

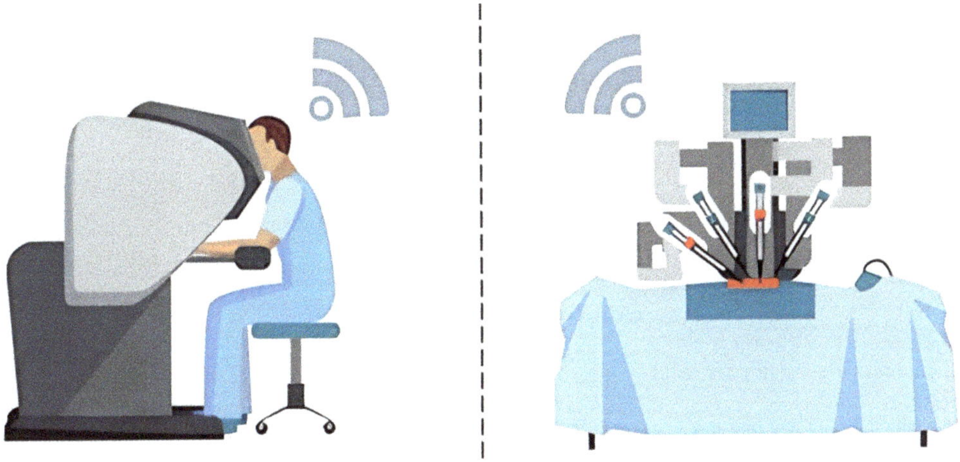

Fig. 2.8 Schematic of robotic surgery without the need of surgeons to be present in the same room.

society that is unable to cater the expensive treatments. The interconnection among all the possible equipment and further automation of the same using CPS will help us write a new chapter on robotic surgeries in the healthcare world. It is important to note the benefits of the automation in surgical procedures:
- Ease of human interaction
- Minimized involvement of human
- Remote access
- Greater accessibility, precision, accuracy, and reliability
- Integration with smart diagnostics thereby fully automating the procedures
- Alerts with live feedback and a tracking system
- Guidance system for surgeons

2.4 Case studies and applications

In this section, studies pertaining to the use of automation in biomedical devices shall be discussed highlighting how the automation has led to enhanced safety, early detection of diseases, robotic surgeries, etc., which are shaping the healthcare industry under the influence of Industry 4.0 (Tables 2.1–2.3).

2.5 Regulatory and safety considerations

Experts when given freedom can generate products which yield outcomes beyond the required working dimensions. However, it can sometimes be fatal for the dedicated application in the long run. Therefore, to try and optimize these boundary conditions,

Table 2.1 Case studies on implantable devices.

Device type	Method of fabrication/ parameter (or disease detected)	Automation used	Reference
Prosthetic hand	Fused deposition modelling	Additive manufacturing	[38]
3D printed medicine	Selective laser melting	Additive manufacturing	[39]
Scaffolds for medical Implants	Selective laser melting and Selective Electron beam melting	Additive manufacturing	[40,41]
Subcutaneous sensor	Glucose level	Continuous glucose monitoring system coupled with artificial neural network to detect glucose level	[42]
Implanted pacemaker	Pacemaker parameters	Remote monitoring using IoT	[43]

Table 2.2 Case studies on wearable devices.

Device used	Parameters/ outcome measured (or disease detected)	Automation used	Reference
Smartwatches	Movement of elderly person	Use of IoT and ML algorithms to analyze movement or fall and to provide actions	[44]
E-textile-based wearable sensor	Invasive blood pressure measurement	Data are collected via the specially designed app and sent to cloud databases for monitoring	[45]
Smartphone and glucometer	Gestational diabetes through glucose level monitoring	ML algorithm used to evaluate the recorded data for suggestions on diet plans and visit to doctors	[46]
Wearable biosensors coupled with imaging and motion sensors	Metabolites and nutrients in biofluids	Cloud-based systems to offer personalized nutrition intake	[47]
Smartphones	Monitoring of symptoms for Alzheimer's disease	IoT and cloud computing to analyze the symptoms and eventually contact doctors	[35]

certain regulations and safety guidelines are put forth by regulatory agencies for biomedical devices. Several cases of risks posed to patients have called for experts to enhance the testing for the safety and effectiveness of new devices [53,54].

The United States (US) and European Union (EU), the two most important markets, have juxtaposing approaches for the approval of biomedical devices for use by the end

Table 2.3 Case studies on equipment for diagnosis and treatment.

Device type	Parameter/data measured (or disease detected)	Automation used	Reference
CT scans	Lung Cancer	AI is used to evaluate CT scan images for detection of cancer	[48]
Minimally Invasive Surgery	Surgical procedure	Robots coupled with AI for suggestion of surgical procedures, and postsurgery care (like recovery time calculation)	[49]
Clinical notes	Conversion of human language in machine-readable format	Natural Language Processing	[50]
Electrocardiogram (ECG)	Heart failure	Use of AI to evaluate ECG data for early detection of heart failure	[51,52]
Da Vinci Surgical System	Robotic Surgery	The surgical system is equipped with technology which allows doctors to perform surgeries remotely and control the arms of robots	[37]

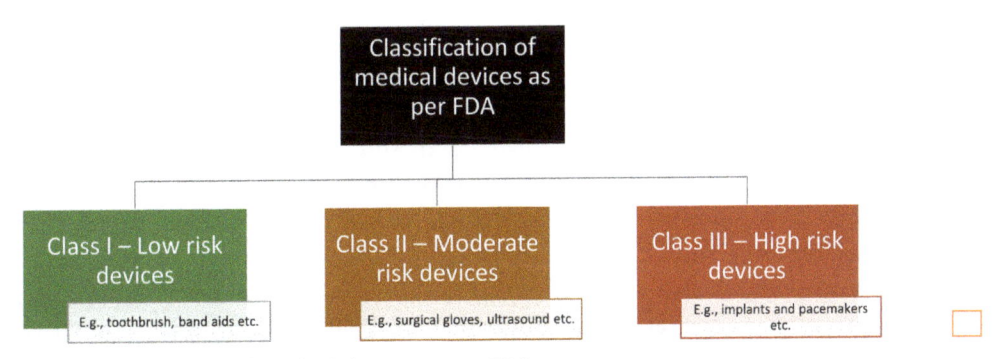

Fig. 2.9 Classification of medical devices as per FDA.

user [55]. The oldest consumer agency in US is the Food and Drug Administration (FDA). It has classified medical devices into three classes as shown in Fig. 2.9. Class I—low-risk devices like toothbrushes, band aids etc., Class II—moderate risk devices like surgical gloves, ultrasound etc., and Class III—high-risk devices like implants and pacemakers. [56]. Each class pertains to a different set of criteria before its sales are allowed. Class III devices are to be subjected to trials by its manufacturer and are approved by the

FDA through a process called premarket approval (PMA) [57]. Similar to the FDA, the Medical Device Directive (MDD) has been regulating medical devices in the EU since the 1990s. In contrast to the US, it has four classes—Class I, Class IIa, Class IIb, and Class III [58]. Affixations of *Conformity "Europe" enne (CE) marking* is one of the regulations of the EU which should be adhered to before marketing of any medical device [59]. Several other agencies from across the globe are Pharmaceuticals Medical Devices Agency (PMDA) in Japan, Therapeutic Goods Administration in Australia, Therapeutic Products Division of Health Canada, Central Drug Standards Control Organization (CDSCO) as part of Ministry of Health and Family Welfare in India, China Food and Drug Administration (CFDA) in China, Roszdravnadzor in Russia, and GOST Standard in Russia.

2.5.1 Compliance with medical device regulations

Specific standards and regulations are already in place and maintained by the bodies of each nation. One such requirement toward compliance is the correct labelling of the devices to highlight their risk class and intent of use. Table 2.4 depicts the requirements of various agencies across the nations.

2.5.2 Standardization and validation

As it is evident from the section above all countries have their local regulating body with different standards for testing, and approval. Therefore, for effective and unanimous automation of biomedical devices, it is especially important to have a standard or central agency that sets the guidelines for regulations, testing, and approval for all biomedical devices across the globe, which will allow us a chance to fully accomplish automation. One such example is the Global Harmonization Task Force (GHTF) which was founded by the US, EU, Japan, Canada, and Australia [66]. GHTF was aimed at integrating and standardizing the regulatory process and supporting the development of technology. This guidance is further shared with member national regulatory authorities which are responsible for implementing them in their regions. GHTF has recommended a four-class system from Class A to Class D and provides 17 rules for the classification of devices. Class A corresponds to low-risk materials and Class D to high-risk materials [60].

2.6 Drawbacks and challenges

As it is important to highlight the advantages, merits, and pros of automation in biomedical devices, it is equally important to lay down their demerits and the areas of special considerations that are to be addressed before the implementation of the above aspects in the future using Industry 4.0. Transparent cost–benefit analysis, infrastructures, lack of skilled workforce, the functionality of existing machines and equipment, and finally

Table 2.4 Medical device regulations/guidelines as stipulated by various countries across the globe.

Country	Regulating/statuary body	Regulation/guidelines	Reference
USA	Food and Drug Administration (FDA)	• Necessary approval to be filed with the FDA before marketing medical devices • PMA process to be followed for all Class III devices • Adherence to the Code of Federal Regulations (CFR) for labelling of medical devices	[60,61]
EU	Medical Device Directive (MDD)	• Devices are to be labeled with the name and address of the manufacturer • Conformity "Europe" (CE) marking is compulsory for all medical devices	[62,63]
Japan	Pharmaceuticals Medical Devices Agency (PMDA) in Japan	• Obtain "shonin" (manufacturing product approval) for marketing a high-risk medical device • "Kyoka" (license) which gives authorization to OEMs to market products • Pharmaceutical Affairs Law (PAL) established guidelines for proper labelling including contact information for the manufacturing site and local office	[61]
China	China Food and Drug Administration (CFDA)	• China Compulsory Certification (CCC) for high-risk devices • All safety information must be in Chinese for high-risk devices	[58]
India	Central Drug Standards Control Organization (CDSCO) as part of the Ministry of Health and Family Welfare	• Various bills and acts like Medical Devices Regulation Bill, 2006, Drugs and Cosmetics Act, 1940, Rules, 1945, and Bill, 2013 have been introduced which defines measure for the manufacture, sale, import and export of medical devices • Devices approved by the FDA and/or with CE Marking are allowed for import without further testing	[64,65]
Russia	Roszdravnadzor and GOST Standard	• Roszdravnadzor is responsible for the registration and assessment of medical devices • GOST-R QC and Hygiene certificate are needed for the import of medical devices	[58,60]

cyber security are some concerns toward automation through Industry 4.0 [67]. The chapter has addressed the above concerns by classifying them into the following categories.

2.6.1 Initial cost and investment

The point requiring the most emphasis is the initial cost and investment. The technology is developed considering a domain of applications; however, to promulgate it to the end user and to make it readily available for the healthcare industry requires huge investment in infrastructure facilities. The investment is required to improve the following facilities:
- Offices and/or workspaces for making it compatible with automation
- Training of workforce on the operation of automated systems
- Upgrading existing hardware and software to equip them with CPS and IoMT
- Installation of hardware and software
- Dedicated cloud storage and required computational power to analyze a large amount of data (big data analytics)
- Updating and making accessible the features of IoMT among the common people
- Maintenance of the system
- Troubleshooting of problems which shall incur at the beginning of trial periods
- Strong, reliable, and fast internet connectivity

It is also very important to note that estimates for initial investments might not be possible, except when the scope and whereabouts of the execution are predefined. It can be understood easily because health and safety regulations are different across the globe. Different agencies responsible in different countries have different norms for biomedical safety. Catering to the very stringent requirement of a certain regulatory body will require higher precision and safety standards, thereby increasing the cost of automation [3]. Analysis as per literature has shown that the payback cost of implementing the CPS is approximately 10 years. A small fluctuation in the initial cost may result in very little recovery or no recovery at all [68]. Therefore, feasibility studies must be performed in advance before automating the field.

2.6.2 Specialized training and workforce adaptation

The development of infrastructure is not the only key to automation of the biomedical devices. The aspect that cannot be avoided at any cost despite 100% automation is the human-machine interaction. Owing to Industry 4.0 leading to the implementation of CPS, AI, and ML algorithms, it is of great importance to have highly skilled workforce which can interact firmly with autonomous systems [69]. This dealing with human factors in implementing Industry 4.0 is termed as "Operator 4.0" [70].

The need not only relies on the implementation of automation but also on training the existing skill pool. It is important to identify the skilled employees among the existing workforce who can take up this new assignment and train them on the needed computational skills associated with the area of implementation [71]. Sectors with a higher degree of automation will also demand higher expertise and better-trained professionals thereby increasing the requirement of basic skill sets and qualifications. As it was also identified that employees involvement also affects the implementation of Industry 4.0 [72]; therefore, it is unavoidable to eliminate the human factor for its implementation. Not only the workforce but also the positions of leadership and/or higher responsibility are also barriers toward the implementation of Industry 4.0 [73] because they nurture vision of the employees by motivating them toward a common goal, proper working culture, and making alliances [74–76].

Steps are required to be taken to integrate the development of technology and humans' hand in hand to achieve relentless growth for the implementation of Industry 4.0.

2.6.3 Technical failures and malfunctions

These are the failures that are expected to occur once the systems are up and running. It is important to understand that failures and malfunctions can occur at any stage and any place in the whole system. However, we will restrict ourselves to some of the important features related to Industry 4.0. Studies have listed quite some challenges on the technical front; however, we have narrowed them down to the following:

2.6.3.1 Internet

As it is impossible to connect all devices using wires, the internet is one of the most important features for achieving automation, i.e., to connect all devices through wireless connections. To understand it easily, it has been divided into three aspects—the logical topology, the communication protocols, and the physical infrastructure [77].

Internet is a decentralized entity and, therefore, it is not in the hands of a single organization or agency to regulate it. This makes it prone to disruptions. The idea of automation is through connecting devices across the globe; therefore, internet disruptions or changes in regulations by any local regulating body will lead to loss of connectivity among the communicating devices thereby refuting the idea of automation and Industry 4.0 [78].

2.6.3.2 Sensor's failure/device malfunction

The implementation of Industry 4.0 relies on the sensor technology which is part of the feedback mechanisms in automating the devices, machines, and/or equipment. This is only possible by using sensors that collect vital data like temperature, pressure, velocity, etc. [79] and send it to the centralized systems where it is processed and further steps to be taken to regulate the process are identified and initiated accordingly. Any failure and mismanagement in sensors can alter the feedback, thereby affecting the device's performance. Hence, it is certainly important that the sensor work efficiently for the effective and correct working of the devices.

2.6.3.3 Connectivity across platforms
Connectivity across platforms has been identified as one of the major issues pertaining to the implementation of IoT [77]. The major guiding attribute is the isolation working of the production units which hinders the flexibility and adaptability of the IoT devices [80] to be able to communicate and establish the features that are beneficial to Industry 4.0. The second important factor under consideration should be the scalability [81], i.e., the capability of the present internet to handle the available and upcoming devices and prevention from cyber-attacks.

2.6.3.4 Software failure
This aspect is relatively untouched or discussed with respect to the requirements of the advancement in software technologies to integrate the devices. Rather, there is a need to understand that once the software is developed and deployed in the market, what general challenges faced if the software fails to realize its functioning. The failure in software may lead to incorrect detection and analysis of signals [82], increased involvement of technicians to run the processes, loss of communication between the physical and cyber-environments [83], and errors in data flow and control flow [84].

2.6.4 Cyber security and cyber-attacks
The exploitation of vulnerable areas through cyber-attacks affecting national and international security has been a major area of concern for the experts and the industries implementing Industry 4.0. This breach of information is a major security threat requiring utmost attention. It has opened new avenues for scammers and attackers to attack, alter and/or control the whole process flow thereby affecting the overall process. In the context of biomedical devices, it is important to understand that data breach is easier because of unavailability of experienced IT professionals in the healthcare sector [85]. The automation in biomedical devices provides them with networking capabilities which in turn allows them to be controlled remotely and opens the areas for attacks and vulnerabilities which is not the case for isolated devices [5]. As biomedical devices are diverse and spread across a spectrum of domains ranging from small implantable stimulators to extremely large, stationary MRI machines, they are more vulnerable, and therefore, each type of device needs its own security measures [86]. Studies have shown that devices could be hacked easily and be altered to launch potentially lethal attacks [87]. The following types of altercations have been suggested by the literature [86,88,89]:
- a. Tampering
- b. Denial of Services
- c. Eavesdropping

d. Power mismanagement
e. Incorrect/artificial sensor readings
f. Unauthorized command
g. Incorrect/altered output signal
h. Repetitive access attempts
i. Information disclosure
j. Reprogramming of the devices etc.

It is also important to understand that not only the biomedical devices but hospitals are also vulnerable to these cyber-attacks. As they are all interconnected, hence, not just patients' data but hospital staff data and other records are also prone to be leaked or tampered with.

2.7 Conclusion

The review provides an in-depth insight into the automation of biomedical devices and how the same can change the way we perceive the present healthcare industry. Biomedical devices were classified into various categories for ease of understanding, and it was concluded that automation is a feature that can be implemented in any of the disciplines. The use of automation through AM, AI, ML, and CPS was discussed for all categories and how the same can be implemented. It was drawn with the help of literature that automating the processes for manufacturing implantable devices gives ease of manufacturing implants followed by their installation using robotics or MIS. Case studies have shown how automation in biomedical devices has led to improved efficiency and early detection of cancers. It was further established that implementation of Industry 4.0 should be done considering the regulations and guidelines that are set forth by various agencies and how there is a need for standard regulations for the implementation of automation in all disciplines. Lastly, this review discussed the drawbacks and challenges by bifurcating them into various subcategories discussing each aspect and its influence on the implementation of automation in the healthcare sector.

References

[1] S. Sahoo, C.-Y. Lo, Smart manufacturing powered by recent technological advancements: a review, J. Manuf. Syst. 64 (2022) 236–250, https://doi.org/10.1016/j.jmsy.2022.06.008.
[2] P. Manickam, et al., Artificial intelligence (AI) and Internet of Medical Things (IoMT) assisted biomedical systems for intelligent healthcare, Biosensors 12 (8) (2022) 562, https://doi.org/10.3390/bios12080562.
[3] Z. Pang, G. Yang, R. Khedri, Y.-T. Zhang, Introduction to the special section: convergence of automation technology, biomedical engineering, and health informatics toward the healthcare 4.0, IEEE Rev. Biomed. Eng. 11 (2018) 249–259, https://doi.org/10.1109/RBME.2018.2848518.
[4] L.R.R. Da Silva, et al., A comprehensive review on additive manufacturing of medical devices, Prog. Addit. Manuf. 6 (3) (2021) 517–553, https://doi.org/10.1007/s40964-021-00188-0.

[5] F. Tettey, S.K. Parupelli, S. Desai, A review of biomedical devices: classification, regulatory guidelines, human factors, software as a medical device, and cybersecurity, Biomed. Mater. Devices (2023), https://doi.org/10.1007/s44174-023-00113-9.

[6] D.B. Kramer, S. Xu, A.S. Kesselheim, How does medical device regulation perform in the United States and the European Union? A systematic review, PLoS Med. 9 (7) (2012) e1001276, https://doi.org/10.1371/journal.pmed.1001276.

[7] R.J. Hemalatha, et al., Biomedical instrument and automation: automatic instrumentation in biomedical engineering, in: Handbook of Data Science Approaches for Biomedical Engineering, Elsevier, 2020, pp. 69–101, https://doi.org/10.1016/B978-0-12-818318-2.00003-9.

[8] A.A. Zadpoor, Design for Additive bio-Manufacturing: from patient-specific medical devices to rationally designed Meta-biomaterials, Int. J. Mol. Sci. 18 (8) (2017) 1607, https://doi.org/10.3390/ijms18081607.

[9] A. Wazeer, A. Das, A. Sinha, K. Inaba, S. Ziyi, A. Karmakar, Additive manufacturing in biomedical field: a critical review on fabrication method, materials used, applications, challenges, and future prospects, Prog. Addit. Manuf. (2022), https://doi.org/10.1007/s40964-022-00362-y.

[10] M. Sekar, et al., Review—towards wearable sensor platforms for the electrochemical detection of cortisol, J. Electrochem. Soc. 167 (6) (2020) 067508, https://doi.org/10.1149/1945-7111/ab7e24.

[11] C. Bergeles, G.-Z. Yang, From passive tool holders to microsurgeons: safer, smaller, smarter surgical robots, IEEE Trans. Biomed. Eng. 61 (5) (2014) 1565–1576, https://doi.org/10.1109/TBME.2013.2293815.

[12] H. Marcus, D. Nandi, A. Darzi, G.-Z. Yang, Surgical robotics through a keyhole: from Today's translational barriers to Tomorrow's 'disappearing' robots, IEEE Trans. Biomed. Eng. 60 (3) (2013) 674–681, https://doi.org/10.1109/TBME.2013.2243731.

[13] J.A. Hawks, J. Kunowski, S.R. Platt, In vivo demonstration of surgical task assistance using miniature robots, IEEE Trans. Biomed. Eng. 59 (10) (2012) 2866–2873, https://doi.org/10.1109/TBME.2012.2212439.

[14] A. Lumsden, J. Bismuth, Current status of endovascular catheter robotics, J. Cardiovasc. Surg. 59 (2018), https://doi.org/10.23736/S0021-9509.18.10447-2.

[15] M. Rueda, C. Riga, M. Hamady, Flexible robotics in pelvic disease: what pathologies? Does the catheter increase applicability of embolic therapy? J. Cardiovasc. Surg. 59 (2018), https://doi.org/10.23736/S0021-9509.18.10422-8.

[16] L.J. De Vries, F. Zijlstra, T. Szili-Torok, Beyond catheter tip and radiofrequency lesion delivery: the role of robotics in ablation of ventricular tachycardia, Neth. Heart J. 23 (10) (2015) 483–484, https://doi.org/10.1007/s12471-015-0737-y.

[17] P.N. Dogra, Current Status of Robotic Surgery in India, 3rd, vol. 25, JIMSA, 2012. http://www.imsaonline.com/june-sep-2012/6.pdf. (Accessed 16 September 2023).

[18] J.M. Chacón, P.J. Núñez, M.A. Caminero, E. García-Plaza, J. Vallejo, M. Blanco, 3D printing of patient-specific 316L–stainless–steel medical implants using fused filament fabrication technology: two veterinary case studies, Bio-Des. Manuf. 5 (4) (2022) 808–815, https://doi.org/10.1007/s42242-022-00200-8.

[19] K.W. Dalgarno, et al., Mass customization of medical devices and implants: state of the art and future directions, Virtual Phys. Prototyp. 1 (3) (2006) 137–145, https://doi.org/10.1080/17452750601092031.

[20] S. Mallakpour, E. Azadi, C.M. Hussain, State-of-the-art of 3D printing technology of alginate-based hydrogels—an emerging technique for industrial applications, Adv. Colloid Interf. Sci. 293 (2021) 102436, https://doi.org/10.1016/j.cis.2021.102436.

[21] W. Aljohani, M.W. Ullah, X. Zhang, G. Yang, Bioprinting and its applications in tissue engineering and regenerative medicine, Int. J. Biol. Macromol. 107 (2018) 261–275, https://doi.org/10.1016/j.ijbiomac.2017.08.171.

[22] S. Santoni, S.G. Gugliandolo, M. Sponchioni, D. Moscatelli, B.M. Colosimo, 3D bioprinting: current status and trends—a guide to the literature and industrial practice, Bio-Des. Manuf. 5 (1) (2022) 14–42, https://doi.org/10.1007/s42242-021-00165-0.

[23] L. Raddatz, et al., Additive manufactured customizable labware for biotechnological purposes, Eng. Life Sci. 17 (8) (2017) 931–939, https://doi.org/10.1002/elsc.201700055.
[24] S.V. Nagar, A.C. Chandrashekar, M. Suvarna, Optimized additive manufacturing technology using digital twins and cyber physical systems, in: M.E. Auer, B.K. Ram (Eds.), Cyber-physical Systems and Digital Twins, Lecture Notes in Networks and Systems, vol. 80, Springer International Publishing, Cham, 2020, pp. 65–73, https://doi.org/10.1007/978-3-030-23162-0_7.
[25] U.M. Dilberoglu, B. Gharehpapagh, U. Yaman, M. Dolen, The role of additive manufacturing in the era of industry 4.0, Procedia Manuf. 11 (2017) 545–554, https://doi.org/10.1016/j.promfg.2017.07.148.
[26] S. Phuyal, D. Bista, R. Bista, Challenges, opportunities and future directions of smart manufacturing: a state of art review, Sustain. Futur. 2 (2020) 100023, https://doi.org/10.1016/j.sftr.2020.100023.
[27] H.S. Kang, et al., Smart manufacturing: past research, present findings, and future directions, Int. J. Precis. Eng. Manuf.-Green Technol. 3 (1) (2016) 111–128, https://doi.org/10.1007/s40684-016-0015-5.
[28] How AI solution Helps empower Smart Manufacturing, Accessed: 16 September 2023. [Online]. Available: https://www.softwebsolutions.com/resources/artificial-intelligence-in-smart-manufacturing.html.
[29] The Growing Influence of AI in Smart Manufacturing, ARC Advisory Group. Accessed: 16 September 2023 [Online]. Available: https://www.arcweb.com/blog/growing-influence-ai-smart-manufacturing.
[30] W.-C. Wang, S.-L. Chen, L.-B. Chen, W.-J. Chang, A machine vision based automatic optical inspection system for measuring drilling quality of printed circuit boards, IEEE Access 5 (2017) 10817–10833, https://doi.org/10.1109/ACCESS.2016.2631658.
[31] H. Atlam, R. Walters, G. Wills, Fog computing and the internet of things: a review, Big Data Cogn. Comput. 2 (2) (2018) 10, https://doi.org/10.3390/bdcc2020010.
[32] T.G. Stavropoulos, A. Papastergiou, L. Mpaltadoros, S. Nikolopoulos, I. Kompatsiaris, IoT wearable sensors and devices in elderly care: a literature review, Sensors 20 (10) (2020) 2826, https://doi.org/10.3390/s20102826.
[33] C. Dilibal, B.L. Davis, C. Chakraborty, Generative design methodology for internet of medical things (IoMT)-based wearable biomedical devices, in: 2021 3rd International Congress on Human-Computer Interaction, Optimization and Robotic Applications (HORA), IEEE, Ankara, Turkey, 2021, pp. 1–4, https://doi.org/10.1109/HORA52670.2021.9461370.
[34] A. Banerjee, C. Chakraborty, A. Kumar, D. Biswas, Chapter 5 - emerging trends in IoT and big data analytics for biomedical and health care technologies, in: V.E. Balas, V.K. Solanki, R. Kumar, M. Khari (Eds.), Handbook of Data Science Approaches for Biomedical Engineering, Academic Press, 2020, pp. 121–152, https://doi.org/10.1016/B978-0-12-818318-2.00005-2.
[35] J. Sharma, S. Kaur, Gerontechnology — The study of alzheimer disease using cloud computing, in: 2017 International Conference on Energy, Communication, Data Analytics and Soft Computing (ICECDS), 2017, pp. 3726–3733, https://doi.org/10.1109/ICECDS.2017.8390159.
[36] N. Jelcic, et al., Feasibility and efficacy of cognitive telerehabilitation in early Alzheimer's disease: a pilot study, Clin. Interv. Aging 9 (2014) 1605–1611, https://doi.org/10.2147/CIA.S68145.
[37] J.J. Rasouli, et al., Artificial intelligence and robotics in spine surgery, Glob. Spine J. 11 (4) (2021) 556–564, https://doi.org/10.1177/2192568220915718.
[38] X. Chen, et al., Scaffold structural microenvironmental cues to guide tissue regeneration in bone tissue applications, Nano 8, no. 11, Art. no. 11 (2018), https://doi.org/10.3390/nano8110960.
[39] W. Jamróz, J. Szafraniec, M. Kurek, R. Jachowicz, 3D printing in pharmaceutical and medical applications—recent achievements and challenges, Pharm. Res. 35 (9) (2018) 176, https://doi.org/10.1007/s11095-018-2454-x.
[40] L.-C. Zhang, H. Attar, M. Calin, J. Eckert, Review on manufacture by selective laser melting and properties of titanium based materials for biomedical applications, Mater. Technol. 31 (2) (2016) 66–76, https://doi.org/10.1179/1753555715Y.0000000076.
[41] X.P. Tan, Y.J. Tan, C.S.L. Chow, S.B. Tor, W.Y. Yeong, Metallic powder-bed based 3D printing of cellular scaffolds for orthopaedic implants: a state-of-the-art review on manufacturing, topological

design, mechanical properties and biocompatibility, Mater. Sci. Eng. C 76 (2017) 1328–1343, https://doi.org/10.1016/j.msec.2017.02.094.

[42] T. Hamdi, et al., Artificial neural network for blood glucose level prediction, in: 2017 International Conference on Smart, Monitored and Controlled Cities (SM2C), 2017, pp. 91–95, https://doi.org/10.1109/SM2C.2017.8071825.

[43] K.G. Tarakji, et al., Performance of first pacemaker to use smart device app for remote monitoring, Heart Rhythm O2 2 (5) (2021) 463–471, https://doi.org/10.1016/j.hroo.2021.07.008.

[44] M. Karakaya, G. Şengül, A. Bostan, Remotely monitoring activities of the elders using smart watches, ISSN 3 (1) (2017).

[45] Y. Fang, et al., Ambulatory cardiovascular monitoring via a machine-learning-assisted textile triboelectric sensor, Adv. Mater. 33 (41) (2021) 2104178, https://doi.org/10.1002/adma.202104178.

[46] M. Rigla, I. Martínez-Sarriegui, G. García-Sáez, B. Pons, M.E. Hernando, Gestational diabetes management using smart Mobile telemedicine, J. Diabetes Sci. Technol. 12 (2) (2018) 260–264, https://doi.org/10.1177/1932296817704442.

[47] J.R. Sempionatto, V.R.-V. Montiel, E. Vargas, H. Teymourian, J. Wang, Wearable and Mobile sensors for personalized nutrition, ACS Sens. 6 (5) (2021) 1745–1760, https://doi.org/10.1021/acssensors.1c00553.

[48] E. Svoboda, Artificial intelligence is improving the detection of lung cancer, Nature 587 (7834) (2020) S20–S22, https://doi.org/10.1038/d41586-020-03157-9.

[49] X.-Y. Zhou, Y. Guo, M. Shen, G.-Z. Yang, Application of artificial intelligence in surgery, Front. Med. 14 (4) (2020) 417–430, https://doi.org/10.1007/s11684-020-0770-0.

[50] J. Carriere, et al., Case report: utilizing AI and NLP to assist with healthcare and rehabilitation during the COVID-19 pandemic, Front. Artif. Intell. 4 (2021). Accessed 16 September 2023. [Online]. Available https://www.frontiersin.org/articles/10.3389/frai.2021.613637. Accessed 16 September 2023. [Online]. Available.

[51] O. Akbilgic, et al., ECG-AI: electrocardiographic artificial intelligence model for prediction of heart failure, Eur. Heart J. Digit. Health 2 (4) (2021) 626–634. Oxford Academic. Accessed 16 September 2023. [Online]. Available https://academic.oup.com/ehjdh/article/2/4/626/6385780.

[52] K.C. Siontis, P.A. Noseworthy, Z.I. Attia, P.A. Friedman, Artificial intelligence-enhanced electrocardiography in cardiovascular disease management, Nat. Rev. Cardiol. 18, no. 7, Art. no. 7 (2021), https://doi.org/10.1038/s41569-020-00503-2.

[53] D.R. Challoner, W.W. Vodra, Medical devices and health — creating a new regulatory framework for moderate-risk devices, N. Engl. J. Med. 365 (11) (2011) 977–979, https://doi.org/10.1056/NEJMp1109150.

[54] M. Thompson, C. Heneghan, M. Billingsley, D. Cohen, Medical device recalls and transparency in the UK, BMJ 342 (2011) d2973, https://doi.org/10.1136/bmj.d2973.

[55] D.B. Kramer, S. Xu, A.S. Kesselheim, Regulation of medical devices in the United States and European Union, N. Engl. J. Med. 366 (9) (2012) 848–855, https://doi.org/10.1056/NEJMhle1113918.

[56] T. Pham, T. Tran, D. Phung, S. Venkatesh, Predicting healthcare trajectories from medical records: a deep learning approach, J. Biomed. Inform. 69 (2017) 218–229, https://doi.org/10.1016/j.jbi.2017.04.001.

[57] W.H. Maisel, Medical device regulation: an introduction for the practicing physician, Ann. Intern. Med. 140 (4) (2004) 296–302, https://doi.org/10.7326/0003-4819-140-4-200402170-00012.

[58] S. Kumar Gupta, Medical device regulations: a current perspective, J. Young Pharm. 8 (1) (2015) 06–11, https://doi.org/10.5530/jyp.2016.1.3.

[59] E. French-Mowat, J. Burnett, How are medical devices regulated in the European Union? J. R. Soc. Med. 105 (Suppl 1) (2012) S22–S28, https://doi.org/10.1258/jrsm.2012.120036.

[60] S. Lamph, Regulation of medical devices outside the European Union, J. R. Soc. Med. 105 (Suppl 1) (2012) S12–S21, https://doi.org/10.1258/jrsm.2012.120037.

[61] R.K. Songara, G.N. Sharma, V.K. Gupta, P. Gupta, Need for Harmonization of Labeling of Medical Devices: A Review, J. Adv. Pharm. Tech. Res. 1 (2010), pp. 127–144.

[62] C. Heneghan, M. Thompson, M. Billingsley, D. Cohen, Medical-device recalls in the UK and the device-regulation process: retrospective review of safety notices and alerts, BMJ Open 1 (1) (2011) e000155, https://doi.org/10.1136/bmjopen-2011-000155.

[63] M. Donawa, New efforts to harmonise clinical evaluation, Med. Device Technol. vol. 17 (2006). pp. 28, 30, 32.
[64] The Drugs And Cosmetics (Amendment) Bill, 2013: Regulations For Medical Devices And Conduct Of Clinical Trial - Food and Drugs Law – India, Accessed 16 September 2023. [Online]. Available: https://www.mondaq.com/india/food-and-drugs-law/264918/the-drugs-and-cosmetics-amendment-bill-2013-regulations-for-medical-devices-and-conduct-of-clinical-trial..
[65] B. Veeranna, P. Kumar, V. Ravi, N. Radhadevi, Regulatory guidelines for medical devices in India: an overview, Asian J. Pharm. 6 (2012) 10, https://doi.org/10.4103/0973-8398.100125.
[66] W.H. Maisel, Semper fidelis- -consumer protection for patients with implanted medical devices, N. Engl. J. Med. 358 (10) (2008) 985–987, https://doi.org/10.1056/NEJMp0800495.
[67] S. Kumar, M. Suhaib, M. Asjad, Narrowing the barriers to industry 4.0 practices through PCA-fuzzy AHP-K means, J. Adv. Manag. Res. 18 (2) (2020) 200–226, https://doi.org/10.1108/JAMR-06-2020-0098.
[68] A.V. Bataev, A. Aleksandrova, Digitalization of the world economy: Performance evaluation of introducing cyber-physical systems, in: 2020 9th International Conference on Industrial Technology and Management (ICITM), IEEE, Oxford, United Kingdom, 2020, pp. 265–269, https://doi.org/10.1109/ICITM48982.2020.9080378.
[69] P. Kumar, R.K. Singh, Application of industry 4.0 technologies for effective coordination in humanitarian supply chains: a strategic approach, Ann. Oper. Res. 319 (1) (2022) 379–411, https://doi.org/10.1007/s10479-020-03898-w.
[70] W.P. Neumann, S. Winkelhaus, E.H. Grosse, C.H. Glock, Industry 4.0 and the human factor—a systems framework and analysis methodology for successful development, Int. J. Prod. Econ. 233 (2021) 107992, https://doi.org/10.1016/j.ijpe.2020.107992.
[71] H. Syed, S.H. Mian, B. Salah, W. Ameen, K. Moiduddin, H. Alkhalefah, Adapting universities for sustainability education in industry 4.0: channel of challenges and opportunities, Sustain. For. 12 (2020) 6100, https://doi.org/10.3390/su12156100.
[72] G. Tortorella, R. Miorando, R. Caiado, D.L. Nascimento, A. Portioli-Staudacher, The mediating effect of employees' involvement on the relationship between industry 4.0 and operational performance improvement, Total Qual. Manag. Bus. Excell. 32 (2018), https://doi.org/10.1080/14783363.2018.1532789.
[73] G.T. Cazeri, L.A. Santa-Eulalia, A.R. Fioravanti, M. Pavan Serafim, I.S. Rampasso, R. Anholon, Main challenges and best practices to be adopted in management training for industry 4.0, Kybernetes (2022), https://doi.org/10.1108/K-03-2022-0365.
[74] S. Helming, F. Ungermann, N. Hierath, N. Stricker, G. Lanza, Development of a training concept for leadership 4.0 in production environments, Procedia Manuf. 31 (2019) 38–44, https://doi.org/10.1016/j.promfg.2019.03.007.
[75] A. Moeuf, R. Pellerin, S. Lamouri, S. Tamayo-Giraldo, R. Barbaray, The industrial management of SMEs in the era of industry 4.0, Int. J. Prod. Res. 56 (3) (2018) 1118–1136, https://doi.org/10.1080/00207543.2017.1372647.
[76] M. Sony, S. Naik, Critical factors for the successful implementation of industry 4.0: a review and future research direction, Prod. Plan. Control 31 (10) (2020) 799–815, https://doi.org/10.1080/09537287.2019.1691278.
[77] G. Aceto, V. Persico, A. Pescape, A survey on information and communication Technologies for Industry 4.0: state-of-the-art, taxonomies, perspectives, and challenges, IEEE Commun. Surv. Tutor. 21 (4) (2019) 3467–3501, https://doi.org/10.1109/COMST.2019.2938259.
[78] C.S. Leberknight, M. Chiang, F.M.F. Wong, A taxonomy of censors and anti-censors: part I-impacts of internet censorship, Int. J. E-Polit. 3 (2) (2012) 52–64, https://doi.org/10.4018/jep.2012040104.
[79] Significance of sensors for industry 4.0: roles, capabilities, and applications, Sens. Int. 2 (2021) 100110, https://doi.org/10.1016/j.sintl.2021.100110.
[80] S. Weyer, M. Schmitt, M. Ohmer, D. Gorecky, Towards industry 4.0 - standardization as the crucial challenge for highly modular, multi-vendor production systems, IFAC-Pap. 48 (3) (2015) 579–584, https://doi.org/10.1016/j.ifacol.2015.06.143.
[81] R. van Kranenburg, A. Bassi, IoT challenges, Commun. Mob. Comput. 1 (1) (2012) 9, https://doi.org/10.1186/2192-1121-1-9.

[82] R. Iqbal, T. Maniak, F. Doctor, C. Karyotis, Fault detection and isolation in industrial processes using deep learning approaches, IEEE Trans. Ind. Inform. 15 (5) (2019) 3077–3084, https://doi.org/10.1109/TII.2019.2902274.

[83] P. O'Donovan, C. Gallagher, K. Bruton, D.T.J. O'Sullivan, A fog computing industrial cyber-physical system for embedded low-latency machine learning industry 4.0 applications, Manuf. Lett. 15 (2018) 139–142, https://doi.org/10.1016/j.mfglet.2018.01.005.

[84] J. Vankeirsbilck, J.V. Waes, H. Hallez, D. Pissoort, J. Boydens, 2019 IEEE international conference on systems, man and cybernetics (SMC), Control flow errors in an industry 4.0 setup: a preliminary study, 2019, pp. 2305–2310, https://doi.org/10.1109/SMC.2019.8914545.

[85] E. Davidson, A. Baird, K. Prince, Opening the envelope of health care information systems research, Inf. Organ. 28 (3) (2018) 140–151, https://doi.org/10.1016/j.infoandorg.2018.07.001.

[86] P. Raj, J.M. Chatterjee, A. Kumar, B. Balamurugan (Eds.), Internet of Things Use Cases for the Healthcare Industry, Springer International Publishing, Cham, 2020, https://doi.org/10.1007/978-3-030-37526-3.

[87] D. Dimitrov, Medical internet of things and big data in healthcare, Healthc. Inform. Res. 22 (2016) 156, https://doi.org/10.4258/hir.2016.22.3.156.

[88] J. Wu, H. Li, L. Liu, H. Zheng, Adoption of big data and analytics in mobile healthcare market: an economic perspective, Electron. Commer. Res. Appl. 22 (2017) 24–41, https://doi.org/10.1016/j.elerap.2017.02.002.

[89] S.V. Kovalchuk, A.A. Funkner, O.G. Metsker, A.N. Yakovlev, Simulation of patient flow in multiple healthcare units using process and data mining techniques for model identification, J. Biomed. Inform. 82 (2018) 128–142, https://doi.org/10.1016/j.jbi.2018.05.004.

CHAPTER 3

Mathematics in biomedical robotics and devices and its role in healthcare delivery

Mo Sadique[a], Sapna Ratan Shah[a], and Sardar M.N. Islam[b]
[a]School of Computational & Integrative Sciences, Jawaharlal Nehru University, New Delhi, India
[b]ISILC, Victoria University, Melbourne, VIC, Australia

3.1 Introduction

Robotics is one of the emerging and innovative fields of research in academia and industry. The robot was first introduced in 1920 by Karl Capek [1]. During the 1920s, Karel Capek coined the term "robot" in his work, *"Rossum's Universal Robots,"* depicting robots as artificial beings designed to assist humanity. In today's context, a robot is described as a programmed and actuated device exhibiting a certain level of autonomy, enabling it to navigate its surroundings and carry out predetermined tasks [2]. In the 1960s, robots emerged in the industrial sector, and these mechanical marvels quickly became indispensable components of automated systems. The robots not only enhance human abilities but also help human workers in monotonous, hazardous, or challenging tasks with an exhibition of impressive speed and precision [3,4]. In recent decades, the intersection of mathematics, robotics, and medicine has given rise to an interesting and emerging field known as biomedical robotics. This emerging discipline utilizes the concepts of mathematical principles to design, develop, and deploy robotic devices and systems that hold great importance in transforming healthcare delivery. With the aging global population, rising prevalence of chronic diseases, and a growing demand for more efficient and precise medical interventions, biomedical robotics has emerged as a key player in addressing these key challenges [5]. The integration of robotics into medicine offers numerous advantages, including enhanced precision, improved patient outcomes, reduced invasiveness, and the ability to overcome the physical limitations of human practitioners, making the healthcare sector a notable beneficiary of the robotic technology [6,7]. The integration of robots in healthcare is not a novel concept. The inaugural instance of robot-assisted surgical intervention dates back to 1985 when a robotic arm was interfaced with a computerized tomography (CT) scanner to perform a CT-guided brain tumor biopsy [8]. The utilization of robotic technology in the field of surgery has sparked the development of a diverse array of innovative methods and devices. There are a number of applications of robotics in healthcare and medical field. These areas encompass robotic surgical systems [9,10], laparoscopic surgery, tele-rounding robots [11], robot-assisted rehabilitation [12–14], as well as caregiver and patient assistance systems [15–17]. Furthermore, the application of robotics extends to various medical fields, including dentistry and bio-prosthetics [18,19]. A wide range of robots has been employed in intricate medical procedures, encompassing fields such as neurosurgery, cardiac surgery, orthopedic surgery, urology, bariatric surgery, prosthetic implantation, and rehabilitation [20]. The field of robotics in healthcare is experiencing rapid and substantial growth. It offers diverse solutions tailored to different healthcare needs, encompassing nursing, surgical procedures, and even minor medical interventions [21]. The role of biomedical robotics in the healthcare field and their types are summarized in Fig. 3.1. The different types of robots used in healthcare fields such as surgical and rehabilitation are shown in Fig. 3.2.

Advancements in mathematics, engineering, and healthcare are helping the rapid evolution of biomedical robots and devices. Mathematics plays a pivotal role in their design, development, and control, ensuring safety, efficacy, and effectiveness [26,27]. Mathematical modeling is crucial for understanding their behavior, enabling simulations of interactions between robots, patients, and the environment [28]. It also optimizes their design, determining materials, shapes, sizes, and motion algorithms [29]. Mathematical optimization plans optimal robot trajectories in surgeries, avoiding critical structures and

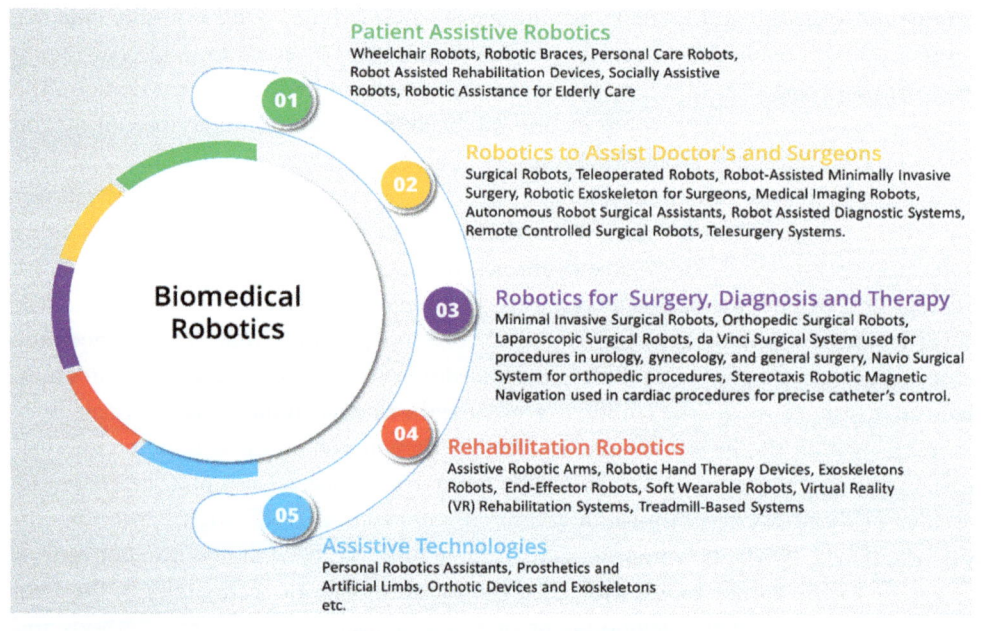

Fig. 3.1 Biomedical Robotics in healthcare field based on their types.

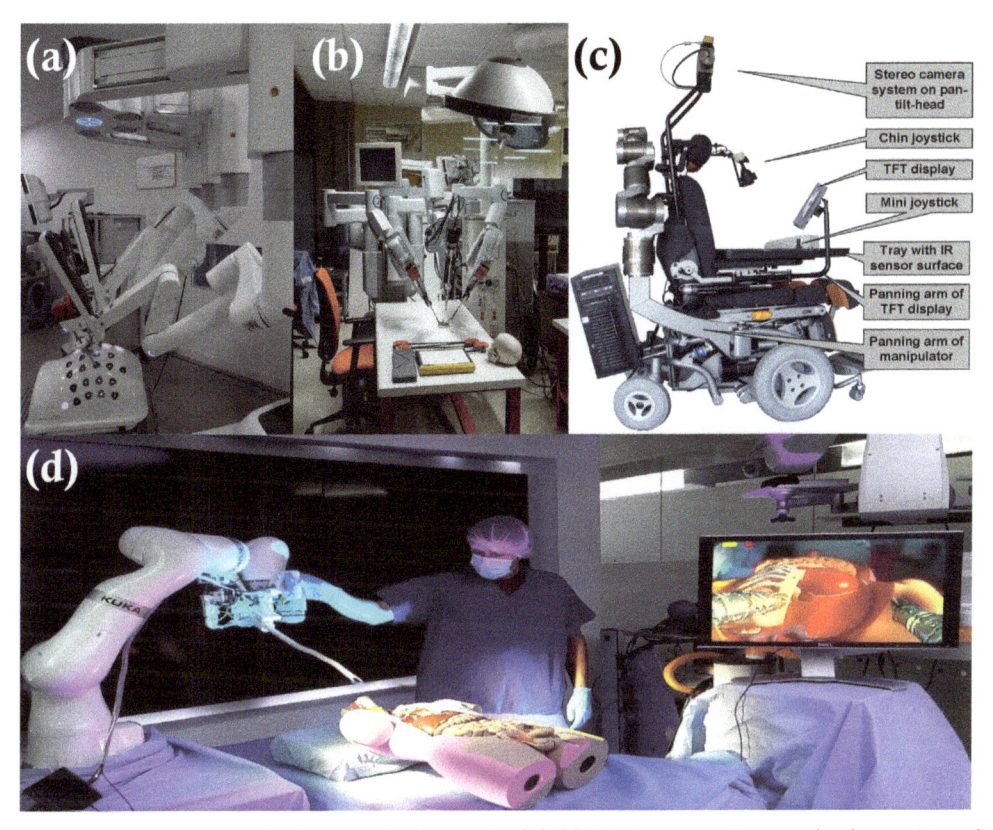

Fig. 3.2 Different types of robots in the biomedical field. (A) Da Vinci Xi surgical robot at Vesoul Hospital Centre. (B) A classroom surgery robot at Johns Hopkins University. (C) Care providing robotic wheelchair, Institute of Automation (IAT), University of Bremen. (D) The i^2 snake robot for endoscopic surgery [22–25]. (All images have been used under Creative Common License.)

ensuring the safety of patients, resulting in the optimization of the efficiency and effectiveness of robot-assisted interventions [30]. Mathematics is also helpful in the development of control algorithms for biomedical robots. Control algorithms, utilizing advanced theories like PID and adaptive control, regulate movements in surgical robots, rehabilitation devices, and teleoperated systems, which is crucial for successful minimally invasive surgery (MIS) [31,32]. Mathematics is essential to processing sensory data, interpreting information from sensors such as force and haptic feedback devices in surgical robotics, and enabling real-time interactions with body tissues [33]. Machine learning, based on mathematical principles, enhances perception and decision-making, making robots adaptive to diverse conditions [34]. Mathematics helps to make decisions in treatment plans based on clinical trial data and identifies potential surgical complications using biomedical robotics and devices [18,35]. In essence, mathematics is

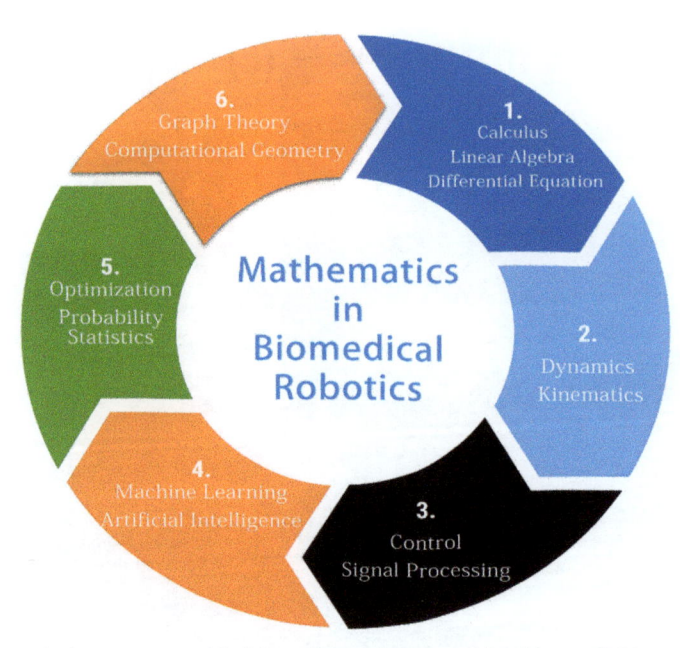

Fig. 3.3 Mathematical concept used in biomedical robotics and healthcare field.

indispensable in biomedical robotics, driving innovation and contributing to improved patient care and outcomes. The role of mathematical principles used in the field of biomedical robotics is demonstrated in Fig. 3.3.

This chapter delves into the fundamental role of mathematics in the field of biomedical robotics. By providing a comprehensive exploration of the mathematical foundations and their applications, this chapter aims to shed light on the potentially transformative impact of this interdisciplinary field on healthcare. The chapter begins by laying the groundwork for understanding the mathematical underpinnings of biomedical robotics. It starts with an introduction to the mathematical principles commonly employed in the field, such as control, motion, and force control. Additionally, the chapter explores how mathematics can be helpful in the development of biomedical robots. How mathematical concepts can form the basis for developing innovative and effective biomedical robotic solutions. Moreover, our aim in this chapter is to highlight the promising opportunities, acknowledge the challenges, and emphasize the transformative potential of mathematics in the field of biomedical robotics. By integrating rigorous mathematical principles with innovative engineering and medical expertise, biomedical robotics stands poised to revolutionize healthcare delivery, improving patient outcomes and enhancing the quality of life for countless individuals worldwide. As research and innovation in this domain continue to flourish, it is crucial to understand and appreciate mathematics' pivotal role in unlocking biomedical robotics' full potential.

3.2 Mathematical foundations of robotics and biomedical robotics

Mathematics is foundational in robotics, shaping the design, modeling, and control of robots, with key principles like linear algebra, kinematics, dynamics, and differential equations playing vital roles [19]. These principles facilitate precise system design for complex tasks, govern robot movements, and enable accurate modeling. Controllers, crafted using mathematical principles like differential equations and control theory, regulate robot motion [36–38]. Besides these foundational concepts, robotics incorporates probability, statistics, and optimization, enhancing capabilities for intricate tasks, with force and motion control being crucial in biomedical robotics applications. In this section we have discussed the concepts of motion and force control in robotics and how these concepts are used in the field of biomedical robotics.

Control is very crucial in robotics, directing robots to achieve the desired purpose by sending signals to their actuators, considering dynamics, forces, and torques. There are two types of control, open loop and closed loop, differing due to sensor feedback use. The objectives of control in robotics include motion, force, hybrid force-motion, and impedance control [39].

3.2.1 Motion control

The dynamic model of rigid robot manipulators for motion control in robotics is described by Lagrange's dynamics. If the robot manipulator has n-links and the vector q of joint variables is given by $q = (q_1, q_2, q_3, \ldots q_n)^T$. Then the following Lagrange's equation gives the dynamic model of the robot's manipulator:

$$H(q)\ddot{q} + C(q,\dot{q})\dot{q} + \tau_g(q) = \tau$$

where $H(q)$ is the inertia matrix, $C(q,\dot{q})$ is the vector of Coriolis and centrifugal forces, $\tau_g(q)$ is the vector of gravity forces, and τ is the vector of the joint control inputs [39].

Various types of motion control govern a robot's manipulators. The important and crucial controls include joint space control, operational space control, independent joint control, PD and PID control, computed torque, and computed torque-like control. While additional control types exist, they are less commonly employed in robotics. Joint space control directly adjusts robot joint angles, aiming to closely track desired motions.

Operational space control, a more indirect approach, sends signals to the end-effector, controlling robot motion by adjusting position, orientation, and velocity. The main objective of the joint space control is to design a feedback controller such that the joint coordinate $q(t) \in \mathbb{R}^n$ tracks the desired motion $q_d(t)$ as closely as possible [40,41]. The dynamics of the robot's manipulator in joint space controls and operational space control are presented by the following equations:

$$H(q)\ddot{q} + C(q,\dot{q})\dot{q} + \tau_g(q) = \tau$$

$$A(q)\ddot{x} + B(q,\dot{q})\dot{x} + C(q) = f_c$$

where the Jacobian matrix $J(q) \in \mathbb{R}^{n \times n}$ transforms the joint velocity $\dot{q} \in \mathbb{R}^n$ to the task velocity $\dot{x} \in \mathbb{R}^n$ by the relation $\dot{x} = J(q)\dot{q}$. The symbol $f_c \in \mathbb{R}^n$ represents the command force in the operational space and A, B, and C are given as follows:

$$A(q) = J^{-T}(q) H(q) J^{-1}(q)$$

$$B(q,\dot{q}) = J^{-T}(q) C(q,\dot{q}) J^{-1}(q) - A(q)\dot{J}(q) J^{-1}(q)$$

$$C(q) = J^{-T}(q) \tau_g(q)$$

Independent joint control is a joint control type where each joint's control input depends only on the measurements of its displacement and velocity. This control involves a single input, single output (SISD) system, and its control's input-output transfer function is defined by,

$$M(s) = \frac{k_m}{s(1 + sT_m)},$$

where k_m and T_m give by $k_m = \frac{G_v}{K_v}$ and $T_m = \frac{R_a J}{K_v K_t}$ are the voltage to velocity gain and time constant. Based on the output transform function the control action with position and velocity feedback are characterized by the following relations:

$$G_p(s) = k_p \text{ and } G_v(s) = k_v \left(\frac{1 + sT_v}{s} \right)$$

where $G_p(s)$ and $G_v(s)$ correspond to the position and velocity control actions. The symbols k_p and k_v represent the constant gain matrices [41,42].

Two widely used feedback control algorithms in robotics are proportional derivative (PD) and proportion-integral-derivative (PID) control. These controllers aim to minimize the error between desired and actual positions, velocities, and forces in robot manipulators. PD control is a simple and effective algorithm that employs proportional and derivative gain terms for trajectory tracking and arm control. It uses a linear control scheme based on system linearization at the operating point. PID control extends PD control by adding an integral gain term to the PD control law to address the impact of gravitational forces. The control scheme for PD and PID controllers used in robotics

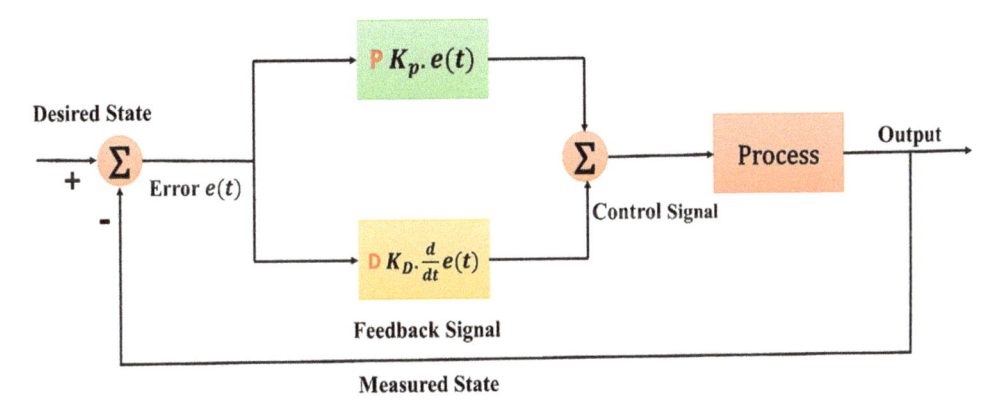

Fig. 3.4 Control scheme for PD controller.

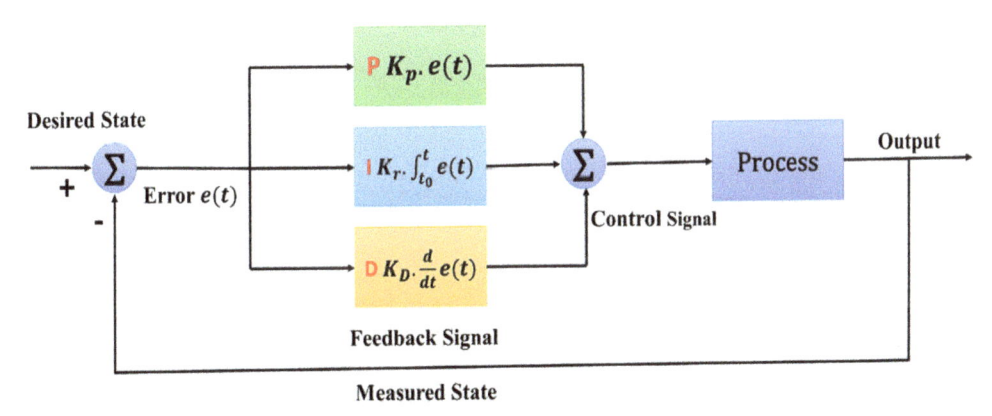

Fig. 3.5 Control scheme for PID controller.

has been given in Figs. 3.4 and 3.5. The equations for PD and PID controllers are given as follows [43–45]:

$$\tau = k_p(q_d - q) - k_v \dot{q} + \tau_g(q)$$

$$\tau = k_p(q_d - q) - k_v \dot{q} + \tau_g(q) + k_I \int f(q_d - q) dt$$

where k_p and k_v are the positive definite gain matrices, q_d is the desired joint trajectory, and k_I is the positive definite gain matrix. When we apply the previously mentioned control equations to the equation of the robotic manipulator's motion, we obtain the closed-loop equation of motion with PD and PID controllers. These equations are given as follows:

$$H(q)\ddot{q} + C(q,\dot{q})\dot{q} + k_v\dot{q} - k_p(q_d - q) = 0$$

$$H(q)\ddot{q} + C(q,\dot{q})\dot{q} + k_v\dot{q} - k_p(q_d - q) + k_I \int f(q_d - q)dt = 0$$

Computed torque control applies feedback linearization to a nonlinear system, comprising an inner nonlinear compensation loop and an outer loop with control signal v. For accuracy, this control requires real-time computation of model parameters and control input. To address this, a computed torque-like control scheme is proposed, achieved by modifying the computed torque-like control. The computed torque-like control transforms a multiinput multioutput system (MIMO) nonlinear robotic system into a simple decoupled linear closed-loop system with a well-established control design. The equations for these two controllers are as follows [41,46]:

$$\tau = H(q)v + C(q,\dot{q})\dot{q} + \tau_g(q)$$

$$\tau = \hat{H}(q)v + \hat{C}(q,\dot{q})\dot{q} + \hat{\tau}(q)$$

where $v = \ddot{q}$ is the auxiliary control input, and the symbol ˆ denotes the computed or nominal value and theoretical uncertainty of exact feedback linearization.

There are less prominent controls in robotics that include adaptive controllers, like adapted computed torque control, adaptive inertia-related control, and adaptive passivity-based control. Stabilizing controllers are designed for nonlinear robotic manipulator systems, and various optimal controllers aim to optimize system stability. Robust control algorithms are also available to overcome the limitations of optimal controllers.

3.2.2 Force control

To perform tasks effectively, robots need to handle physical contact with their surroundings. Pure motion control is inadequate as it does not consider modeling errors and uncertainties, leading to increased contact forces and instability. Force feedback and control are crucial for robots to operate safely and effectively in unstructured environments, around humans, and in open-ended settings. Force control is pivotal for achieving robust and versatile robotic as well as biomedical robotics behavior, significantly enhancing human-robot interaction in healthcare applications [41,47].

Successful manipulation of tasks in robotics depends on precise manipulator-environment interaction. The contact force at the manipulator signifies these interactions, which are crucial for manipulating objects. Constrained motion, where the end-effector follows geometric path constraints, is common during interactions. Achieving successful robot-environment interaction requires accurate modeling of robot and environment, with environment modeling being challenging. Planning errors can result in contact forces deviating from the robot's trajectory, leading to issues. To address this, maintaining compliant behavior during interaction is paramount [41,48]. Interaction control is further categorized into passive and active interaction controls. Passive interaction control utilizes a robot's inherent compliance to adjust its end-effector's path in response to interaction forces, avoiding the need for force/torque sensors and ensuring faster reactions. In contrast, active interaction control employs a dedicated control system that measures contact forces and modifies the robot's end-effector trajectory. While active control addresses passive control limitations, it tends to be slower, more expensive, and more complex, and these two can be combined for effective task execution speed and disturbance rejection [49,50]. Active interaction control is further categorized into indirect force control, focusing on motion control without force feedback, and direct force control, utilizing a force feedback loop. Impedance control and stiffness control are examples of indirect force control, and hybrid force/motion control is direct force control [48,49].

Hybrid force-motion control (HFC) merges motion and force control in robotics for precise interaction with the environment. Approaches like acceleration-resolved, velocity-based, and passivity-based ensure stable robot contact. Acceleration-resolved and passivity-based methods suit both rigid and compliant environments [51,52]. The operational space formulation of the dynamic model of a robot manipulator in contact with the environment for indirect force control is as follows [41,50]:

$$A(q)\dot{v} + B(q,\dot{q})v_e + \eta(q) = h_c - h_e$$

where $v_e = J(q)\dot{q} = \left(\dot{P}_e^T, w_e^T\right)$ is the velocity of the end-effector, P_e and w_e are the translational and angular velocity, $A(q)$ is the inertia matrix, $B(q,\dot{q})$ is the wrench including centrifugal and Coriolis effect, $\eta(q)$ is the wrench of the gravitational effect, h_c is the equivalent end-effector wrench corresponding to the input joint torques.

Stiffness control specifies a desired position and orientation, establishing a relationship between end-effector deviations from the desired motion and the applied force on the environment. The equation of motion for stiffness control law is given by [47,48]:

$$A^{-T}(\varphi_e)k_p\Delta x_{de} - k_p v_e + \eta(q) = h_e$$

where T is the matrix of the mapping $w_e = T(\varphi_e)\dot{\varphi}_e$, φ_e is the set of Euler's angles obtained from the rotation matrix, the symbols $\Delta x_{de} = x_d - x_e$, and $\Delta \dot{x}_{de} = -\dot{x}_e = -A^{-T}(\varphi_e)v_e$ are end-effector and velocity error, k_p and k_p^{-1} are the matrices of active stiffness and active compliance, $h_e = \left(P_e^T, \varphi_e^T\right)^T$ represents the orientation of the end-effector's position, and the matrix A is defined by $A(\varphi_e) = \begin{pmatrix} I_3 & 0 \\ 0 & T_{3\times 3}(\varphi_e) \end{pmatrix}$.

Impedance control regulates force interaction, enabling the robot to adapt more compliantly to its environment. It achieves the desired position-force relation by considering the robot's mass, stiffness, and damping. The control law for impedance control in environmental interaction is derived from the inverse dynamics control law. The impedance control law is given by;

$$A(q)\alpha + B(q,\dot{q})\dot{q} + h_e = h_c,$$ Where α is the properly designed input.

To obtain the dynamic behavior of the controlled end-effector interpreted as the generalized impedance, let us suppose that $\dot{v}_e = \overline{R}_e^T \dot{v}_e^e + \dot{\overline{R}}_e^T v_e^e$, where $\overline{R}_e$ is the matrix given by $\overline{R}_e = \begin{bmatrix} R_e & 0 \\ 0 & R_e \end{bmatrix}$. Now we choose the relation $\alpha = \dot{v}_e$ and $\alpha = \overline{R}_e^T \alpha^e + \dot{\overline{R}}_e^T v_e^e$ from control law to obtain $\alpha^e = \dot{v}_e^e$, moreover, we suppose the expression of α^e by $\alpha^e = k_m^{-1}(\dot{v}_d^e + k_D \Delta v_{de}^e + h_d^e - h_e^e)$ to obtain the expression for the closed-loop system for the dynamic behavior of the controlled end-effector, which is given by;

$$k_m \Delta \dot{v}_{de}^e + k_D \Delta v_{de}^e + h_\Delta^e = h_e^e$$

where k_m and k_D are the positive definite matrix, $\Delta \dot{v}_{de}^e = \dot{v}_d^e - \dot{v}_e^e$, and $\Delta v_{de}^e = \Delta v_d^e - \Delta v_e^e$ are the acceleration and velocity differences of the desired frame. The symbols v_d^e and $\dot{v}_d^e$ denotes the velocity and acceleration of the desired frame, respectively, and h_Δ^e represents the elastic wrench [47,53].

3.2.3 Mathematics in biomedical robotics

The force and motion control in biomedical robotics has been used in prostatectomy, neurosurgery, nephrectomy, cholecystectomy, orthopedics, and radiosurgery reviewing algorithms for interventional systems and highlighting the role of force sensors for enhanced human-machine interaction and safety in medical applications [54]. Active constraints control in surgical robots is implemented as an admittance controller, achieving force control via motion control, without the explicit closure of a force feedback loop, and to achieve the desired velocity, the torques are multiplied by an admittance gain [54]. The velocity of the joint vector in this control is given by:

$$\dot{q} = J^{-1}(q).K(d).G_f.[F_w, T_w]^T$$

where q is the joint vector, J is the Jacobian matrix resolved at the robot's tooltip, $K(d)$ and G_f are the diagonal matrix of scale factors and admittance gains, and F_w and T_w are the measured force and vector of the torques.

Verma et al. discussed the impact of robotic technology in revolutionizing the medical domain, focusing on the application of the Selective Compliant Assembly Robot Arm (SCARA) for surgical tasks, with detailed mathematical modeling, kinematics equations, and evaluation of CTC for trajectory tracking compared to PD and PID controllers [55]. Active control utilizing RCM-constrained Jacobian resolves the remote center of motion constraint by the derivation of a kinematic control formulation for surgical robotic systems in minimally invasive robotic surgeries [56]. A hybrid force-magnetic control scheme has been used for a magnetically actuated flexible surgical robot that minimizes energy consumption and reduces the system size, ensuring safety and maintaining compliant contact with the human body [57]. An adaptive motion-force control scheme has been introduced for a networked ultrasound robotic manipulator, demonstrating superior efficiency in robot-assisted ultrasound imaging [58]. Bajo et al. [59] proposed a unified framework for multi-backbone continuum robots to achieve hybrid motion/force control and concluded that these robots overcome challenges in surgical applications, ensuring safety without the need for dedicated sensors.

The dynamic model for the robot-assisted ultrasound imaging system is given by;

$$M_r(q)\ddot{q} + C_r(q,\dot{q})\dot{q} + G_r(q) + B_r(\dot{q}) = \tau_a - \tau_{int} + d; \text{ and } M_r(q) = Ge^2 J_m + M_l(q)$$

The symbols $q, \dot{q}, \ddot{q}$, represents the joint angle, velocity, and acceleration vectors. $M_r(q)$ and $C_r(q,\dot{q})$ denotes the total inertia matrix and matrix of Coriolis and centrifugal forces, $G_r(q)$ and $B_r(\dot{q})$ are the gravitational and friction effects, τ_a and τ_{int} are the actuator and joint torque, d denotes the external disturbance, Ge and J_m represents the ratio of motor gear and inertia of motor, and $M_l(q)$ denotes the inertia matrix of robot links.

The backpropagation (BP) neural network algorithm, a multilayer feedforward network trained according to an error BP algorithm, has been used to develop a robotic catheter manipulation system. It has been shown that the BP neural network PID controller is more efficient than the traditional PID controller [60]. The control system of the BP neural network PID controller is given in Fig. 3.6. The dynamic model of the axial motion of the surgical robot for the BP neural network PID controller is given by the following equation:

$$M\ddot{q} + C\dot{q} + kq = f(t)$$

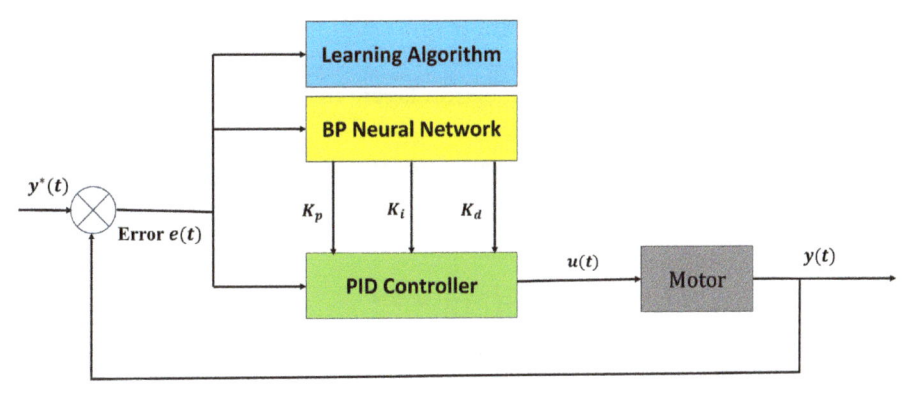

Fig. 3.6 Control system of BP neural network PID controller [60].

The symbol *M* denotes the mass of the overall axial movement of the push platform, *C* is the overall damping coefficient of the push platform, and *k* is the overall elastic coefficient of the push platform.

3.3 Applications of mathematics in biomedical robotics and devices

3.3.1 Mathematics in surgical robotics

Surgical robotics has emerged as a cutting-edge field within biomedical robotics, revolutionizing the base of surgical procedures and medical interventions. Mathematics plays an important role in enhancing the capabilities of surgical robots, enabling precise, minimally invasive, and patient-specific procedures.

3.3.1.1 Image processing and analysis

Medical imaging methods, such as X-rays, CT scans, MRI, and ultrasound, provide critical visual information to guide surgical interventions. Mathematics plays a fundamental role in image reconstruction, filtering, and enhancement, ensuring the clarity and accuracy of the captured images [61]. Techniques such as Fourier transforms, wavelet analysis, and image registration are utilized to improve the quality and interpretability of medical images, aiding surgeons in diagnosing diseases and planning surgical procedures effectively. Precise surgical planning and execution depend on identifying and delineating relevant structures from medical images [62]. Mathematical algorithms for image segmentation, including region-growing, active contours, and level sets, enable the extraction of anatomical regions of interest. This process facilitates surgical navigation and provides crucial information for robot-assisted surgical systems to accurately interact with targeted tissues [63]. Convolutional neural network (CNN) is a deep learning method that uses deep neural networks for end-to-end feature extraction and image classification, automating the process of extracting high-level semantic features and enabling recognition [64]. The CNN model usually consists of a convolution layer, a pooling layer, a full connection layer, and an activation function. The pooling layer reduces feature map dimensions and enhances feature extraction, often employing Max Pooling, and the fully connected layer links convolutional and pooling layer outputs for classification or regression tasks [65]. These are given by the following equations:

$$O[i,j] = f\left(\sum(m,n)\left(I[i+m, i+n] * [m,n] + b\right)\right)$$

$$P[i,j] = max\left(I[2i,2], [2i,2], [2i+1,2], [2i+1,2j], [2i+1,2j+1]\right)$$

$$O = f(Wx + b)$$

where $O[i,j]$ and $P[i,j]$ represent the pixel value of the output feature map, $I[i,j]$ represents the pixel value of the input image, K is the weight of the convolution kernel, b is the offset term, f is the activation function, $\sum(m,n)$ represents the summation of all elements of the convolution kernel, O is the output of the full connection layer, and W is the weight matrix.

Smoothing and segmentation are the most important parts of biomedical image processing and analysis. Smoothing is the process of the simplification of a biomedical image while preserving important information. There are a number of methods to smooth a biomedical image but Naïve or linear smoothing, anisotropic smoothing, and regularized anisotropic smoothing are more prevalent [62–64]. The following diffusion equation makes the image smooth for linear smoothing at any time t.

$\frac{\partial S^t}{\partial t} = \Delta S^t$, $S^0 = I$, where I represent the original image at time $t=0$.

The anisotropic and regularized anisotropic smoothing of biomedical images is done by solving the following equations:

$$\text{Anisotropic Smoothing, } \frac{\partial S}{\partial t} = div\{g|\nabla S|\nabla S\} = \sum_{i,j} a_{ij}(\nabla S)\nabla_{ij}^2 S$$

$$\text{Regulersied Anisotropic Smoothing, } \frac{\partial S}{\partial t} = h|(G_\sigma * \nabla S)||\nabla S|\sum_{i,j} b_{ij}(\nabla S)\nabla_{ij}^2 S$$

where g represents the stopping function, G_σ is the smoothing kernel, and a_{ij} and b_{ij} are the matrices of diffusion coefficients.

3.3.1.2 Surgical navigation and path planning

Surgical robots are often equipped with advanced motion planning algorithms to determine optimal paths for instruments and robotic arms. Mathematics underpins these algorithms, enabling the planning of safe, collision-free paths that minimize tissue damage and ensure precise targeting of surgical sites [66]. Techniques like rapidly exploring random trees (RRT) and Dijkstra's algorithm are employed to find efficient paths in complex anatomical structures. Optimal control theory plays a significant role in enhancing the performance of surgical robots. By formulating surgical tasks as optimization problems, mathematical optimization techniques can be applied to achieve optimal motion trajectories, minimize energy consumption, and optimize surgical outcomes. Optimal control also aids in overcoming physical constraints, such as joint limits and workspace boundaries, ensuring smooth and efficient robot movements during surgery [67,68]. Kinematics and optical constraints criteria can be applied to robot-assisted surgical procedures for precise path planning and optimization of the position of the surgical robot [68]. The kinematic criteria for optimal placement and optical constraints of the surgical robot are given by the following equations:

$$w = \sqrt{det(J.J^T)}$$

$$f_{mv} = \begin{cases} 1, (M_i \cap FOV) = 1 \\ 0, Otherwise \end{cases}$$

where J is the Jacobian matrix of robot, computed from the kinematics description of robot, M_i is the marker attached to the patient and robot, and FOV is the field of view of the optical tracking camera.

3.3.1.3 Robotic-assisted MIS

Mathematics is integral to developing the control algorithms for robotic platforms used in MIS. These algorithms compensate for the limited dexterity of minimally invasive instruments, providing surgeons with enhanced maneuverability and stability during complex procedures [69]. The success of robotic-assisted surgery relies on the accuracy and precision of the robotic system. Mathematical models are employed to calibrate robotic arms, end-effectors, and surgical tools, ensuring precise control and alignment during surgery. Feedback control systems, including proportional-integral-derivative (PID) controllers and adaptive control, enable real-time adjustments to maintain the desired level of precision and stability [70,71]. Kapsalyamov et al. [72] introduced a compliant, seven degrees-of-freedom, pneumatically actuated robotic surgical system designed for MIS, including a remote center of motion for the laparoscopic camera. Simulation results confirm that the system meets the design requirements, paving the way for the development of a supportive surgical robot in MIS. The TMR-MRS, a three-arm surgical robot system for mandible reconstruction, employs spatial registration and hand-eye coordination to enhance accuracy. Experimental validations, including positioning accuracy tests and skull model experiments, confirm the system's feasibility and alignment with preoperative planning [73]. The control scheme for this surgical robotic system is given in Fig. 3.7. The trajectory of the robotic arm during minimal invasive neurological surgery

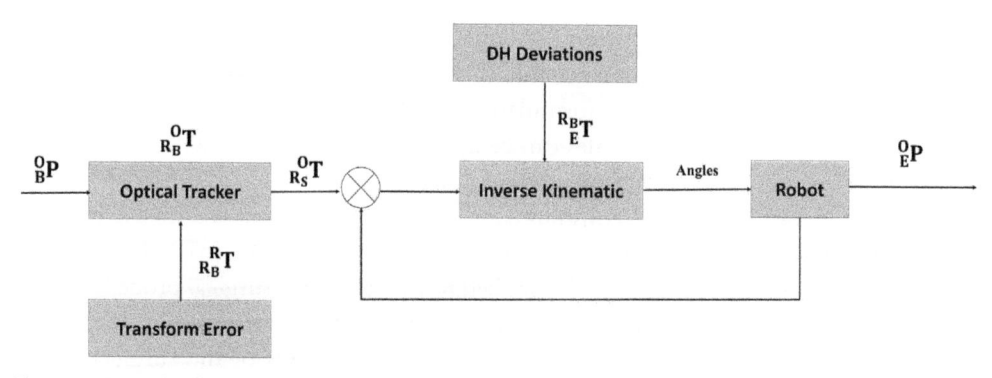

Fig. 3.7 Control scheme for TMR-MRS system [73].

can be optimized using an adaptive approach through cost-functionality dependent on the position error, trajectory speed, and brain tissue force, and optimal control methods are efficient in robotic neurological surgery to enhance the trajectory speed and avoid the damage during surgery [74]. The control law and speed of the robotic arm during surgery in this control are given by:

$$\ddot{x} = \frac{(x_d - x)}{2\lambda_v}\left[-2\lambda_F F^2(x) - 2\lambda_{err} + 2\lambda_F(x_d - x)\frac{\partial F}{\partial x}\right]$$

$$v(x) = \sqrt{\frac{\lambda_F(x_d - x)^2 F^2(x) + \lambda_{err}(x_d - x)^2}{2\lambda_v}}$$

The symbol $\ddot{x}$ denotes the speed of the robot's arm, x_d is the displacement, λ_F and λ_v are square terms of force and speed, λ_{err} is the square position error, and F is the applied force brain retractor.

An interesting mathematical model has also been developed to find out the effectiveness of the robotic surgery, and further, it has been applied to laparoscopic and robot-assisted surgeries and concluded that robotic surgery is favored for lung lobectomies and prostatectomies, while laparoscopy is the preferred option for various other procedures, with a strong preference for gastric bypass and marginal preference for hysterectomies and ventral hernia repairs [75]. In this model, the score of morbidity and mortality is given by:

$$\text{Score of Morbidity Rate} = 1.5 \times \sqrt[9]{\frac{\text{Morbidity Rate}}{4}}, \text{Score of Mortality}$$

$$= 1.5 \times (9.898)^{\text{Mortality Rate}}$$

Mathematics enhances surgical robotics, improving outcomes and the overall experience. By enabling real-time navigation and feedback, surgical robots enhance precision, reduce complications, and ensure patient safety, emphasizing mathematics' foundational role in accurate image analysis, surgical planning, and robotic control [75]. In conclusion, with the integration of complex and advanced mathematical techniques in biomedical robotics, mathematics plays a foundational role in surgical robotics, enabling accurate image analysis, surgical planning, and robotic control.

3.3.2 Mathematics in rehabilitation robotics

Rehabilitation robotics has emerged as a transformative field within biomedical engineering, aiming to enhance the rehabilitation process for individuals with mobility impairments. By integrating mathematical principles, rehabilitation robots offer personalized and effective therapeutic interventions, promoting motor recovery and improving the quality of life for patients with impairments.

3.3.2.1 Assistive devices for motor rehabilitation

In rehabilitation robotics, human-robot interaction is crucial to creating a seamless and intuitive experience for the patient. Mathematical models of human biomechanics and dynamics help in understanding how patients interact with robotic devices [76]. These models, coupled with control algorithms, enable the design of assistive devices that can adapt to the user's movements, providing targeted assistance and promoting active engagement during therapy. Mathematical control algorithms play a central role in rehabilitation robotics to facilitate smooth and coordinated movements of robotic devices. Advanced control techniques, such as impedance control and adaptive control, allow rehabilitation robots to provide the appropriate level of assistance based on the patient's abilities and needs. By continuously adjusting the level of assistance, these algorithms optimize the therapeutic impact, maximizing patient recovery [77,78]. In rehabilitation robotics, an omnidirectional walker (ODW) aids in walking rehabilitation for individuals with disabilities by storing training programs. To enhance accuracy, an adaptive control strategy with automatic parameter adjustment via a genetic algorithm can be used to address issues from users' arm forces during training. Walk-assist robots with an efficient, improved genetic algorithm can optimize parameters and help people with disabilities. The kinetics analysis of the ODW and other similar walk-assisted robots is carried out with the help of the following set of equations:

$$(M + m)\ddot{x}_G = -f_1 sin\theta + f_2 cos\theta - f_3 sin\theta + f_4 cos\theta$$

$$(M + m)\ddot{y}_G = -f_1 cos\theta + f_2 sin\theta - f_3 cos\theta + f_4 sin\theta$$

$$(I + mr_0^2)\ddot{\theta} = L(f_1 - f_2 - f_3 + f_4)$$

where M and m are the mass of the ODW and imposed by user to the ODW by the armrest. I is the inertia of mass, f_1, f_2, f_3 and f_4 are the input of the system, x_G, y_G are the output of the system, and the orientation angle of the walker is θ. Here, m and r_0 are uncertain due to the user-imposed pressure on walker.

3.3.2.2 Neural interfaces and brain-machine interactions

Brain-machine interfaces (BMIs) have opened new frontiers in rehabilitation robotics, allowing direct communication between the human brain and robotic devices. Mathematics is fundamental in analyzing neural signals, such as electroencephalography (EEG) or electrocorticography (ECG), to decode the patient's intentions and control robotic prosthetics or exoskeletons [79]. Signal processing techniques, including time-frequency analysis and machine learning algorithms, enable extracting relevant information from neural signals and translating them into control commands for robotic devices. Mathematical decoding algorithms interpret neural activity and map it to specific movements of the robotic devices [80]. These algorithms use statistical models and pattern recognition techniques to identify the patient's intended actions, allowing for precise control of assistive devices or robotic limbs. By continuously learning and adapting to the patient's neural patterns, rehabilitation robots provide natural and intuitive control, empowering patients to regain functional movements [81,82].

3.3.2.3 Quantitative assessment and personalized therapy
Mathematics enables the quantification of patient progress and performance during rehabilitation sessions. Metrics such as joint angles, forces, and movement patterns are captured and analyzed using mathematical algorithms, providing objective and quantitative assessments of a patient's functional abilities and progress [83]. These objective measures offer valuable feedback to clinicians, assisting in treatment planning and decision-making. Machine learning techniques can be employed to personalize rehabilitation therapies based on individual patient characteristics and progress. By analyzing data from multiple patients, machine learning algorithms can identify patterns and correlations that inform personalized therapy plans [84,85]. Mathematics in rehabilitation robotics revolutionizes treatment by continuously adapting plans to the patient's response, optimizing outcomes. It enables personalized and adaptive therapies, utilizing mathematical models and algorithms for efficient, tailored interventions, offering innovative solutions for those with mobility impairments in neurorehabilitation.

3.3.3 Mathematics in medical robotics for diagnosis and monitoring
3.3.3.1 Medical robot-assisted diagnosis, monitoring, and intervention
Medical robotics has benefited surgical interventions and rehabilitation and made significant advancements in medical diagnosis and continuous monitoring. By harnessing mathematical principles, medical robots offer innovative tools for precise diagnosis, early detection, and real-time monitoring of patients' health [86]. Medical robots equipped with artificial intelligence algorithms provide valuable decision support to healthcare professionals. These algorithms assist in accurate and timely diagnosis by analyzing patient data, medical images, and other diagnostic information. Mathematical techniques, such as pattern recognition, statistical analysis, and machine learning, can be used to identify patterns and correlations within vast datasets, aiding in the early detection of diseases and improving diagnostic accuracy [87]. Medical robots are integrated with diagnostic imaging modalities to enhance imaging and obtain more precise and detailed images. Mathematics plays a vital role in image registration, where images from different modalities or time points are aligned to facilitate accurate comparison and analysis [88]. Additionally, image fusion techniques merge information from multiple imaging sources, providing a comprehensive view of the patient's condition. Closed-loop control systems, driven by mathematical algorithms, enable medical robots to continuously monitor patients and deliver appropriate interventions as needed. For instance, closed-loop infusion pumps can regulate drug dosages based on real-time physiological measurements, ensuring optimal drug delivery and minimizing the risk of adverse events [89]. Medical robotics has the

potential to revolutionize diagnostic accuracy and monitoring capabilities in healthcare. By leveraging mathematical algorithms, medical robots can rapidly process vast amounts of data, enabling precise and timely diagnoses. Additionally, continuous monitoring through closed-loop control ensures prompt interventions and personalized treatment, enhancing patient outcomes and reducing the burden on healthcare professionals. Mathematics is crucial in medical robotics, facilitating accurate decision support, integration with diagnostic imaging, continuous monitoring, promising advancements in diagnostic accuracy, early disease detection, and personalized healthcare delivery.

3.4 Future perspectives and limitations

Due to the current and future advancements in mathematics and robotics, biomedical robotics will play a very important role in transforming healthcare delivery. Machine learning algorithms, especially deep and reinforcement learning, promise to enhance medical decision support, robot control, and personalized therapies. As medical robots gain autonomy, prioritizing their explainability becomes crucial for healthcare professionals to trust and validate their reasoning. The collaboration between robots and healthcare experts, leveraging AI-driven automation and human intuition, holds the promise of more precise, efficient, and patient-centered care across various medical domains. Medical robots can anticipate patient needs and potential health issues with the help of predictive analytics, which may enable proactive interventions. The future envisions cognitive robots displaying human-like understanding and empathy, improving patient experiences. Predictive analytics, enabled by mathematical models, allows medical robots to anticipate patient needs and intervene proactively. Virtual reality integration aids preoperative planning, medical training, and patient education. Future biomedical robotics developments will hinge on converging technologies, including AI, nanotechnology, and biotechnology, accelerating innovation and creating integrated healthcare solutions. A focus on cost-effective and scalable robotics for resource-limited regions is crucial for supporting global health initiatives. However, ethical considerations, including patient consent, data privacy, robot autonomy, and accountability, must be addressed comprehensively. A flexible regulatory framework, developed collaboratively with researchers and industry stakeholders, is essential to ensure the responsible and ethical deployment of medical robots.

Despite exciting advances in healthcare robotics, addressing inherent challenges is crucial. The safety-critical nature of healthcare, with vulnerable individuals, demands careful consideration. Mathematics in biomedical robotics presents solutions, but obstacles such as usability, acceptability, safety, reliability, capability, functioning, clinical effectiveness, and cost-effectiveness must be tackled. Ethical concerns, regulatory hurdles, and adoption barriers further may also complicate the integration of robots into healthcare. Strategies to reduce costs and improve accessibility, such as shared facilities or public-private partnerships, need to be explored to make medical robotics more widely available. Ensuring the accuracy and reliability of robotic systems in medical applications is the first and foremost priority. Real-time processing, balancing accuracy with speed, during surgical interventions is an ongoing challenge. Computational efficiency is also critical to avoid delays that could compromise patient safety. Embracing medical robots as a part of healthcare delivery relies on patient acceptance and trust. Patient acceptance relies on safety, reliability, autonomy, privacy, and communication with robotic systems. Autonomy raises ethical concerns, necessitating a delicate balance between robotic actions and human oversight for trust and transparency. Ensuring that patients feel comfortable and confident in the capabilities of robotic devices is crucial for successful integration. Safety and reliability are incredibly important when biomedical robots and patients are proximately located as clinicians and surgeons rely extensively on robots to help the patients. Addressing concerns related to patient autonomy, privacy, and communication with robotic systems is essential to garner patient trust. Medical robotics must also adhere to stringent regulatory standards and safety requirements to be approved for clinical use. Ensuring compliance with these standards adds complexity to the design and testing processes, prolonging the time to market for new robotic technologies. Successful integration of mathematics requires collaboration between engineering and medical professionals, bridging disciplinary gaps due to differences in terminology, priorities, and approaches. The effective use of medical robots demands specialized training for healthcare professionals, including surgeons, therapists, and medical technicians, to achieve optimal outcomes and patient safety. The integration of mathematics in biomedical robotics holds immense promise for advancing healthcare delivery, but several challenges and limitations must also be navigated. Addressing accuracy, safety concerns, ethical considerations, and patient acceptance requires robust research and collaboration between engineers, clinicians, and policymakers. Overcoming regulatory hurdles and improving accessibility will enhance the broader adoption of these transformative technologies. Proactive collaboration and research between engineers, clinicians, and policymakers are essential to harness the full potential of mathematics in biomedical robotics, leading to a new era of precision medicine and transformative healthcare delivery.

3.5 Conclusion

The integration of mathematics in biomedical robotics has led to a new era of transformative healthcare delivery. By combining the concepts of mathematical principles, robotics, and artificial intelligence, medical robots have the potential to enhance medical treatments, diagnostics, and patient monitoring. Throughout this chapter, we have explored the critical role of mathematics in various facets of biomedical robotics, from surgical interventions to rehabilitation and medical diagnostics. Mathematics forms the backbone of biomedical robotics, providing the foundation for accurate spatial representations, dynamic modeling, and control algorithms. Through mathematical modeling of human anatomy and physiology, medical robots can interact seamlessly with biological systems, enabling personalized and effective treatments. Sensor fusion and signal processing techniques allow for the integration and interpretation of complex data, empowering robots to make informed decisions and respond to real-time changes in the patient's condition. In surgical robotics, mathematics has facilitated minimally invasive procedures. This can help enhance surgical precision and can enable complex operations with smaller incisions. Rehabilitation robotics, driven by mathematical models, can offer personalized therapies, assisting patients in their motor recovery. Medical robots also play a crucial role in medical diagnosis and monitoring. Mathematical algorithms can be used in biomedical robotics to aid in early stage disease identification that can help clinicians with decision support systems and optimization of patient care. Biomedical robots can be integrated with telemedicine for remote consultation and home-based monitoring and will help in accessing better healthcare for a larger section of the population. Emerging mathematical techniques, such as advanced machine learning and artificial intelligence, may enhance the capabilities of medical robots, making them more autonomous and human-centric in the future. The convergence of technologies, interdisciplinary research, and global health initiatives will advance the development of cost-effective and extensive robotic solutions, benefiting a wider range of patients and healthcare setups. However, this transformation also has some limitations and is not without challenges. Ensuring accuracy, safety, and ethical considerations remain key priorities in the further development and deployment of medical robots.

References

[1] R. Raj, A. Kos, A comprehensive study of Mobile robot: history, developments, applications, and future research perspectives, Appl. Sci. 12 (14) (2022) 6951, https://doi.org/10.3390/app12146951.
[2] A. Gasparetto, L. Scalera, A brief history of industrial robotics in the 20th century, AHS 08 (01) (2019) 24–35, https://doi.org/10.4236/ahs.2019.81002.
[3] T. Brito, J. Queiroz, L. Piardi, L.A. Fernandes, J. Lima, P. Leitão, A machine learning approach for collaborative robot smart manufacturing inspection for quality control systems, Procedia Manuf. 51 (2020) 11–18, https://doi.org/10.1016/j.promfg.2020.10.003.
[4] D.M. West, The Future of Work: Robots, AI, and Automation, First Printing in Paperback, Brookings Institution Press, Washington, D.C, 2019.
[5] Z. Li, C. Yang, E. Burdet, Guest editorial an overview of biomedical robotics and bio-mechatronics systems and applications, IEEE Trans. Syst. Man Cybern, Syst. 46 (7) (2016) 869–874, https://doi.org/10.1109/TSMC.2016.2571786.
[6] T. Ashuri, A. Armani, R. Jalilzadeh Hamidi, T. Reasnor, S. Ahmadi, K. Iqbal, Biomedical soft robots: current status and perspective, Biomed. Eng. Lett. 10 (3) (2020) 369–385, https://doi.org/10.1007/s13534-020-00157-6.
[7] C. Hu, Q. Shi, L. Liu, U. Wejinya, Y. Hasegawa, Y. Shen, Robotics in biomedical and healthcare engineering, J. Healthc. Eng. 2017 (2017) 1–2, https://doi.org/10.1155/2017/1610372.
[8] Y.S. Kwoh, J. Hou, E.A. Jonckheere, S. Hayati, A robot with improved absolute positioning accuracy for CT guided stereotactic brain surgery, IEEE Trans. Biomed. Eng. 35 (2) (1988) 153–160, https://doi.org/10.1109/10.1354.

[9] K. Khandalavala, T. Shimon, L. Flores, P.R. Armijo, D. Oleynikov, Emerging surgical robotic technology: a progression toward microbots, Ann. Laparosc. Endosc. Surg. 5 (2020) 3, https://doi.org/10.21037/ales.2019.10.02.

[10] S. Najarian, M. Fallahnezhad, E. Afshari, Advances in medical robotic systems with specific applications in surgery—a review, J. Med. Eng. Technol. 35 (1) (2011) 19–33, https://doi.org/10.3109/03091902.2010.535593.

[11] M. Iftikhar, M.J. Majid, M. Muralindran, G. Thayabaren, R. Vigneswaran, T.T.K. Brendan, OTOROB: Robot for Orthopaedic Surgeon - Roboscope: Non-interventional Medical Robot for Telerounding, 2011 5th International Conference on Bioinformatics and Biomedical Engineering, IEEE, Wuhan, China, 2011, pp. 1–5, https://doi.org/10.1109/icbbe.2011.5780335.

[12] S. Balasubramanian, J. Klein, E. Burdet, Robot-assisted rehabilitation of hand function, Curr. Opin. Neurol. 23 (6) (2010) 661–670, https://doi.org/10.1097/WCO.0b013e32833e99a4.

[13] T. Nef, M. Mihelj, R. Riener, ARMin: a robot for patient-cooperative arm therapy, Med. Bio. Eng. Comput. 45 (9) (2007) 887–900, https://doi.org/10.1007/s11517-007-0226-6.

[14] M. Kaczmarski, G. Granosik, Rehabilitation robot RRH1, Arch. Civ. Mech. Eng. 58 (1) (2011), https://doi.org/10.2478/v10180-011-0007-5.

[15] M. Mariappan, T. Ganesan, V. Ramu, M. Iftikhar, Safety system and navigation for Orthopaedic robot (OTOROB), in: S. Jeschke, H. Liu, D. Schilberg (Eds.), Intelligent Robotics and Applications, Lecture Notes in Computer Science, vol. 7102, Springer, Berlin Heidelberg, Berlin, Heidelberg, 2011, pp. 358–367, https://doi.org/10.1007/978-3-642-25489-5_35.

[16] T. Mukai, et al., Development of a nursing-care assistant robot RIBA that can lift a human in its arms, in: 2010 IEEE/RSJ International Conference on Intelligent Robots and Systems, IEEE, Taipei, 2010, pp. 5996–6001, https://doi.org/10.1109/IROS.2010.5651735.

[17] P.E. Hsu, Y.L. Hsu, K.W. Chang, C. Geiser, Mobility assistance Design of the Intelligent Robotic Wheelchair, Int. J. Adv. Robot. Syst. 9 (6) (2012) 244, https://doi.org/10.5772/54819.

[18] M.J. Iqbal, et al., Clinical applications of artificial intelligence and machine learning in cancer diagnosis: looking into the future, Cancer Cell Int. 21 (1) (2021) 270, https://doi.org/10.1186/s12935-021-01981-1.

[19] F. Valero, M. Ceccarelli, A. Ghosal, Applied mathematics to Mobile robotics and their applications, Math. Probl. Eng. 2017 (2017) 1–2, https://doi.org/10.1155/2017/8706164.

[20] B. Morris, Robotic surgery: applications, limitations, and impact on surgical education, MedGenMed 7 (3) (2005) 72.

[21] S. Aggarwal, D. Gupta, S. Saini, A Literature Survey on Robotics in Healthcare, 2019 4th International Conference on Information Systems and Computer Networks (ISCON), IEEE, Mathura, India, 2019, pp. 55–58, https://doi.org/10.1109/ISCON47742.2019.9036253.

[22] A. BourgeoisP, CC BY-SA 4.0 <https://creativecommons.org/licenses/by-sa/4.0>, via Wikimedia Commons. (https://commons.wikimedia.org/wiki/File:2023-09_-_Robot_chirurgien_Da_Vinci_Xi_-_Centre_hospitalier_de_Vesoul_-_13.jpg.)..

[23] Jason Knauer, CC BY 3.0 <https://creativecommons.org/licenses/by/3.0>, via Wikimedia Commons. (https://upload.wikimedia.org/wikipedia/commons/0/00/Domo_Origato_Surgeon_Roboto_%28230350985%29.jpeg)..

[24] Institute of Automation (IAT), University of Bremen, GFDL <http://www.gnu.org/copyleft/fdl.html>, via Wikimedia Commons. (https://commons.wikimedia.org/wiki/File:FRIEND-III_klein.png#file)..

[25] P. Berthet-Rayne, G. Gras, K. Leibrandt, P. Wisanuvej, A. Schmitz, C. A. Seneci, G.-Z. Yang, CC BY 4.0 https://creativecommons.org/licenses/by/4.0, via Wikimedia Commons. (https://upload.wikimedia.org/wikipedia/commons/6/6e/The_i%C2%B2Snake_Robot.png)..

[26] D. Gupta, M. Sharma, V. Chaudhary, A. Khanna, Robotic Technologies in Biomedical and Healthcare Engineering, first ed., CRC Press, Boca Raton, 2021, https://doi.org/10.1201/9781003112273.

[27] G.P. Soriano, et al., Robots and robotics in nursing, Healthcare 10 (8) (2022) 1571, https://doi.org/10.3390/healthcare10081571.

[28] I.A. Baba, B.A. Baba, P. Esmaili, A mathematical model to study the effectiveness of some of the strategies adopted in curtailing the spread of COVID-19, Comput. Math. Methods Med. 2020 (2020) 1–6, https://doi.org/10.1155/2020/5248569.

[29] F. Stroppa, A. Soylemez, H.T. Yuksel, B. Akbas, M. Sarac, Optimizing exoskeleton design with evolutionary computation: an intensive survey, Robotics 12 (4) (2023) 106, https://doi.org/10.3390/robotics12040106.
[30] J. Colan, J. Nakanishi, T. Aoyama, Y. Hasegawa, Optimization-based constrained trajectory generation for robot-assisted stitching in Endonasal surgery, Robotics 10 (1) (2021) 27, https://doi.org/10.3390/robotics10010027.
[31] Q. Wu, X. Wang, B. Chen, H. Wu, Z. Shao, Development and hybrid force/position control of a compliant rescue manipulator, Mechatronics 46 (2017) 143–153, https://doi.org/10.1016/j.mechatronics.2017.08.003.
[32] M.T. Thai, P.T. Phan, T.T. Hoang, S. Wong, N.H. Lovell, T.N. Do, Advanced intelligent systems for surgical robotics, Adv. Intell. Syst. 2 (8) (2020) 1900138, https://doi.org/10.1002/aisy.201900138.
[33] R.V. Patel, S.F. Atashzar, M. Tavakoli, Haptic feedback and force-based teleoperation in surgical robotics, Proc. IEEE 110 (7) (2022) 1012–1027, https://doi.org/10.1109/JPROC.2022.3180052.
[34] M. Soori, B. Arezoo, R. Dastres, Artificial intelligence, machine learning and deep learning in advanced robotics, a review, cognitive, Robotics 3 (2023) 54–70, https://doi.org/10.1016/j.cogr.2023.04.001.
[35] Z. Ahmed, K. Mohamed, S. Zeeshan, X. Dong, Artificial intelligence with multi-functional machine learning platform development for better healthcare and precision medicine, Database 2020 (2020) baaa010, https://doi.org/10.1093/database/baaa010.
[36] M.G. Abd Elfatah, H.N. Zaky, M. Gharib, Mobile robot position estimation using Euler-Maruyama algorithm, IOP Conf. Ser.: Mater. Sci. Eng. 610 (1) (2019) 012074, https://doi.org/10.1088/1757-899X/610/1/012074.
[37] R. Featherstone, D. Orin, Robot dynamics: Equations and algorithms, in: Proceedings 2000 ICRA. Millennium Conference. IEEE International Conference on Robotics and Automation. Symposia Proceedings (Cat. No.00CH37065), IEEE, San Francisco, CA, USA, 2000, pp. 826–834, https://doi.org/10.1109/ROBOT.2000.844153.
[38] T. Alsultan, H.M. Ali, Q.Y. Hamid, A numerical approach for solving problems in robotic arm movement, Prod. Manuf. Res. 6 (1) (2018) 385–395, https://doi.org/10.1080/21693277.2018.1525326.
[39] C.C. de Wit, B. Siciliano, G. Bastin (Eds.), Theory of Robot Control, Communications and Control Engineering, Springer, London, London, 1996, https://doi.org/10.1007/978-1-4471-1501-4.
[40] R. Kelly, V.S. Davila, A. Loría, Control of Robot Manipulators in Joint Space, Advanced Textbooks in Control and Signal Processing, Springer-Verlag, London, 2005, https://doi.org/10.1007/b135572.
[41] B. Siciliano, O. Khatib (Eds.), Springer Handbook of Robotics, Springer, Berlin Heidelberg, Berlin, Heidelberg, 2008, https://doi.org/10.1007/978-3-540-30301-5.
[42] T.C.S. Hsia, T.A. Lasky, Z. Guo, Robust independent joint controller design for industrial robot manipulators, IEEE Trans. Ind. Electron. 38 (1) (1991) 21–25, https://doi.org/10.1109/41.103479.
[43] J. Alvarez-Ramirez, I. Cervantes, R. Kelly, PID regulation of robot manipulators: stability and performance, Syst. Control Lett. 41 (2) (2000) 73–83, https://doi.org/10.1016/S0167-6911(00)00038-4.
[44] K.J. Åström, T. Hägglund, P.I.D. Controllers, Theory, Design, and Tuning, second ed., Instrument Society of America, Research Triangle Park, NC, 1995.
[45] D. Angeli, Input-to-state stability of PD-controlled robotic systems, Automatica 35 (7) (1999) 1285–1290, https://doi.org/10.1016/S0005-1098(99)00037-0.
[46] A. Datta, M.-T. Ho, Computed torque adaptive control of rigid robots with improved transient performance, American Control Conference, 1993, IEEE, San Francisco, CA, USA, 1993, pp. 1418–1422, https://doi.org/10.23919/ACC.1993.4793104.
[47] R.J. Schilling, Fundamentals of Robotics: Analysis and Control, Prentice Hall, Englewood Cliffs, N.J, 1990.
[48] M.W. Spong, M. Vidyasagar, Robot Dynamics and Control, Wiley, New York, 1989.
[49] F.L. Lewis, C.T. Abdallah, D.M. Dawson, F.L. Lewis, Robot Manipulator Control: Theory and Practice, second ed., Marcel Dekker, New York, 2004 (Expanded in Control engineering series).
[50] R.M. Murray, Z. Li, S.S. Sastry, A Mathematical Introduction to Robotic Manipulation, first ed., CRC Press, 2017, https://doi.org/10.1201/9781315136370.

[51] A. De Luca, C. Manes, Hybrid force-position control for robots in contact with dynamic environments, IFAC Proc. 24 (9) (1991) 177–182, https://doi.org/10.1016/S1474-6670(17)51052-6.
[52] M.H. Raibert, J.J. Craig, Hybrid position/force control of manipulators, J. Dyn. Syst. Meas. Control. 103 (2) (1981) 126–133, https://doi.org/10.1115/1.3139652.
[53] P. Song, Y. Yu, X. Zhang, Impedance Control of Robots: An Overview, 2017 2nd International Conference on Cybernetics, Robotics and Control (CRC), IEEE, Chengdu, 2017, pp. 51–55, https://doi.org/10.1109/CRC.2017.20.
[54] T. Haidegger, B. Benyó, L. Kovács, Z. Benyó, Force sensing and force control for surgical robots, IFAC Proc. 42 (12) (2009) 401–406, https://doi.org/10.3182/20090812-3-DK-2006.0035.
[55] V. Verma, A. Gupta, M.K. Gupta, P. Chauhan, Performance estimation of computed torque control for surgical robot application, JMES 14 (3) (2020) 7017–7028, https://doi.org/10.15282/jmes.14.3.2020.04.0549.
[56] H. Sadeghian, F. Zokaei, S. Hadian Jazi, Constrained kinematic control in minimally invasive robotic surgery subject to remote center of motion constraint, J. Intell. Robot. Syst. 95 (3–4) (2019) 901–913, https://doi.org/10.1007/s10846-018-0927-0.
[57] Y. Huang, R. Ma, H. Liu, A hybrid force-magnetic control scheme for flexible medical device steering, Mechatronics 95 (2023) 103072, https://doi.org/10.1016/j.mechatronics.2023.103072.
[58] M. Abbas, S. Al Issa, S.K. Dwivedy, Event-triggered adaptive hybrid position-force control for robot-assisted ultrasonic examination system, J. Intell. Robot. Syst. 102 (4) (2021) 84, https://doi.org/10.1007/s10846-021-01428-9.
[59] A. Bajo, N. Simaan, Hybrid motion/force control of multi-backbone continuum robots, Int. J. Robot. Res. 35 (4) (2016) 422–434, https://doi.org/10.1177/0278364915584806.
[60] X. Ma, J. Zhou, X. Zhang, Q. Zhou, Development of a robotic catheter manipulation system based on BP neural network PID controller, Appl. Bionics Biomech. 2020 (2020) 1–11, https://doi.org/10.1155/2020/8870106.
[61] M. Vashisht, M. Bhatia, Role of mathematics in image processing, in: 2019 International Conference on Machine Learning, Big Data, Cloud and Parallel Computing (COMITCon), IEEE, Faridabad, India, 2019, pp. 538–543, https://doi.org/10.1109/COMITCon.2019.8862438.
[62] K. Bredies, D. Lorenz, Mathematical image processing, applied and numerical harmonic analysis, Birkhäuser, Baseline (2018), https://doi.org/10.1007/978-3-030-0458-2.
[63] P.B. Henderson, The role of mathematics in computer science and software engineering education, Adv. Comput. 65 (2005) 349–395, https://doi.org/10.1016/S0065-2458(05)65008-5. Elsevier.
[64] Q. Li, W. Cai, X. Wang, Y. Zhou, D.D. Feng, M. Chen, Medical image classification with convolutional neural network, in: 2014 13th International Conference on Control Automation Robotics & Vision (ICARCV), IEEE, Singapore, 2014, pp. 844–848, https://doi.org/10.1109/ICARCV.2014.7064414.
[65] S.S. Yadav, S.M. Jadhav, Deep convolutional neural network based medical image classification for disease diagnosis, J. Big Data 6 (1) (2019) 113, https://doi.org/10.1186/s40537-019-0276-2.
[66] A. Falcó, L. Hilario, N. Montés, M.C. Mora, E. Nadal, A path planning algorithm for a dynamic environment based on proper generalized decomposition, Mathematics 8 (12) (2020) 2245, https://doi.org/10.3390/math8122245.
[67] J.R. Sánchez-Ibáñez, C.J. Pérez-del-Pulgar, A. García-Cerezo, Path planning for autonomous Mobile robots: a review, Sensors 21 (23) (2021) 7898, https://doi.org/10.3390/s21237898.
[68] Q.C. Nguyen, Y. Kim, H. Kwon, Optimization of layout and path planning of surgical robotic system, Int. J. Control. Autom. Syst. 15 (1) (2017) 375–384, https://doi.org/10.1007/s12555-015-0418-z.
[69] V. Vitiello, K.-W. Kwok, G.-Z. Yang, Introduction to robot-assisted minimally invasive surgery (MIS), in: Medical Robotics, 2012, pp. 1–P1, https://doi.org/10.1533/9780857097392.1. Elsevier.
[70] P.J. From, On the kinematics of robotic-assisted minimally invasive surgery, MIC 34 (2) (2013) 69–82, https://doi.org/10.4173/mic.2013.2.3.
[71] M.N. Huda, H. Yu, S. Cang, Robots for minimally invasive diagnosis and intervention, Robot. Comput. Integr. Manuf. 41 (2016) 127–144, https://doi.org/10.1016/j.rcim.2016.03.003.
[72] A. Kapsalyamov, S. Hussain, P.K. Jamwal, A novel compliant surgical robot: preliminary design analysis, Math. Biosci. Eng. 17 (3) (2020) 1944–1958, https://doi.org/10.3934/mbe.2020103.

[73] Y. Wang, X. Duan, Spatial registration for a three-arm robot assisted mandible reconstruction surgery, Math. Probl. Eng. 2015 (2015) 1–10, https://doi.org/10.1155/2015/689278.
[74] I. Inziarte-Hidalgo, I. Uriarte, U. Fernandez-Gamiz, G. Sorrosal, E. Zulueta, Robotic-arm-based force control in neurosurgical practice, Mathematics 11 (4) (2023) 828, https://doi.org/10.3390/math11040828.
[75] H.G. Dandapani, K. Tieu, The contemporary role of robotics in surgery: a predictive mathematical model on the short-term effectiveness of robotic and laparoscopic surgery, Laparosc. Endosc. Surg. Sci. 2 (1) (2019) 1–7, https://doi.org/10.1016/j.lers.2018.11.003.
[76] A. Alamdari, V. Krovi, Robotic assistive devices for motor disability rehabilitation, in: J.G. Webster (Ed.), Wiley Encyclopedia of Electrical and Electronics Engineering, first ed., Wiley, 2016, pp. 1–14, https://doi.org/10.1002/047134608X.W6603.pub2.
[77] S. Khalid, F. Alnajjar, M. Gochoo, A. Renawi, S. Shimoda, Robotic assistive and rehabilitation devices leading to motor recovery in upper limb: a systematic review, Disabil. Rehabil. Assist. Technol. 18 (5) (2023) 658–672, https://doi.org/10.1080/17483107.2021.1906960.
[78] S. Zhang, H. Hu, H. Zhou, An interactive internet-based system for tracking upper limb motion in home-based rehabilitation, Med. Biol. Eng. Comput. 46 (3) (2008) 241–249, https://doi.org/10.1007/s11517-007-0295-6.
[79] J.P. Donoghue, Bridging the brain to the world: a perspective on neural Interface systems, Neuron 60 (3) (2008) 511–521, https://doi.org/10.1016/j.neuron.2008.10.037.
[80] L.R. Hochberg, et al., Neuronal ensemble control of prosthetic devices by a human with tetraplegia, Nature 442 (7099) (2006) 164–171, https://doi.org/10.1038/nature04970.
[81] D.J. Bakkum, Z.C. Chao, S.M. Potter, Spatio-temporal electrical stimuli shape behavior of an embodied cortical network in a goal-directed learning task, J. Neural Eng. 5 (3) (2008) 310–323, https://doi.org/10.1088/1741-2560/5/3/004.
[82] A. Novellino, P. D'Angelo, L. Cozzi, M. Chiappalone, V. Sanguineti, S. Martinoia, Connecting neurons to a Mobile robot: an in vitro bidirectional neural Interface, Comput. Intell. Neurosci. 2007 (2007) 1–13, https://doi.org/10.1155/2007/12725.
[83] C. Spalletti, et al., A robotic system for quantitative assessment and Poststroke training of forelimb retraction in mice, Neurorehabil. Neural Repair 28 (2) (2014) 188–196, https://doi.org/10.1177/1545968313506520.
[84] M. Alghamdi, N. Alhakbani, A. Al-Nafjan, Assessing the potential of robotics technology for enhancing educational for children with autism Spectrum disorder, Behav. Sci. 13 (7) (2023) 598, https://doi.org/10.3390/bs13070598.
[85] M.J. Johnson, Recent trends in robot-assisted therapy environments to improve real-life functional performance after stroke, J. Neuroeng. Rehabil. 3 (1) (2006) 29, https://doi.org/10.1186/1743-0003-3-29.
[86] T. Habuza, et al., AI applications in robotics, diagnostic image analysis and precision medicine: current limitations, future trends, guidelines on CAD systems for medicine, Inform. Med. Unlocked 24 (2021) 100596, https://doi.org/10.1016/j.imu.2021.100596.
[87] S. Huang, et al., MRI-guided robot intervention—current state-of-the-art and new challenges, Med-X 1 (1) (2023) 4, https://doi.org/10.1007/s44258-023-00003-1.
[88] K. Kumar, P. Kumar, D. Deb, M.-L. Unguresan, V. Muresan, Artificial intelligence and machine learning based intervention in medical infrastructure: a review and future trends, Healthcare 11 (2) (2023) 207, https://doi.org/10.3390/healthcare11020207.
[89] E.D. Oña, J.M. Garcia-Haro, A. Jardón, C. Balaguer, Robotics in health care: perspectives of robot-aided interventions in clinical practice for rehabilitation of upper limbs, Appl. Sci. 9 (13) (2019) 2586, https://doi.org/10.3390/app9132586.

CHAPTER 4

Advancing ankle–foot orthosis design through biomechanics, robotics, and additive manufacturing: A review

Vidyapati Kumar, Pushpendra Gupta, and Dilip Kumar Pratihar
Department of Mechanical Engineering, Indian Institute of Technology Kharagpur, Kharagpur, West Bengal, India

4.1 Introduction

In our world today, nearly one billion individuals, constituting approximately 15% of the global population, grapple with various forms of disabilities, encompassing muscle weakness, partial or full paralysis, and loss of lower limb functionality [1]. These conditions, often stemming from degenerative diseases that predominantly affect the elderly or sudden muscle weakness and paralysis resulting from strokes, significantly impede the affected individuals from carrying out their daily activities without substantial physical assistance. The existing orthotic and exoskeleton devices, although undeniably revolutionary in their application, are often marked by their prohibitively high costs due to their sophisticated embedded technologies [2]. This stark reality underscores the pressing need for the development of affordable devices that can empower individuals in their day-to-day activities, assist in their rehabilitation journeys, and enhance their overall mobility. Orthotic and exoskeleton devices are mechanical wearable solutions designed to support the human body in an anthropomorphic manner, understanding and responding to the wearer's motion intentions [3]. When these devices encompass the lower limb, they are aptly termed lower limb exoskeleton systems. A defining feature of exoskeleton devices is their close alignment with the anatomical structure of the human limb, resulting in a significant interaction between the joints of the device and the wearer's body. The genesis of research in orthotic and exoskeleton devices can be traced back to the late 1960s when pioneering research groups in the United States and Yugoslavia initiated studies in lower limb exoskeletons to provide motion assistance, primarily for military and rehabilitation purposes [3,4]. Subsequent years witnessed the evolution of orthotic and exoskeleton devices, with research encompassing diverse mechanical structures, actuators, and control interfaces. Researchers have delved into the intricacies of actuation modes, hardware, sensor technologies, and varied control strategies, with the pioneering work by Dollar and Herr in 2008 serving as a pivotal milestone [3]. Herr's classification of exoskeleton and orthotic devices based on parallel and series arrangements with the human lower limb laid the foundation for the physical and cognitive interfaces that these devices establish with individuals, providing mobility support and receiving critical user mobility information [5].

The applications of orthotic and exoskeleton devices are manifold, with the core objective being strengthening weakened muscles to facilitate the recovery of locomotion capabilities. These devices have been harnessed for diverse purposes, including empowering healthy individuals to carry heavy loads, enhancing mobility for elderly individuals by aiding in walking and climbing stairs, and assisting paraplegic or quadriplegic individuals in their locomotion [6–9]. For the healthcare community, orthotic and exoskeleton devices like LokoMat and LOPES have offered valuable tools to prevent the physical strain of repetitive work over extended periods [10,11]. In light of demographic shifts, with approximately 11.5% of the global population aged 60 or above, a figure projected to double by 2050 [1], the development and application of these devices hold immense significance for improving the lives of impaired and elderly individuals.

Lower limb orthotic devices, specifically ankle–foot orthoses (AFOs) and knee–ankle–foot orthoses (KAFOs), constitute indispensable assistive tools for individuals with spinal cord injuries, stroke, and various neurological or musculoskeletal conditions that impact lower limb mobility. These orthoses offer external support and joint stabilization, substantially enhancing ambulation, balance, and overall quality of life. Nonetheless, current orthotic devices present limitations that include discomfort, excessive weight, misalignment with natural joint axes, and suboptimal control of limb movements.

This chapter serves as a profound exploration of research-based approaches aimed at propelling orthotic device design for lower limb rehabilitation toward greater heights. Focusing on the objective of improving mobility, it meticulously reviews the biomechanical underpinnings, design principles, manufacturing techniques, and emerging technologies that have the potential to revolutionize orthosis functionality. The chapter introduces innovative perspectives on the integration of state-of-the-art additive manufacturing (AM), smart materials, robotics, and computational tools to craft highly customized, high-performance orthoses. It further addresses the challenges associated with user acceptance, power requirements, and the transition from laboratory-based innovations to real-world clinical applications.

The ultimate goal of this chapter is to inspire the development of next-generation lower limb orthoses, meticulously tailored to individual user requirements through a data-driven approach. This endeavor necessitates the seamless convergence of knowledge from fields, such as biomechanics, ergonomics, mechatronics, and material sciences, all working in concert to engineer superior solutions. The research-based insights and perspectives offered have the potential to significantly advance the design of assistive devices while enhancing rehabilitation outcomes and the quality of life for individuals grappling with mobility impairments.

4.2 Biomechanics of biological ankle and foot

A comprehensive understanding of the biomechanics of the human ankle and foot is vital when designing orthotic devices. Human body biomechanics, as depicted in Fig. 4.1, are typically analyzed in three planes: the sagittal plane, coronal plane, and transverse plane [12].

To develop effective ankle prostheses, it is essential to grasp how a healthy ankle functions. The inverted pendulum model [13] explains that during walking, one leg controls landing while the other propels the body upward, following a parabolic trajectory. Synchronization between both legs is vital to maintaining this trajectory. Lower limb prosthetics and orthotics help to bridge the gap, with the ankle playing a critical role in maintaining the parabolic trajectory during walking.

Human walking has five primary objectives: moving forward in the sagittal plane at a specific speed and direction, minimizing energy expenditure, minimizing discomfort from painful foot ailments, adapting to uneven terrain, and imparting forward momentum to the body. These objectives require an understanding of foot movements like dorsiflexion, plantarflexion, eversion, inversion, and internal–external axial rotation, as exhibited in Fig. 4.2 [14].

Human walking consists of two primary phases: the stance phase, which comprises approximately 60% of the walking cycle, and the swing phase. Within the stance phase, ankle biomechanics are characterized by several stages, notably focusing on controlled dorsiflexion and powered plantarflexion. During controlled dorsiflexion, ankle torque

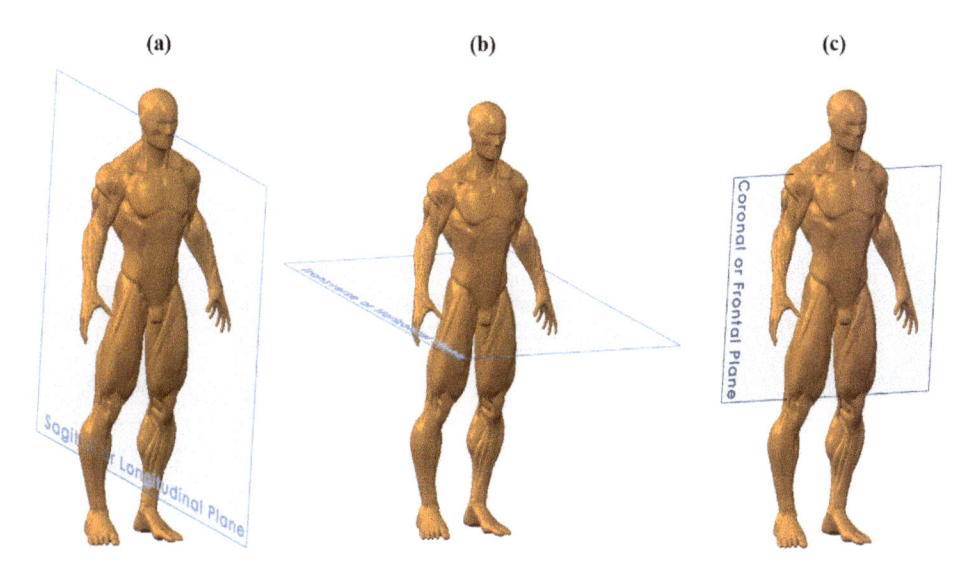

Fig. 4.1 Various planes of motion such as sagittal, transverse, and coronal [12].

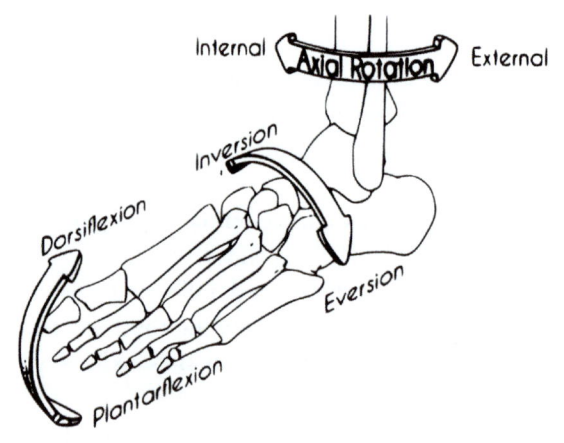

Fig. 4.2 Various movements of foot [14].

gradually increases to support the body weight, while the opposite leg carries the body's load. The powered plantarflexion phase involves the ankle's effort to move the body's center of mass against gravity to maintain a parabolic trajectory. The gait cycle consists of distinct phases. It begins with the heel strike, progresses to early flatfoot, then late flatfoot, and concludes with heel rise. The transition from early to late flatfoot is crucial, marking the shift from shock absorption to forward propulsion. The heel rise is the push-off phase, with the foot enduring significant forces. Taking thousands of steps daily, the toe-off phase begins, initiating the swing phase of the biological foot. This repetitive stress can lead to various foot conditions. This movement concludes, when the ankle returns to its initial position during the swing phase, as depicted in Fig. 4.3 [15]. Furthermore, the stance phase comprises five sub-phases, including heel strike, early flatfoot, late flatfoot, heel rise, and toe-off. A profound understanding of these sub-phases is crucial for the development of prosthetic and orthotic devices aimed at optimizing mobility and minimizing discomfort.

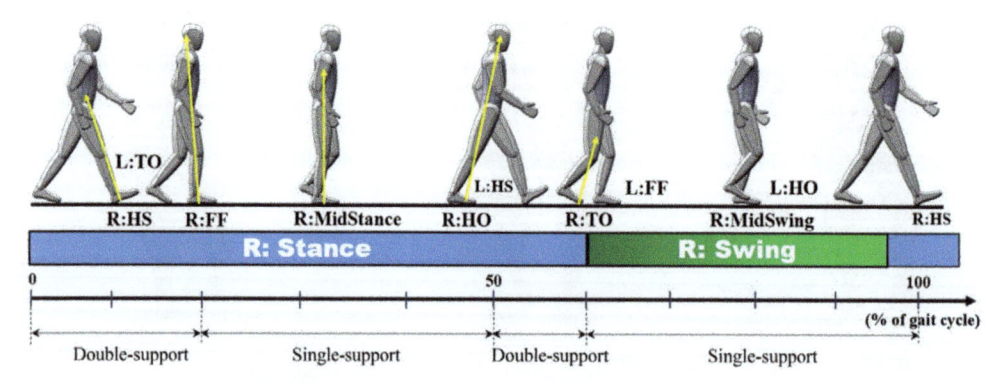

Fig. 4.3 Gait cycle of the biological right foot with different phases [15].

4.3 Design of Orthoses for lower limb

In this section, a variety of orthotic devices, each meticulously designed to address distinct needs and conditions, are explored. These encompass AFOs, KAFOs, HKAFOs, as well as advanced alternatives, such as hydraulic, pneumatic, and electrically powered orthoses. The objective is to provide valuable insights into the attributes and applications of these orthotic devices, serving as a resource for practitioners and individuals in pursuit of orthotic solutions to enhance their lower limb rehabilitation experiences.

4.3.1 Ankle–foot orthoses

AFOs play a crucial role in the rehabilitation of individuals dealing with conditions, such as incomplete spinal cord injury (ISCI) or lower limb lesions spanning from L4 to S2. These specialized devices are intricately engineered to enable safe and efficient ambulation by offering support to the weakened musculature surrounding the ankle joint. Their principal objectives encompass addressing challenges like excessive plantarflexion during initial contact, ensuring stability in the late stance for effective push-off, and averting toe-drag during the swing phase of walking [16–18]. The recommendation for AFOs is guided by principles that focus on controlling ankle joint movements, promoting safe joint mechanics, reducing the risk of falls, and enhancing overall mobility and efficiency [16,19]. The commonly prescribed AFOs types are listed as follows:

- Solid-ankle AFO: This AFO variant is crafted from sturdy materials, including plastics or advanced substances like carbon fiber. It offers exceptional support and stability, effectively restricting both dorsiflexion and plantarflexion. This results in comprehensive joint control. However, due to its bulk and rigidity, it may not be suitable for everyone's comfort [20].
- Posterior leaf spring AFO: A more flexible and prefabricated device, the posterior leaf spring AFO is typically constructed from thermoplastic materials. It maintains the ankle and foot in a specific position while allowing for a degree of ankle flexibility [20]. It is particularly beneficial for individuals with isolated ankle dorsiflexor weakness.
- Articulated AFO: This innovative design incorporates hinge joints that closely mimic the anatomical ankle joint. Its primary goal is to stabilize the ankle while permitting the ankle motion on the sagittal plane. There are two varieties of motion-articulated AFOs: one with limited motion allowing ankle plantarflexion and free dorsiflexion, and the other with limited motion allowing ankle dorsiflexion and free plantarflexion. These AFOs offer specific advantages for individuals with conditions such as drop foot, knee hyperextension, and ankle instability [20] (Fig. 4.4).

4.3.2 Knee–ankle–foot orthosis

The prescription of a knee–ankle–foot orthosis (KAFO) is a collective endeavor, involving a rehabilitation team with essential participants, including the patient, physician,

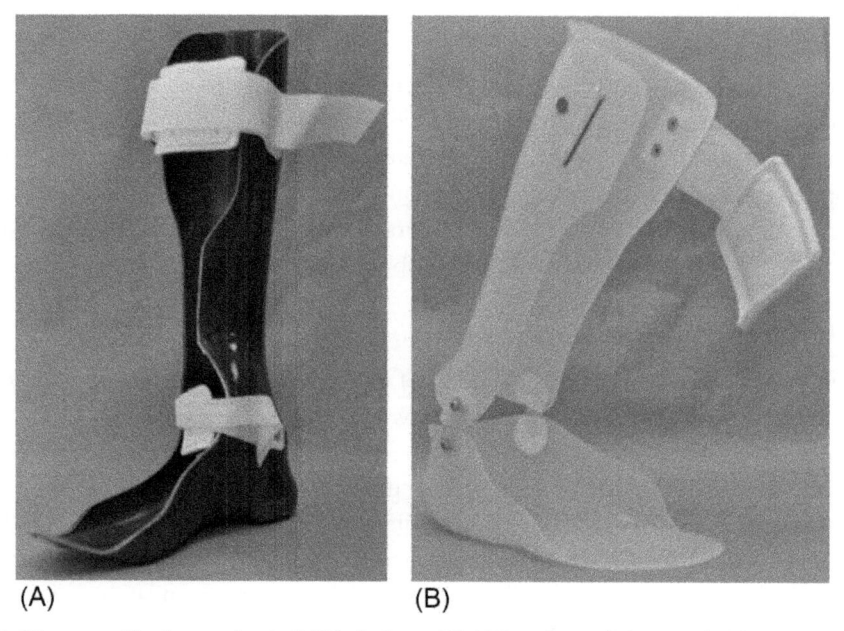

Fig. 4.4 Diverse ankle–foot orthosis (AFO) designs. (A) AFO with medial control: A laminated ankle–foot orthosis designed for medial control [20]. (B) Articulating ankle–foot orthosis [20].

orthopedist, therapist, and family or caregiver. This multidisciplinary collaboration is crucial to ascertain that the KAFO's objectives and functionalities harmonize with the patient's individual requirements and circumstances. The decision to endorse a KAFO should only be made by following an extensive clinical assessment conducted by each specialist within the rehabilitation team.

KAFOs are often prescribed when AFOs alone cannot adequately control knee instability from quadriceps weakness, laxity, or other issues. KAFOs have several potential benefits, including managing abnormal involuntary movements like spasticity, stabilizing weak ankle and knee segments, and avoiding painful or problematic joint positions. They are frequently provided for spinal cord injury patients with paraplegia from lesions at T9 through L1 spinal levels [21,22].

Various KAFO designs exist, utilizing specialized knee joints and locks tailored to patients' specific needs. These orthopedic braces play a primary role in providing stability to the knee and ankle. Their secondary impact involves affecting hip stability through the interaction with ground reaction forces. A KAFO, as illustrated in Fig. 4.5, typically consists of proximal thigh bands or thermoplastic thigh and calf shells. These are connected to upright metal sidebars, which, in turn, are linked by a footplate [20].

To attain ideal standing stability, it is essential to maintain a specific posture. This involves keeping the ankle in a neutral or dorsiflexed position, locking the knees in full extension, and allowing for passive hip extension. This posture, often referred to as "parastance," generates an extension moment at the hips, which effectively prevents

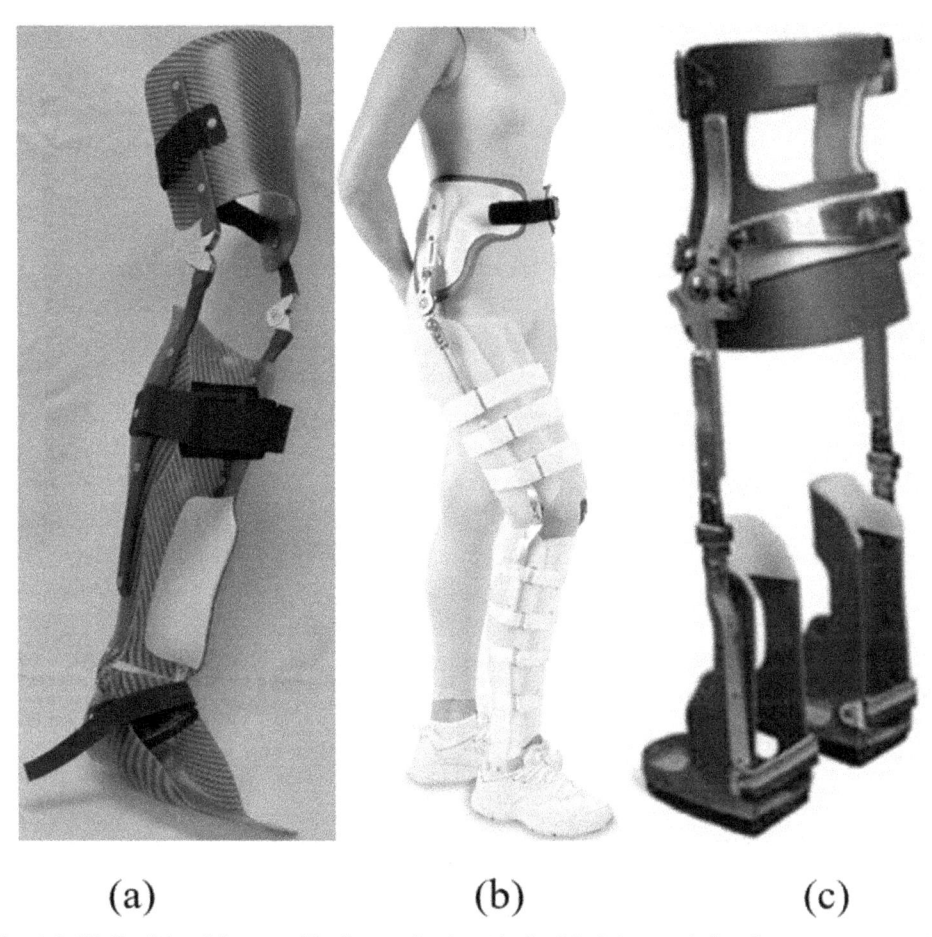

Fig. 4.5 (A) Traditional knee–ankle–foot orthosis with flexible joints and dorsiflexion assistance [20]. (B) Innovative hip–knee–ankle–foot orthosis design [20]. (C) Reciprocating gait orthosis configuration [20].

the body from leaning forward. Simultaneously, it ensures the preservation of passive hip extension, primarily facilitated by the anterior capsular ligaments. However, hips require flexion during gait, necessitating assistive devices like crutches to maintain stability [21]. Some of the commonly prescribed KAFOs are listed as follows [23]:

- The Craig–Scott orthosis, often prescribed bilaterally for patients with paraplegia from T7 to L1 [24], aims to enable functional gait with maximal stance stability. It incorporates thigh and knee straps, upright metal sidebars, and a rigid ankle–foot section. This lightweight brace facilitates swing-to gait with crutches in complete paraplegics.
- The New England Regional Spinal Cord Injury Center (NERSCIC) KAFO is another lightweight option combining upright metal sidebars with a custom molded ankle–foot orthosis (AFO). It suits complete spinal cord injury patients below T6 able to stand. The molded AFO integrates the ankle–foot support [25].

- The lightweight modular orthosis offers quick prefabricated assembly for children with muscular dystrophy. Its plastic thigh shell and AFO connect via a modular metal knee joint system with automatic locks. This extends ambulation in these patients [26].

4.3.3 Hip–knee–ankle–foot orthosis

The hip–knee–ankle–foot orthosis, commonly known as HKAFO, is a remarkable orthotic device designed to stabilize or lock the hip, knee, and ankle joints. An HKAFO typically consists of two knee–ankle–foot orthoses (KAFOs) connected above the hip with a pelvic band, lumbosacral orthosis, or thoracolumbosacral orthosis (TLSO). This orthotic solution becomes essential when an individual requires hip component stabilization due to factors like level of injury (LOI), hip, knee, or ankle contractures, balance issues, or diminished motor control [20].

The hip component provides critical stability in the transverse plane for knee–ankle–foot orthoses (KAFOs), especially when the hip joints are locked. This configuration enables a swing-to or swing-through gait pattern, where hip motion is limited. Some patients can unlock their hip joints through positioning and weight shifting to achieve a more natural reciprocal gait. A prime example is the Orthotic Research and Locomotor Assessment Unit (ORLAU) Parawalker [20], also called a hip-guidance orthosis, with free-moving hip joints enabling reciprocity.

A subset of KAFOs called reciprocating gait orthoses (RGOs) uses a mechanical system linking both brace sides through an isocentric bar, cables, or other mechanisms. This allows a reciprocal gait by the patient shifting their weight forward and sideways, extending the hips and trunk to advance the contralateral leg. RGO ambulation relies on weight shifting versus lifting the orthosis itself, unlike swing-to gait [20].

RGO variations like the hip-and-ankle linked orthosis (HALO) and RGOs with stance control have emerged [20]. The HALO connects the ankle joints via a medial hip cable, assisting leg swing, when the opposite ankle flexes. This maintains foot parallelism, reducing excessive pelvic rotation needs. RGOs with stance control have cam-locking knee joints for stability in stance, yet allow free swing-through motion with knee flexion.

Commonly prescribed HKAFOs include a range of models, such as reciprocating braces, ortho-walk pneumatic orthoses, adjustable ARGO orthosis, IRGO, HALO, and more [20]. These orthotic solutions aim to provide individuals with comprehensive joint stability and enable improved mobility, particularly in cases where standard orthoses may not suffice.

4.3.4 Advancements in mobility-enhancing orthotic systems

In the quest to improve mobility for individuals with spinal cord injuries (SCI), the field has witnessed the development of advanced orthotic systems that employ cutting-edge technologies, such as both hydraulic and pneumatic control systems, as well as electrical power sources, to facilitate forward leg movement during the swing phase [20]. Although many of these innovations have primarily undergone evaluation in controlled laboratory environments, they offer promising strides in the realm of lower limb rehabilitation. Here, we present a selection of noteworthy examples:

- Electronic KAFO: This orthosis, as shown in Fig. 4.6, employs electronic mechanisms to support the advancement of the legs during the swing phase, offering an innovative approach to knee–ankle–foot orthosis design.
- Hydraulic reciprocating gait hip–knee–ankle foot orthosis (HRGO): Designed with hydraulic components, this orthosis facilitates reciprocating gait, emphasizing the coordinated movement of the hip, knee, and ankle. It provides a dynamic solution for individuals with SCI.
- Pneumatic active gait orthosis (PAGO): Utilizing pneumatic control systems, the PAGO is engineered to actively assist in the gait of individuals with lower limb impairments. Pneumatic technology contributes to dynamic movement and support.

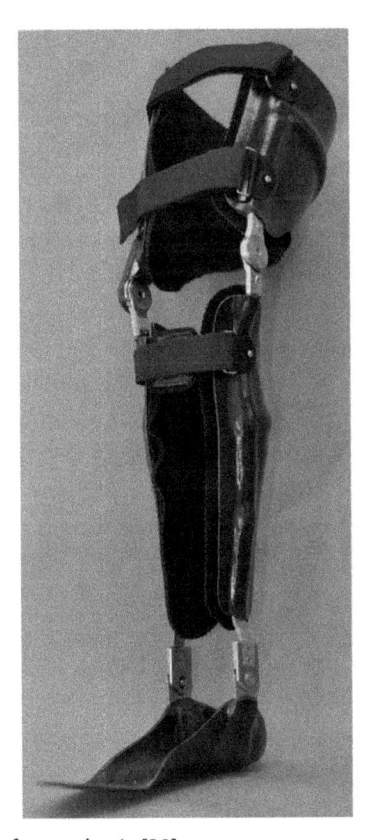

Fig. 4.6 Electronic knee–ankle–foot orthosis [20].

- Powered gait orthosis (PGO): As the name suggests, the PGO harnesses electrical power sources to provide assistance during gait. This electrically powered orthosis offers a new dimension of mobility support, potentially increasing the efficiency of leg movement.
- Weight-bearing control (WBC) orthosis: The WBC orthosis focuses on controlling and distributing the weight-bearing load during gait, enhancing stability, and ensuring safe and balanced leg advancement.
- Powered gait orthosis: This orthosis incorporates advanced two-degree-of-freedom motorized systems to facilitate the movement of the legs during gait. It is a significant technological advancement in the quest for improved mobility solutions.
- Driven gait orthosis (DGO): The DGO is engineered to offer powered assistance during gait. With innovative mechanisms, it seeks to optimize leg movement, especially for individuals with SCI.

These orthotic innovations represent a convergence of technology and rehabilitation, promising greater mobility and independence for individuals with SCI. While they have been primarily assessed in laboratory settings, they hold great potential for improving the daily lives of those in need of advanced lower limb mobility support.

4.4 Advances in orthotic manufacturing

Presently, the creation of rehabilitation devices predominantly relies on the craftsmanship of orthopedic specialists. The quality of these devices is, therefore, intricately linked to the expertise and experience of these specialists. Crafting these products is a time-intensive process, heavily contingent on the specialist's skills to ensure the devices align with the unique gait dynamics of each individual. Consequently, the demand for tailor-made solutions, such as orthoses and assistive devices, has grown considerably, spurred by technological advancements in the early 21st century [27]. In orthoprosthetic manufacturing, the first step is to capture the body segment's morphology. Traditional techniques typically employ foam or plaster molds for this purpose. A prototype is then fashioned using computerized numerical control (CNC) or a milling machine, based on the thermosetting polyurethane model derived from the mold. Subsequently, the specialist makes numerous adjustments to the device to achieve a precise fit for the individual as depicted in Fig. 4.7.A. However, CNC and milling methods present certain limitations, as they struggle to replicate intricate surface designs or accommodate varying thicknesses and materials.

In contrast, the emerging rapid prototyping technology (RPT) approach initiates the manufacturing process differently as illustrated in Fig. 4.7.B. It commences with 3D scanning technologies to capture the individual's morphology. Computer-aided design (CAD) and computer-aided engineering (CAE) tools are then employed to formulate designs tailored to the specific subject, taking into account functionality through experimentation with different materials and structures [28]. Finally, the design seamlessly

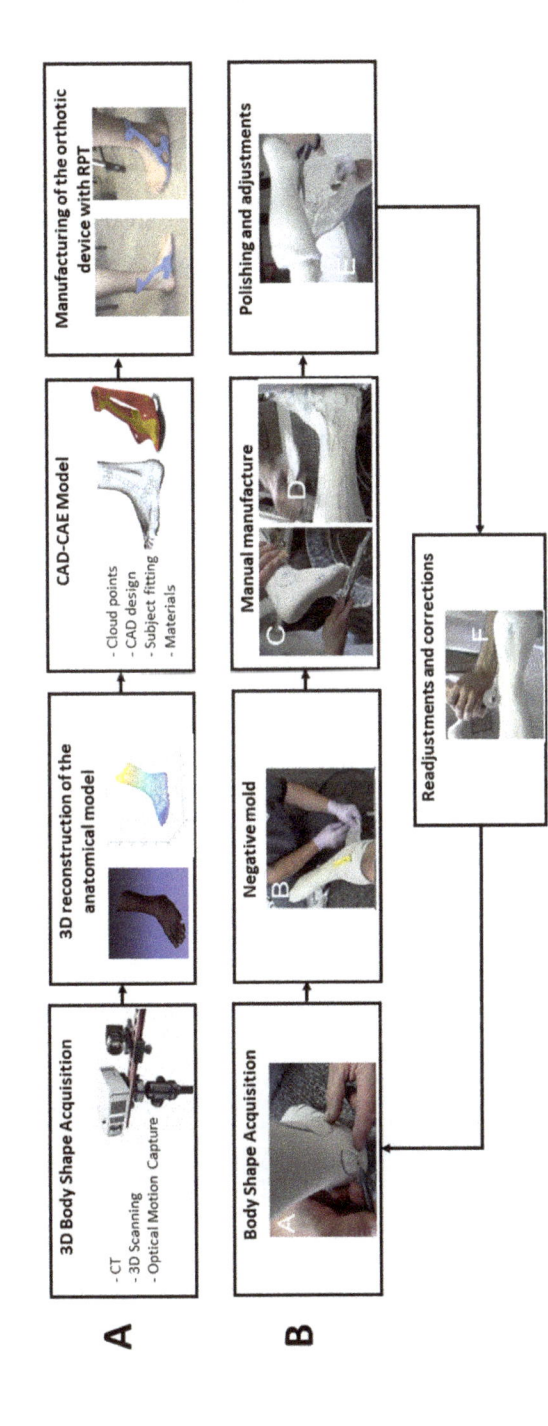

Fig. 4.7 Key stages in the production of custom-fit orthotic devices [27]. (A) Utilizing rapid prototyping techniques (RPT) methodology. (B) Traditional approach involving computer-aided design (CAD), computer-aided engineering (CAE), and computed tomography (CT) imaging.

transfers to an AM machine, culminating in the prototype. This transformative process significantly reduces manufacturing time, transitioning from several weeks in the traditional approach to merely a couple of days in RPT [29]. Consequently, RPT, coupled with novel 3D acquisition methods, serves as a compelling alternative within the orthoprosthetic industry.

The application of AM and RPT extends beyond orthotic devices into various medical spheres, encompassing the creation of medical instruments, drug delivery systems, engineered tissues, bone regeneration scaffolds, dental implants, prosthetic sockets, and surgical applications [29,30]. This review provides a comprehensive examination of advancements in orthotic device manufacturing, with a specific focus on the integration of RPT to improve quality and expedite production within the field of rehabilitation. It delves into devices, such as splints, AFOs, and arm prostheses, elucidating the diverse methodologies available for use in the orthotic and prosthetic domains [31]. Additionally, it highlights novel 3D data acquisition techniques and material considerations. This work aims to serve as an authoritative resource for practitioners and researchers seeking further exploration in this area.

4.4.1 3D anatomical data acquisition technologies in orthotic device design

In the field of orthotic device design, the integration of RPT with advanced anatomical data acquisition techniques has created innovative opportunities. These technologies facilitate the creation of custom orthotic devices tailored to individual patients' needs.

- Computed tomography (CT): CT scans, with their high-resolution imaging capabilities, have proven invaluable in the development of orthotic devices. They aid in diagnostics and surgical planning, offering detailed insights into anatomical structures. Recent studies have harnessed CT to produce insoles for diabetes patients and prosthetic devices with remarkable precision [27]. However, concerns about radiation exposure and the partial pixel effect persist.
- 3D scanning: 3D scanning technologies offer a practical and efficient means of capturing human body shape. These systems use various techniques, including lasers and structured light, to generate precise point cloud data, which is then converted into CAD models. This approach reduces processing time, lowers data file sizes, and is known for its cost-effectiveness and accessibility [27].
- Optical motion capture systems: To cater to dynamic conditions, orthotic devices need to account for the human body's movements. Optical motion capture systems, employing reflective markers and cameras, are pivotal in capturing body kinetics. While marker-based technologies are commonly used for assessing the performance of orthotic devices, markerless systems, and emerging 4D scanning methods hold promise for capturing intricate body shape changes during dynamic activities like walking [27].

The fusion of RPT with these data acquisition technologies is redefining orthotic device design by enhancing accuracy, efficiency, and the ability to create patient-specific solutions. Further research and comparisons between these technologies will continue to drive progress in the orthotic and prosthetic industry, benefiting both practitioners and patients seeking customized, high-quality devices.

4.4.2 Rapid prototyping technologies transforming orthotic device manufacturing

The evolution of orthotic device manufacturing is experiencing a significant shift, primarily due to the integration of CAD and computer-aided manufacturing (CAM) processes, popularly known as RPT. This shift from traditional craft practices is aimed at delivering tailor-made orthotic devices by following a structured approach of custom manufacturing keeping the user-centric needs into consideration.

The process of custom manufacturing via RPT follows a structured sequence of steps. It commences with a 3D scan of the anatomical surface, followed by 3D surface reconstruction and CAD modeling. Subsequently, the CAD model is transformed into the commonly used stereolithography (STL) file format. This STL file serves as the blueprint for creating the physical orthotic device with the assistance of a specialized rapid prototyping machine, often referred to as a 3D printer. The advantages of this approach are manifold and encompass greater design flexibility, the ability to incorporate functional elements, heightened precision, cost-effectiveness, shorter production times, and an improved end-user experience with the final product. Some of the primary RPT manufacturing techniques preferably employed in this context are as follows:

- Fused deposition modeling (FDM): FDM entails the extrusion of semi-molten material through an extrusion head, which moves along the X and Y axes to build each two-dimensional layer of the orthotic device. This process employs two extrusion nozzles: one for the primary building material and the other for support material. FDM is known for its use of economical materials such as polycarbonate (PC), acrylonitrile butadiene styrene (ABS), or combinations thereof [31]. While FDM offers the advantage of cost-effective materials, the production times can be relatively extended. Nevertheless, it finds applications in upper and lower limb orthoses, hand prostheses, and various other domains.
- Selective laser sintering (SLS): SLS systems create three-dimensional objects by selectively fusing powdered polymer materials using a CO_2 laser. This process transforms the powder into solid objects, layer by layer. SLS typically employs materials like polyamide 12 (PA), ABS, and PC, offering a significant reduction in weight, which is crucial in orthotic devices. SLS has been used for AFOs and various custom orthotic and prosthetic devices, maintaining a remarkable accuracy that aligns with clinical standards [27].

- Powder bed and inkjet head 3D printing (3DP): In the 3DP process, a layer of powder is spread on a build platform, followed by the selective deposition of liquid adhesive through an inkjet printhead. The process repeats for each layer. Though it offers lower accuracy than SLS, 3DP is favored for its low cost and quickness [29]. It employs thermoplastics, such as ABS, and has seen applications in the production of functional prostheses, patient-specific maxillofacial implants, and tissue engineering.

These RPT methods have significantly transformed orthotic device manufacturing and offered unprecedented flexibility, accuracy, and efficiency while adhering to cost constraints. This shift empowers healthcare providers and patients to benefit from custom orthotic devices that are perfectly tailored to individual needs and deliver superior comfort and functionality.

4.5 Technical challenges

While recent advances in orthotic device design show great promise, translating these innovations into effective clinical solutions requires overcoming key technical challenges. The areas that need particular focus include improving device ergonomics, reducing weight, enhancing safety and reliability, managing power requirements, and ensuring user acceptance. Specifically, issues around human–robot interaction (HRI), sensors and control, structural design, actuators and batteries, materials selection, and overall usability persist. Careful consideration of these challenges is critical during the design process to create orthotic devices that are comfortable, intuitive, and able to withstand repeated use in real-world settings. A human-centered approach should be employed, gathering end-user perspectives to refine the technology. Additionally, continued materials research and engineering are needed to balance often competing priorities like strength, weight, power efficiency, and cost. By systematically addressing these technical barriers through an interdisciplinary effort, the next generation of orthotic devices can fulfill their potential to restore mobility and transform rehabilitation outcomes. The main challenges are elaborated as follows:

4.5.1 HRI challenges

- The cognitive and physical interaction between the human operator and the exoskeleton needs to be carefully studied and designed based on the intended application. Mismatches can occur between human joint frequencies and gait patterns compared to the exoskeleton, which can cause discomfort for the user.
- Mechanical transparency refers to how seamlessly the exoskeleton can follow the movements of the human operator without introducing resistive forces. It is an important desired characteristic but is affected by many factors like overall mass, inertia, structural design, actuators used, etc. Lighter exoskeletons with backdrivable actuators can help to improve transparency.

- The interaction forces between the human and the exoskeleton are the basis for generating assistive/restorative torques by the control system. However, these forces can be difficult to accurately estimate and model during the design phase. In practice, force sensors have measurement uncertainties affecting control.
- Backdrivability allows physical interaction between the human and the exoskeleton by allowing bidirectional transfer of mechanical power. However, commonly used electric motors with high gear reductions increase joint impedance and reduce backdrivability. Compliant actuators like series elastic actuators (SEAs) can help to overcome this.
- The fixtures used for attaching the exoskeleton to the human body can be rigid or flexible. If designed poorly, tight fixtures can cause discomfort and skin abrasions and affect muscle diameter during use. The attachments need to balance stability with ergonomics.

4.5.2 Sensors and controllers challenges

- Several different sensors are used in exoskeletons to measure positions, forces, EMG signals, etc. Sensor accuracy, noise, calibration, cost, and reliable data rates are issues. EMG sensors need electrodes attached to the skin and are user-specific.
- The control strategy depends heavily on the physical quantities being measured by the sensors for feedback. Mismatch in sensors vs control approach can cause problems. EMG signals cannot be used for patients with muscle disorders necessitating hybrid control approaches.
- For rehabilitation exoskeletons, the controller needs to adapt to changes in the patient's condition and progression of recovery, which continuously alters the sensed physical quantities. Machine learning can potentially help with personalized control.
- The performance of exoskeletons can vary significantly based on the environment these are operated in like walking on stairs, slopes, uneven terrain, etc. This may necessitate designing different control algorithms and modes for robust performance.

4.5.3 Structural design challenges

- The biomechanics and range of motion of human joints and limbs need to be carefully studied and matched in the exoskeleton structural design. Significant mismatches in joint velocities, degrees of freedom, and range of motions can make the exoskeleton ineffective.
- While stiffer exoskeleton structures are aimed to provide effective force transmission and controllability, if misaligned with human joints, they can overly restrict or even break human joints during use. Kinematic compliance needs to be ensured.
- Over-simplifying the degrees of freedom in human joints while designing exoskeleton joints can cause structural misalignments and overly restrict the operator's natural workspace and movements.

4.5.4 Actuators and batteries challenges

- The type of actuator used, such as hydraulic, pneumatic, electric, SEA, etc. significantly impacts parameters like power output, precision, efficiency, and controllability. Actuators must be selected based on the requirements.
- The location of actuators relative to the joints also affects power transmission efficiency and the complexity of control methods. Geared motors add torque regulation challenges. Direct drive motors could simplify control.
- Onboard batteries add significant weight to the exoskeleton structure which can adversely affect the biomechanics and performance, and consequently, more energy-dense batteries or external power sources are required.

4.5.5 Materials and safety challenges

- Lightweight and stiff materials are needed to maintain the mechanical efficiency of power transmission, while not overly increasing total exoskeleton mass. Heavyweight exoskeletons can negatively impact human biomechanics.
- Ensuring safety is critical in exoskeletons since these are in direct physical contact with the users. High reliability and mechanical robustness are needed to avoid injuries from component failures or fall hazards.

4.5.6 Ergonomics challenges

- Donning and doffing the exoskeleton should take very little time to maximize usability. For shared exoskeletons in rehabilitation clinics, proper sanitization between users is a must.
- The exoskeleton must be designed to properly fit the user and the specific tasks for which it will be used to avoid discomfort and risk of injury. A mismatch can reduce effectiveness.
- The user experience must be studied carefully and enhanced via design iterations. Feedback from the users and ergonomic testing is critical.

4.6 Summary

This comprehensive chapter has elucidated the tremendous potential of lower limb orthotic devices to transform rehabilitation outcomes through an interdisciplinary approach unifying biomechanics, mechatronics, materials science, and human-centered design. By providing a thorough grounding in joint biomechanics, gait analysis, orthosis types, manufacturing methods, actuator technologies, and control systems, this research-backed resource aims to propel assistive device innovation. The path ahead necessitates systematically tackling key challenges around device weight, cost, safety, power, and user experience while drawing inspiration from emerging areas like biomimetics, smart materials, AM, and AI-enabled personalization. With the sustained, collaborative efforts across engineering, medicine, and ergonomics focused on human empowerment, the next generation of lightweight, intelligent orthoses can arise, fulfilling the promise of restoring mobility and independence for millions with physical impairments. This future compels us to combine technological capabilities with a profound understanding of human comfort and dignity. Using science to uplift the human spirit is the vital mission and immense opportunity at the heart of orthotic device research.

4.7 Future directions

While recent advances offer immense promise, realizing the full potential of orthotic devices requires continued research across multiple fronts.

- Safety and risk management: Additional studies are required to thoroughly evaluate the physical and psychological risks associated with the use of orthotic devices, especially for home/personal use without medical supervision [32,33]. Developing comprehensive safety standards and risk mitigation guidelines through rigorous testing and research can aid regulatory approval processes. Investigating safety systems like fall detection, airbags, and sensors to detect issues early (e.g., heat, abrasions) could help mitigate risks and improve overall safety [34].
- End-user experience and needs: Further research through surveys, focus groups, and ethnographic studies is needed to analyze end-user satisfaction, difficulties, preferences, and needs across demographics, impairment types, and applications [35]. Gathering user feedback is vital for optimizing device ergonomics, comfort, perceived usefulness, emotional response, ease of use, independence, and other aspects of the human–technology interaction. Additionally, studying device abandonment, refusal to use, and related behaviors can provide insights into human–technology integration challenges that should be addressed through universal design thinking.
- Power systems and energy storage: One key priority is developing more energy-dense, compact, lightweight, fast-charging batteries to improve usable time for portable orthotic devices. Exploring alternative power sources like compact hydrogen fuel cells and solar panels integrated into the device structure seems promising. Energy-efficient mechanical, electrical, and control system designs (motors, transmissions, power electronics, etc.) are required, along with kinetic energy harvesting from gait motions [36]. Advanced battery management encompassing charge monitoring, thermal regulation, and safety protocols are also important. Quick battery swapping modules could enhance the convenience.
- Smart materials and design: In terms of materials and design, harnessing smart materials like shape memory alloys and electro-rheological fluids to create adaptable assistive properties and sensing capabilities holds potential. Customized, 3D-printed, flexible orthotic components using advanced polymers and composites can improve fit and

function [37]. Strong, lightweight materials like carbon fiber composites are especially valuable. Pursuing biomimetic designs for better movement synergy between user and device is another avenue, along with softer, less rigid structures to boost safety and reduce strain injuries. Integrating wearable sensor systems can enable more intuitive control, tactile feedback, injury prevention, and environment sensing [37].
- Artificial intelligence and autonomy: Significant opportunities exist for applying AI techniques to enable more individualized, intuitive control that adapts to user physiology, preferences, and disabilities by leveraging neural networks and big data analytics. Semi-autonomous operation can reduce the cognitive burden on users, while mix-initiative interaction allowing user and robot initiation of actions seems promising [38]. Analytics applied to sensor data using AI could also detect improvements or deterioration in patient conditions and therapy effectiveness over time, informing treatment.
- Teleoperation and wireless control: Leveraging wireless control over 5G/6G networks can potentially enable remote operation and cloud-based processing for more compact, portable orthotic devices [39]. Teleoperation may allow expert guidance and supervision remotely, while also assisting in case of emergencies like falls. Remote monitoring of patient biometrics and device status data can further aid professionals [40]. Wireless software and capability upgrades are also enabled through connectivity.

References

[1] B. Kalita, J. Narayan, S.K. Dwivedy, Development of active lower limb robotic-based orthosis and exoskeleton devices: a systematic review, Int. J. Soc. Robot. 13 (4) (2021) 775–793.
[2] A. Kapsalyamov, P.K. Jamwal, S. Hussain, M.H. Ghayesh, State of the art lower limb robotic exoskeletons for elderly assistance, IEEE Access 7 (2019) 95075–95086.
[3] A.M. Dollar, H. Herr, Lower extremity exoskeletons and active orthoses: challenges and state-of-the-art, IEEE Trans. Robot. 24 (1) (2008) 144–158.
[4] H. Herr, Exoskeletons and orthoses: classification, design challenges and future directions, J. Neuroeng. Rehabil. 6 (1) (2009).
[5] J.L. Pons, Rehabilitation exoskeletal robotics, IEEE Eng. Med. Biol. Mag. 29 (3) (2010) 57–63.
[6] Y. Sankai, HAL: Hybrid assistive limb based on cybernics, Springer Tracts Adv. Robot. 66 (STAR) (2010) 25–34.
[7] L. Wang, S. Wang, E.H.F. Van Asseldonk, H. Van Der Kooij, Actively controlled lateral gait assistance in a lower limb exoskeleton, in: IEEE International Conference on Intelligent Robots and Systems, 2013, pp. 965–970.
[8] P.D. Neuhaus, J.H. Noorden, T.J. Craig, T. Torres, J. Kirschbaum, J.E. Pratt, Design and evaluation of Mina: A robotic orthosis for paraplegics, in: IEEE International Conference on Rehabilitation Robotics, 2011.
[9] A. Esquenazi, M. Talaty, A. Packel, M. Saulino, The Rewalk powered exoskeleton to restore ambulatory function to individuals with thoracic-level motor-complete spinal cord injury, Am. J. Phys. Med. Rehabil. 91 (11) (2012) 911–921.
[10] G. Colombo, M. Joerg, R. Schreier, V. Dietz, Treadmill training of paraplegic patients using a robotic orthosis, J. Rehabil. Res. Dev. 37 (6) (2000) 693–700.
[11] J.F. Veneman, R. Kruidhof, E.E.G. Hekman, R. Ekkelenkamp, E.H.F. Van Asseldonk, H. Van Der Kooij, Design and evaluation of the LOPES exoskeleton robot for interactive gait rehabilitation, IEEE Trans. Neural Syst. Rehabil. Eng. 15 (3) (2007) 379–386.

[12] P. Chauhan, A.K. Singh, N.K. Raghuwanshi, The state of art review on prosthetic feet and its significance to imitate the biomechanics of human ankle-foot, Mater. Today Proc. 62 (P12) (2022) 6364–6370.

[13] A.D. Kuo, J.M. Donelan, A. Ruina, Energetic consequences of walking like an inverted pendulum: step-to-step transitions, Exerc. Sport Sci. Rev. 33 (2) (2005) 88–97.

[14] J. Zagoya-López, L.A. Zúñiga-Avilés, A.H. Vilchis-González, J.C. Ávila-Vilchis, Foot/ankle prostheses design approach based on Scientometric and Patentometric analyses, Appl. Sci. 11 (12) (2021) 5591.

[15] A. Alamdari, V.N. Krovi, A review of computational musculoskeletal analysis of human lower extremities, in: Human Modeling for Bio-Inspired Robotics: Mechanical Engineering in Assistive Technologies, 2017, pp. 37–73.

[16] W. Bunch, D.R. Wenger, American Academy of Orthopaedic Surgeons' atlas of orthotics—biomechanical principles and application, J. Pediatr. Orthop. 7 (1) (1987) 109.

[17] D.J. Maxwell, M.H. Granat, G. Baardman, H.J. Hermens, Demand for and use of functional electrical stimulation systems and conventional orthoses in the spinal lesioned community of the UK, Artif. Organs 23 (5) (1999) 410–412.

[18] J.W. Middleton, P.J. Sinclair, R.M. Smith, G.M. Davis, Postural control during stance in paraplegia: effects of medially linked versus unlinked knee-ankle-foot orthoses, Arch. Phys. Med. Rehabil. 80 (12) (1999) 1558–1565.

[19] J.F. Lehmann, Biomechanics of ankle-foot orthoses: prescription and design, Arch. Phys. Med. Rehabil. 60 (5) (1979) 200–207.

[20] T.D. Lavis, L. Codamon, Lower limb orthoses for persons with spinal cord injury, in: Atlas of Orthoses and Assistive Devices, fifth ed., 2018, p. 247. 255.e4.

[21] M.B. Atrice, Lower extremity orthotic management for the spinal-cord-injured client, Top. Spinal Cord Inj. Rehabil. 5 (4) (2000) 1–10.

[22] G.K. Rose, The principles and practice of hip guidance articulations, Prosthetics Orthot. Int. 3 (1) (1979) 37–43.

[23] M.J. DeVivo, R.M. Shewchuk, S.L. Stover, K.J. Black, B.K. Go, A cross-sectional study of the relationship between age and current health status for persons with spinal cord injuries, Paraplegia 30 (12) (1992) 820–827.

[24] M.J. DeVivo, K.J. Black, S.L. Stover, Causes of death during the first 12 years after spinal cord injury, Arch. Phys. Med. Rehabil. 74 (3) (1993) 248–254.

[25] J.G. Doherty, A.S. Burns, D.M. O'Ferrall, J.F. Ditunno, Prevalence of upper motor neuron vs lower motor neuron lesions in complete lower thoracic and lumbar spinal cord injuries, J. Spinal Cord Med. 25 (4) (2002) 289–292.

[26] R. Douglas, P.F. Larson, R. D'Ambrosia, R.E. McCall, The LSU reciprocation-gait orthosis, Orthopedics 6 (7) (1983) 834–839.

[27] J. Barrios-Muriel, F. Romero-Sánchez, F.J. Alonso-Sánchez, D.R. Salgado, Advances in orthotic and prosthetic manufacturing: a technology review, Materials 13 (2) (2020).

[28] A. Babbar, Y. Tian, V. Kumar, A. Sharma, 3D bioprinting in biomedical applications, in: Additive Manufacturing of Polymers for Tissue Engineering, CRC Press, Boca Raton, 2022, pp. 1–16.

[29] V. Kumar, A. Babbar, A. Sharma, R. Kumar, A. Tyagi, Polymer 3D bioprinting for bionics and tissue engineering applications, in: Additive Manufacturing of Polymers for Tissue Engineering, CRC Press, Boca Raton, 2022, pp. 17–39.

[30] V. Kumar, C. Prakash, A. Babbar, S. Choudhary, A. Sharma, A.S. Uppal, Additive manufacturing in biomedical engineering, Addit. Manuf. Process. Biomed. Eng. (2022) 143–164.

[31] A. Babbar, et al., Additive manufacturing for the development of biological implants, scaffolds, and prosthetics, Addit. Manuf. Process. Biomed. Eng. (2022) 27–46.

[32] Y. He, D. Eguren, T.P. Luu, J.L. Contreras-Vidal, Risk management and regulations for lower limb medical exoskeletons: a review, Med. Devices: Evidence Res 10 (2017) 89–107.

[33] I. Tijjani, S. Kumar, M. Boukheddimi, A survey on design and control of lower extremity exoskeletons for bipedal walking, Appl. Sci. 12 (5) (2022).

[34] P.V. Er, K.K. Tan, Wearable solution for robust fall detection, in: Assistive Technology for the Elderly, 2020, pp. 81–105.

[35] P.M. Kuber, M. Abdollahi, M.M. Alemi, E. Rashedi, A systematic review on evaluation strategies for field assessment of upper-body industrial exoskeletons: current practices and future trends, Ann. Biomed. Eng. 50 (10) (2022) 1203–1231.
[36] S. Toxiri, et al., Back-support exoskeletons for occupational use: an overview of technological advances and trends, IISE Trans. Occup. Ergon. Hum. Factors 7 (3–4) (2019) 237–249.
[37] A. Esquenazi, M. Talaty, Future trends and research in orthoses, in: Atlas of Orthoses and Assistive Devices, fifth ed., 2018, p. 448. 450.e1.
[38] D. David, Aging Changes in the Nervous System: MedlinePlus Medical Encyclopedia, MedlinePlus, 2020, pp. 1–4. no. January.
[39] W. Saad, M. Bennis, M. Chen, A vision of 6G wireless systems: applications, trends, technologies, and open research problems, IEEE Netw. 34 (3) (2020) 134–142.
[40] P.K. Padhi, F. Charrua-Santos, 6G enabled industrial internet of everything: towards a theoretical framework, Appl. Syst. Innov. 4 (1) (2021) 1–30.

CHAPTER 5

Application of multibistatic frequency-domain measurements for enhanced medical sensing and imaging

Behnaz Sohani[a], Amir Rahmani[b], and Aliyu Aliyu[b]

[a]Wolfson School of Mechanical, Electrical & Manufacturing Engineering, Loughborough University, Loughborough, United Kingdom
[b]School of Engineering, University of Lincoln, Lincoln, United Kingdom

5.1 Introduction

The urgency of immediate medical attention is paramount in the management of patients afflicted with brain injuries, a condition fraught with the rapid degeneration of brain cells and the potential for dire consequences, ranging from enduring neurological impairment to fatality. The timely detection of brain injuries, such as strokes, and the prompt administration of appropriate pharmacological interventions within a crucial window of a few hours from symptom onset wield a profound influence on patient outcomes. Thus, the development and deployment of a portable diagnostic system tailored for rapid on-site detection of brain injuries emerge as an imperative within the contemporary healthcare landscape.

In the context of conventional diagnostic modalities, medical practitioners predominantly depend on magnetic resonance imaging (MRI) and computed tomography (CT) imaging scans to assess brain injuries. While these imaging techniques provide invaluable insights into the extent and nature of brain injuries, they are characterized by inherent limitations that impede their utility in certain clinical contexts. Specifically, the substantial size and immobility of CT and MRI machines render them impractical for point-of-care applications, particularly in resource-constrained environments and small medical centers. Consequently, there exists an imperative need for innovative diagnostic approaches that combine the diagnostic precision of CT and MRI with the portability and speed required to address the exigencies of acute brain injury management [1]. The concept of employing microwave imaging (MWI) as a method for detecting brain abnormalities has recently been introduced in the literature [2,3]. MWI capitalizes on disparities in the dielectric properties exhibited by various tissues, rendering it a promising avenue for diagnostic innovation [3].

Evidence has substantiated the impact of hemorrhagic stroke on the alteration of tissue dielectric properties [4]. Notably, hemorrhagic stroke induces a marked escalation in dielectric properties, reaching levels up to 20% higher in comparison to white and gray matter tissue's dielectric characteristics [5]. In contrast, ischemic stroke is associated with a decline in dielectric in comparison to white and gray matter tissue's dielectric characteristics relative to those observed in white and gray matter tissues [2,6].

MWI techniques fall under various classifications, including radar methods and microwave tomography (MT) [7]. MT seeks to reconstruct the dielectric characteristic distribution within a cranial region by addressing a complex and inherently challenging inverse scattering problem, which is characterized by nonlinearity and ill-posedness [8,9].

One of the notable challenges inherent in MT lies in the susceptibility to solution instability, which arises due to the intricate mathematical formulations involved. In contrast, radar imaging presents a comparatively simpler problem focused on the detection of scattering patterns based on disparities in dielectric properties. Various radar imaging techniques have been proposed to address this simplified problem [10].

From a hardware perspective, MWI encounters the challenge of effectively integrating multiple antennas to cover the target area within human tissues for investigation [11]. While the coupling substance has the capability to enhance antenna infiltration, it introduces significant complications [12]. Additionally, achieving wideband functionality and efficient energy linking with the head necessitates engaging the antenna in a 90% glycerine-water mixture [13].

Furthermore, within the domain of Medical Sensing and Imaging, the utilization of frequency-domain measurements—using multiple bistatic configurations—offers an avenue to acquire the transfer function (S21) that links a pair of antennas. Multibistatic frequency-domain measurements represent a technique employed in the realm of electromagnetic and radio frequency research and applications. This approach entails the deployment of multiple antennas for the transmission and reception of electromagnetic signals distributed across various frequencies within the frequency-domain spectrum. Typically, these antennas are strategically arranged, with the first antenna functioning as a transmitter and the second antenna acting as a receiver, facilitating the assessment of signal propagation dynamics between them across diverse frequencies.

The principal objective of multibistatic frequency-domain measurements is to glean insights into the transfer function or response characteristics of a system spanning a spectrum of frequencies. This method necessitates a straightforward hardware setup involving the transmitting and receiving antennas (interconnected via a vector network analyzer (VNA)) that rotate in free space around the target object, collecting signals using a multibistatic configuration [14]. This versatile approach holds considerable value across various applications, encompassing radar systems, wireless communication networks, and electromagnetic imaging methodologies [14–21]. It facilitates a comprehensive analysis of signal interactions with objects or materials throughout the entire frequency spectrum, promising significant advancements in sensing and imaging techniques.

5.2 Advantages of integrating multibistatic antennas in the development of detecting hemorrhagic brain strokes using a scanner

Severe brain injuries constitute a spectrum of conditions, encompassing both obtained and traumatic injuries induced by external factors like falls or accidents, alongside internal occurrences like strokes and tumors. Of particular concern are brain strokes, wherein cerebral blood circulation is compromised either by an obstructed blood passage or ruptured one, culminating in ischemic or hemorrhagic events, respectively. It is noteworthy that certain symptoms exhibit overlap among transient ischemic attacks, strokes, and various other prevalent medical conditions, including syncope, migraines, cardiac ailments, and seizures [22]. Thus, the accurate differentiation of strokes from these unrelated health conditions is of paramount importance.

The urgency of timely medical intervention in cases of brain injury cannot be overstressed, for every fleeting moment following a brain injury precipitates the irreversible loss of millions of vital brain cells, potentially resulting in enduring damage or fatality [23]. Consequently, the expeditious diagnosis of brain injuries, particularly strokes, necessitates access to a portable diagnostic system capable of swiftly providing assessments. Initially, a clinical evaluation, administered by a general practitioner (GP), constitutes of this diagnostic journey [23]. Nevertheless, clinical assessments may not invariably distinguish strokes from nonvascular conditions manifesting similar symptoms. Consequently, healthcare practitioners frequently depend on CT imaging and MRI scans for a definitive diagnosis. Regrettably, the substantial dimensions of CT and MRI machines render them neither swift nor portable, thus making them unsuitable for deployment in smaller medical facilities.

In stark contrast to conventional imaging methodologies, MWI proffers a promising solution. MWI offers portability and the capacity for swift initial diagnoses of life-threatening conditions, such as strokes, even during a patient's transit to a hospital via an ambulance, thereby saving precious time [1]. Recent strides in MWI have been directed toward its suitability for detecting brain abnormalities by leveraging disparities in the dielectric properties of tissues [2,3]. Studies have revealed that hemorrhagic strokes provoke substantial changes in tissue dielectric properties, leading to a marked increase of up to 20% compared to those of white and gray matter [4]. Conversely, ischemic strokes engender a failure in dielectric characteristics relative to white and gray matter [2,6].

MWI encompasses radar techniques and MT [7], with the latter striving to reconfigure the dielectric characteristic profile of the head by addressing a notably nonlinear and ambiguous inverse scattering challenge [8,9]. Nonetheless, MT confronts challenges stemming from solution instability resulting from intricate mathematical expressions. Conversely, radio detection and ranging imaging centers on identifying scattering maps predicated on disparities in dielectric properties, thereby offering a more straightforward approach [10].

From a hardware perspective, MWI encounters intricacies concerning the configuration of multiple antennas to cover the area of interest within human tissues [11]. While the application of a coupling medium can optimize antenna penetration, it introduces complexity [12]. Additionally, achieving broadband operation and efficient energy coupling often mandates the immersion of antennas in a solution consisting of 90% glycerine and water [13].

To streamline the hardware, this study introduces an innovative approach employing transmitting and receiving antennas (interconnected via a VNA) functioning in unobstructed airspace. These antennas circumnavigate the area of interest, collecting signals using a multibistatic configuration. Subsequently, an algorithm grounded on the Huygens principle is harnessed to identify significant scatterers, reminiscent of radar-based imaging. This Huygens principle (HP)-based approach enables the revealing of dielectric inconsistencies within the frequency spectrum [24,25]. While HP has hitherto been deployed in the detection of cancer, particularly focusing on breast and skin malignancies [26–28], this study centers on appraising its efficacy exclusively in the detection of hemorrhagic strokes. This assessment involves simulations and experimental measurements conducted within the context of a head model with multiple layers, wherein a pair of custom-built wideband (WB) antennas function as both the transmitter and receiver within the MWI framework derived from HP.

A stroke ensues when blood flow to a specific brain region is obstructed or diminished (cerebral ischemia) or when a blood vessel bursts, causing bleeding in brain tissues (brain hemorrhage). Forecasts indicate a substantial increase in global stroke incidence, primarily attributable to the growing population aged 65 and above, particularly nations with modest to moderate incomes [29]. A stroke constitutes a critical medical situation, and swift treatment is imperative. Early detection holds the potential to mitigate cerebral injury and associated complexities. Therefore, patient outcome hinges on a prompt diagnosis facilitated by an effective imaging technique.

While MWI was formerly primarily centered on advancements in breast cancer diagnosis endeavors, it has expanded its scope to encompass alternative uses, notably neuroimaging. This transition is motivated by several advantages offered by MWI [2]. First, it is a nonintrusive method employing nonionizing, low-power electromagnetic waves, rendering it entirely harmless. Furthermore, its brief data collection times, varying from milliseconds to several seconds, enable rapid stroke assessments, a critical factor in ensuring timely drug administration [30]. Additionally, MWI demonstrates economic viability for healthcare systems. Advances in the realm of mobile technology and microwave devices in recent times have made it possible for electromagnetic imaging to offer portable, cost-effective imaging platforms tailored to the requirements of the medical industry.

Nonetheless, the development of a robust MWI device for brain analysis and imaging constitutes a formidable challenge. To develop a functioning MWI device for the detection of intracranial bleeding, a delicate balance of resolution and depth of penetration within cerebral tissue must be struck. Consequently, maximizing the incoming power transmitted into the brain and ensuring images with satisfactory spatial resolution become imperative considerations [31]. To optimize the level of incoming power permeating brain tissue, the microstrip antenna is operated within the 1 to 2 GHz range, owing to the pronounced attenuation of electromagnetic waves traversing the head [1]. Moreover, it is evident that WB technology can enhance lesion detection performance [32]. Consequently, a WB antenna operating effectively across this spectrum represents a critical component in the success of the proposed system. Numerous potential MWI head scanner configurations may be contemplated to meet this requirement, including headbands, helmet structures, or specialized chambers [33].

5.2.1 Advancement of a microwave cerebral imaging trial product for the detection of stroke

Fig. 5.1 displays the bespoke MWI configuration, meticulously crafted by London South Bank University (LSBU) and situated within the confines of an anechoic chamber. This meticulously designed setup has been specifically tailored for radar configurations, as elucidated in our prior publications [14–21]. Within this setup, both antennas used for transmission and reception are intricately linked to A VNA with multiple ports produced by Anritsu EMEA Ltd., denoted as the Anritsu MS2028C VNA Master.

The suggested antennas, aligned parallel to the y-axis of the reference system and featuring omnidirectional coverage in the azimuthal plane, were employed following thorough verification of S-parameters. Vertical and horizontal mounts (as shown in Fig. 5.2) are employed to finely tune the position of the antennas with accuracy and precision. It is

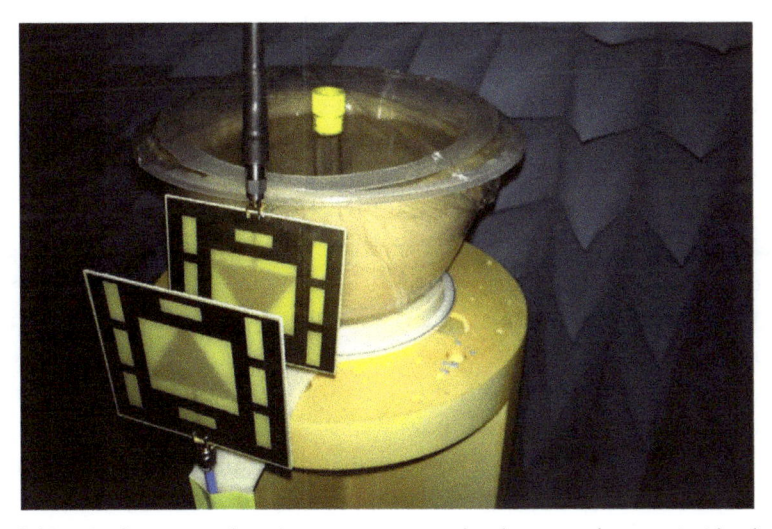

Fig. 5.1 Multibistatic frequency-domain measurements hardware and setup inside the anechoic chamber [14].

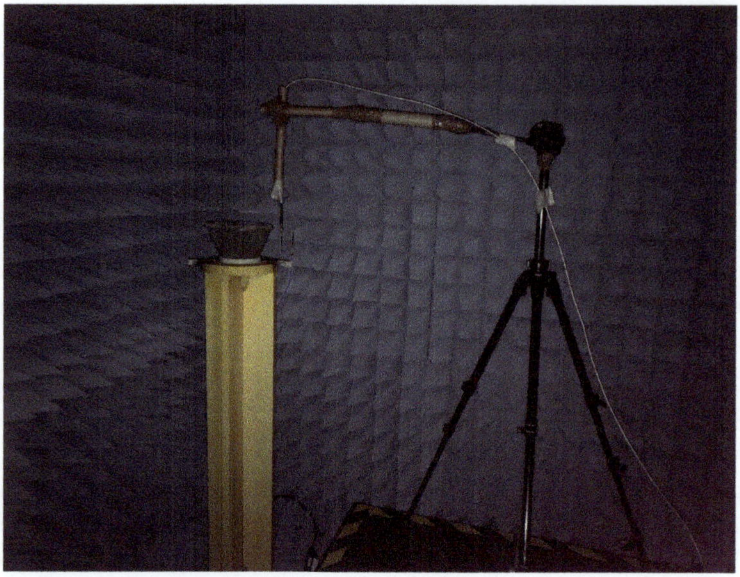

Fig. 5.2 The measurements setup in the anechoic chamber [14].

worth emphasizing that the suggested microstrip patch antennas serve as the means for conducting experiments within the anechoic chamber.

The multibistatic frequency-domain experiments were executed to gather the transfer function (S21) among these two antennas, within the confines of the anechoic chamber, by applying the multitiered phantom model designed to mimic a human head during the measurement procedures. It is crucial to note that these microstrip patch antennas are utilized for conducting measurements within the anechoic chamber.

In the anechoic chamber, frequency-domain experiments were executed to gather the transfer function (S21) among the two antennas. These experiments involved using a multilayered phantom designed to emulate a human head as part of the measurement procedures.

A typical radar system consists of a transmitting component and a receiving component. The transmitter emits a signal, which is then scattered by objects in its path. Subsequently, the receiver detects and gathers the scattered signal, however, in research focusing on electromagnetic scattering mechanisms, conventional terms such as transmitters and receivers are disregarded and substituted. Instead of a transmitter, an incident wave is utilized, while an observation point replaces the role of the receiver.

For the simulation, a microstrip antenna and a three-dimensional model of the Ella head (ITIS Foundation, Switzerland) were employed. The antenna has been simulated using Computer Simulation Technology (CST) Microwave Studio. Moreover, it is oriented such that its axis of symmetry, which forms an isosceles triangle, is aligned with the y-axis of the coordinate system reference. Similarly, the model of Ella's head is situated in such a way that its longitudinal axis aligns parallel to the y-axis of the coordinate system reference.

For frequency-domain measurements, two vertically polarized antennas have been positioned and utilized in a free-space environment. These two omnidirectional WB dipole antennas, one serving as the transmitting antenna and the other as the receiving antenna, were both connected to the VNA device. The antennas are positioned at an equivalent vertical elevation. The ultrawideband (UWB) frequency-domain measurements were conducted employing the VNA to procure the transfer function (S21) within the specified frequency range. To elaborate further, the VNA was configured with the transmitter linked to port 1, while the receiver was securely fastened to port 2 for data collection. The parameter S21 denotes the intricate transfer function from the transmitter antenna to the receiver antenna. The term S21 characterizes the intricate transfer function extending from the transmitter to the receiver (antennas). The prepared phantom was centrally positioned on a rotating table. The phantom under preparation was placed at the center of rotation on the table.

With each transmitter position, the receiving antenna undergoes a radial rotation (counterclockwise) in 5-degree increments, scanning the electromagnetic field outside the phantom at eight distinct receiver locations. In each measurement set, the transmitter was situated 17 cm from the central point of the rotating table, mirroring the configuration employed in the simulations. The separation among the rotating table's center and the receiver measures 14 cm. The antennas are positioned in the air, with no medium used for matching.

The realistic head model is constructed to closely mimic both the physical characteristics of the head and its authentic dielectric properties. To enable practical construction, the phantom has been created with three distinct layers that replicate different aspects of the human head:

(a) The first-layer simulates the properties of skull bone, encompassing both cancellous and cortical bone. This layer mimics the dielectric characteristics of real bone found in the human skull, providing a realistic representation.

(b) The second layer is a composite representing both gray matter and white matter. This composite layer simulates the electrical properties of brain tissue, capturing the intricate nature of these tissues within the head.

(c) The third layer incorporates properties similar to blood. This layer emulates the dielectric characteristics of blood to include the effects of vascular structures within the head.

These three layers together construct a realistic head phantom, allowing for accurate and controlled testing and measurement in various applications, such as electromagnetic simulations and medical imaging research. The proposed phantom is specifically crafted to emulate the characteristics of the skull bone, featuring an approximate thickness of

10 mm, a consistent conductivity of 0.24 S/m, and a relative permittivity of 12 at a frequency of 1.6 GHz. These parameter values are assumed to represent an average approximation for both cancellous and cortical bone properties. Adjacent to the innermost stratum of the cranial bone, the phantom replicates the dominance of gray and white tissues, possessing a typical conductivity rating of 1.01 S/m and a permittivity value of 44 at the frequency of 1.6 GHz. Employing this arrangement for simulating a hemorrhagic stroke involves the insertion of a cylindrical target measuring 35 mm in diameter into the gel-based brain phantom. This process involves isolating a portion of the brain mixture using a cylindrical mold with a 35 mm diameter, leading to the formation of a cylindrical void. Subsequently, this void is infused with gel-based phantoms designed to mimic the appearance of hemorrhaging in cases of a hemorrhagic stroke. This composition accurately mimics the electrical properties of brain tissue. Furthermore, to introduce a discernible contrast, blood is incorporated into the phantom, contributing a distinctive electrical profile with a conductivity with a conductivity of 1.79 S/m and a permittivity of 60 at a frequency of 1.6 GHz.

5.2.2 HP in imaging: Algorithms and procedures

Following the procedures, the antennas perform rotational maneuvers encompassing the object to gather signals employing a multibistatic approach. Subsequently, an algorithm rooted in the HP is employed to pinpoint robust scatterers, akin to radar imaging techniques. To elaborate further, the HP-based method enables the identification of dielectric irregularities within the frequency domain [24,25]. Historically, HP has been harnessed across various cancer detection applications, with particular prominence in breast and skin cancer detection [26–28]. This methodology facilitates the differentiation between distinct tissue types or varying tissue conditions, ultimately yielding a composite image that serves as a map of dielectric property homogeneity, encompassing parameters such as dielectric constant and conductivity. The radar-based Huygens algorithm, originally introduced in reference [32], has demonstrated its promising applicability in medical contexts as illustrated in references.

As a consequence of the discrepancy between the properties of two distinct media, a mismatch arises within the transition zone. This discrepancy presents an opportunity to capture the contrast, which can then be utilized to identify, detect, and localize the inhomogeneities.

This assertion holds validity based on the HP: "Each locus of a wave excites the local matter which re-radiates secondary wavelets, and all wavelets superpose to a new, resulting wave (the envelope of those wavelets), and so on" [34]. Fig. 5.3 represents the description of the HP for Hemorrhagic stroke detection measurements.

Fig. 5.3 illustrates the diagram of the measurement configuration, with the hemiellipsoidal head phantom emulating the brain with a light blue hue. The circular outlines in green and black are represented as dashed lines, marking the area where the positioning

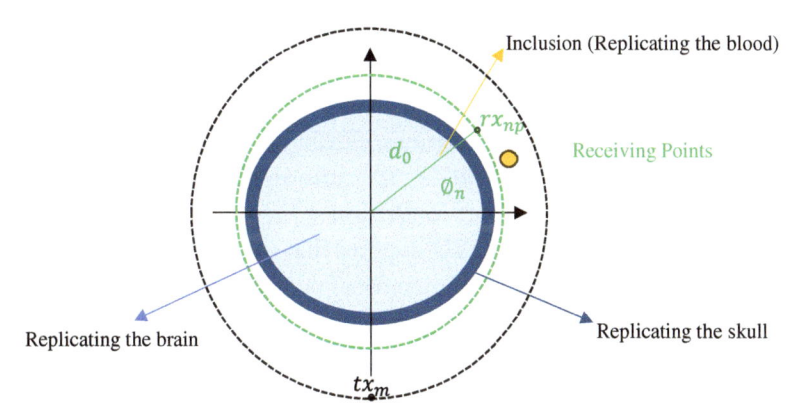

Fig. 5.3 Pictorial description of the Huygens principle for hemorrhagic stroke detection measurements [14].

of the transmitter and receiver is adjustable in a circular manner within the azimuthal plane. This movement allows for the irradiation and subsequent reception of signals from various directions. We obtain S21 measurements at specific points denoted as rx_{np}, defined as (d_0, $\varnothing_{np}$), where $\varnothing_{np}$ represents angular displacements along a circular surface with a radius of d_0. The value of d_0 corresponds to the separation between the central point of the revolving platform and the antenna designated for reception, as indicated in Fig. 5.3.

$$\text{S21}_{tx_m}\big|_{rx_{np}} = \text{S21}_{np,tx_m} \text{ With } np = 1, \ldots, N_{PT} \tag{5.1}$$

The subscript "m" is used to denote the transmitting positions, represented as "tx," and "np" ranges from 1 to N_{PT}, indicating the receiving positions. It is important to highlight that, rather than physically relocating the transmitter, adjusting the transmission points is created through controlled rotation of the phantom. In total, there are eight transmitting positions that have been synthesized, which are organized into four pairs, each separated by 90° and comprising two closely spaced transmitting positions differing by 5°. In summary, the synthesized transmitting positions are as follows: 0 and 5°, 90 and 95°, 180 and 185°, 270 and 275°. To explore the signal variations across frequencies, comprehensive S21 values were logged across the entire frequency spectrum ranging from 1 to 2 GHz, with frequency samples taken at intervals of 5 MHz.

The opportunity to apply Huygens's Principle by employing $E_{HP,2D}^{rcstr}$ as the locus of a wave has been investigated [14–21]. To be exact, it is a consideration of what happens if the HP reconstructs the internal field of the medium. This involves engaging the field measured or simulated on the external surface of the medium as the locus of a wave. Consequently, it is deduced that adopting such an approach enables the calculation of the internal field as the summation of the fields radiated by the N_{PT} receiving points in:

$$E_{HP,2D}^{rcstr}(\rho, \varnothing; tx_m; f) = \Delta_S \sum_{np=1}^{N_{PT}} \text{S21}_{np,tx_m} \, G\left(k_1 \left|\overrightarrow{\rho_{np}} - \overrightarrow{\rho}\right|\right) \tag{5.2}$$

In this context, where $\vec{\rho} \equiv (\rho, \varnothing)$ denotes the observation point, k_1 represents the wave number of the medium within the imaging zone, and Δ_S signifies the spatial sampling. Additionally, the subscript m denotes the transmitting positions tx, while $np = 1, 2, \ldots, N_{PT}$, N_{PT} indicates the receiving positions. Furthermore, in Eq. (5.2), f denotes the frequency. The term S21 corresponds to the transmission coefficient depicting the transmission of waves from port 1 to port 2. Within $E_{HP,2D}^{rcstr}$, the term $rcstr$ signifies the "reconstructed" internal electric field, 2D denotes that the analysis and artifact removal algorithms are developed using a two-dimensional configuration, and HP indicates the utilization of a Huygens Principle-based approach.

Moreover, it is observed that the resulting electric field is influenced by both the frequency of the incident waves and the characteristics of the illuminating source, as indicated by $E_{HP,2D}^{rcstr}$ dependency on these parameters. In Eq. (5.2), the utilization of Green's function G for homogeneous media facilitates the forward propagation of the field.

It is important to emphasize that while the HP technique is useful in addressing homogeneous problems, it does not accurately determine the internal field. This limitation stems from the principle's focus on far-field phenomena, specifically propagating wavefronts. However, for our purposes, a precise measurement of the internal field is unnecessary; rather, our goal is to image the shape of the inclusion. What we seek is the ability to detect contrast between different tissues. To achieve this, we only need knowledge of the E-field to capture the far field, as it involves plane wavefronts. Conversely, to capture and recover the near field, for accurate reconstruction, familiarity with either the normal derivative of the electric field or the magnetic field is essential.

In this specific scenario, the objective is not to evaluate the internal field; rather, it is to determine whether HP can effectively capture the boundaries of mismatch (termed as contrast) and consequently distinguish inclusions within a volume. The capability to capture contrast arises from the disparities in properties between two distinct media [35], which Eq. (5.1) fails to account for. Consequently, the reconstructed field exhibits mismatches within the transitional region between the two media. This contrast presents an opportunity for a novel approach to detecting and positioning. To elaborate, if we consider irradiating the external cylinder from various sources (points) with a range of frequencies, the reconstructed fields would consistently depict mismatches, always situated in the transitional region between the two media. Thus, by summing up all solutions incoherently. In other words, by aggregating the reconstructed fields, we could identify, detect, and precisely locate the inclusion.

This suggested technique may be considered a practical use of the theory of holography, which was initially suggested by A. J. Devaney and R. P. Porter in the 80-decade [36,37]. These researchers proved that the determination of an inverse source problem can be achieved by considering the field's value and its normal derivative over any closed surface completely surrounding the volume of interest. Anyhow, in [37], they mainly concentrated on recovering the image from the dielectric properties within the volume.

In a contrary manner, here, the proposed procedure solves an easier computational problem by pursuing the goal of identifying the prominent scatterers; to fulfill this aim, the field would be analyzed across a closed surface of arbitrary shape. With the aim of pursuing this goal, in [38], it has been proved that in particular circumstances, a precise solution could come from applying just the field on the arbitrary closed surface.

In this context, we exploit the HP to reconstruct the field. Employing Green's function in conjunction with a homogeneous medium for the reconstruction process, mismatches emerge when transitioning between different media. The capability to detect these mismatch boundaries suggests that this proposed method enables the identification of abnormalities.

Now, assuming the exploitation of N_F is the frequencies, f_i is the final image intensity, I is obtained through Eq. (5.3) by summing all solutions incoherently [35]:

$$I(\rho, \emptyset) = \sum_{i=1}^{N_F} \left| E_{HP}^{rcstr}(\rho, \emptyset; tx_m; f_i) \right|^2 \qquad (5.3)$$

Eq. (5.3) can be employed to generate a map of intensity.

5.2.3 Design (methodology)

5.2.3.1 Description of human head phantom

The design of the artificial human head model is suggested in this chapter. Recently, various methods have been proposed for representing human tissue [39,40]. Numerous studies in the literature have garnered attention by advocating the use of MWI systems for detecting abnormalities in the human head. However, a majority of these experiments have employed relatively simple human head phantoms [41,42], often neglecting the intricacies of head tissue properties. While some recent research endeavors have attempted to define human head phantoms by incorporating electrical properties [43,44], they still lack comprehensive details about brain tissue compositions.

Hence, to obtain accurate and scientifically valuable results in head imaging experiments, it has become imperative to design and fabricate a human head phantom that simulates brain hemorrhage alongside other essential characteristics. Key criteria for this phantom fabrication include durability, simplicity in production, and cost-effectiveness. To validate experimental procedures for microwave exploration of brain hemorrhages, a lifelike three-dimensional model of a human head is introduced and created in this chapter, serving the purpose of validating the proposed imaging technique.

Due to the pragmatic choice of exclusively modeling the upper portion of the cranium (half), we opted for a straightforward hemiellipsoidal structure with external horizontal dimensions of 210 mm (front to back), 195 mm (side to side), and a height of 120 mm. In addition, the brain mold is filled with materials emulating white and gray substances, with horizontal dimensions of 190 mm (front to back) and 165 mm (side

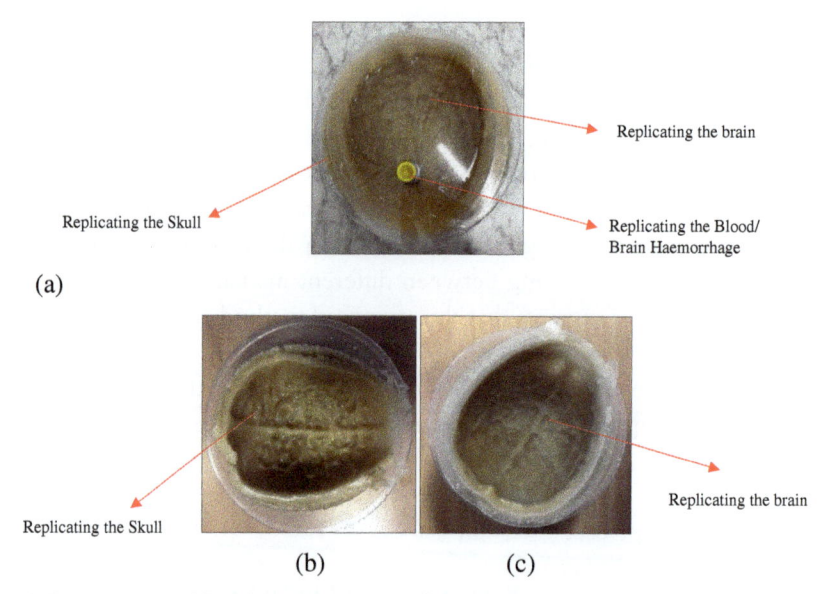

Fig.5.4 (A) The constructed head model consists of three distinct strata replicating the skull (bone), human brain, and brain hemorrhage; (B) the skull replicates the phantom, and (C) the brain replicates the phantom [14].

to side), with a height of 90 mm. Within the brain mold is a small tube containing a substance simulating blood, characterized by a circular cross-sectional radius measuring 5 millimeters and a height of 35 millimeters. As illustrated in Fig. 5.4, three containers with different volumes are subsequently nested inside one another. Every stratum of the head model is constructed with blends of component substances in the appropriate proportions.

The dielectric constant of tissue-mimicking ingredients for the human head is specified in Tables 5.1 and 5.2, obtained from [45,46]. In simulating the dielectric characteristics of the human head, various materials were employed to approximate reported values. The proposed phantom comprises a solid component representing the skull, filled with a blend of liquids to mimic white and gray tissue. Additionally, material selection was influenced by cost-effectiveness, accessibility (readily available off-the-shelf), and long-term stability for storage.

The dielectric characteristics of the tissue mixture simulating the skull were determined using the Epsilon dielectric measurement device, specifically the Biox Epsilon Model E100, manufactured by Biox System Company Ltd. For the mixtures imitating brain and blood tissues, the electrical properties were measured at room temperature utilizing a dielectric probe (model: Keysight Technologies, M9370A) linked to a network analyzer.

Table 5.1 Tissue mimicking ingredients for skull [45].

Component (g)	Skull
Sunflower oil	35
Deionized water	15
Corn flour	55
Salt	0.3
Sugar	11

Table 5.2 Conductivity and permittivity values at a frequency of 1.6 GHz [45–47].

Tissue	Conductivity (S/m)	Relative permittivity
Human brain model (incorporating both white and gray matter components)	1.01	44
Blood	1.79	60
Skull	0.24	12

5.2.3.2 Description of microstrip antenna design

Utilization of WB technology can significantly enhance performance when it comes to lesion detection [32]. This chapter offers a comprehensive examination of developing and crafting a WB microstrip antenna, tailored for operation in the 1–2 GHz frequency range, which has been demonstrated as the ideal choice for imaging of the head, as referenced in Ref. [1]. Hence, the importance of a WB antenna that operates efficiently across that frequency range cannot be overstated when considering the success of the proposed system. In pursuit of broadening the antenna's bandwidth to achieve improved imaging capabilities, the antenna has been configured to create an equilateral triangular patch antenna with a fractal ground plane inspired by Ref. [48].

The antenna was simulated applying CST Microwave Studio and crafted utilizing FR-4 substrate material, featuring a dielectric constant (ε_r) 4.7. A discrete microstrip feeding structure, designed for a 50-Ω impedance, is employed on the lower section of the patch.

The envisioned microstrip antenna follows a monolithic configuration and comprises four key components: an isosceles triangular patch, a microstrip feed line, a substrate, and a fractal ground plane. Fig. 5.5 illustrates the physically constructed antenna intended for our brain imaging scanner project. The triangular antenna shape is responsible for the antenna's shape, and it is fed through an SMA connector linked to a transmission line, as depicted in Fig. 5.5.

The triangular antenna design, as depicted in Fig. 5.5, was constructed internally at LSBU. Enhancing the frequency range over which the antenna exhibits suitable

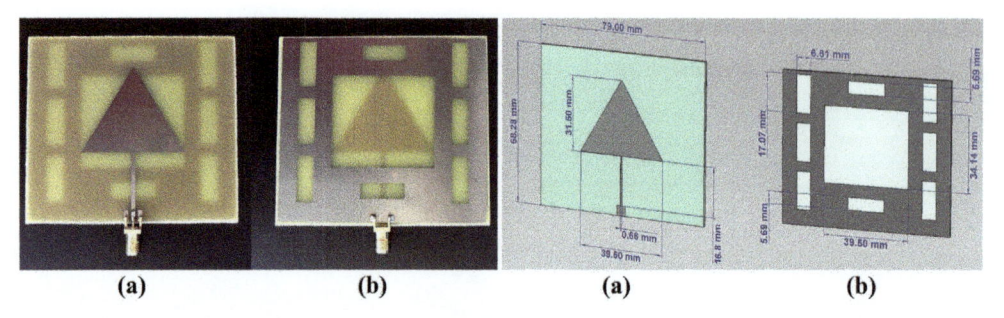

Fig. 5.5 The triangular patch microstrip antenna that was designed, along with the antennas that were physically manufactured, features a fractal ground plane: (A) front and (B) back [14].

impedance characteristics involves optimizing both the shape and dimensions of the slots within the ground plane and the antenna design featuring a triangular configuration. The simulated and fabricated antennas are evaluated under two conditions: in free space and in proximity to a head model. For the simulation, a three-dimensional model featuring the head tissues of the Ella model from the ITIS Foundation in Switzerland is utilized. This model has a resolution of 2 mm × 2 mm × 2 mm isotropic voxels, as depicted in Fig. 5.2. Notably, the Ella model offers comprehensive data on electric conductivity and relative permittivity for various tissues of a young and healthy 26-year-old female [47,49].

The antenna is situated in this model with its axis of symmetry aligned with the y-axis of the coordinate system reference. In order to replicate the presence of a condition characterized by hemorrhaging in the brain within the head model, we introduced a spherical region with dielectric properties matching those of blood. This region has a radius of 10 mm and exhibits relative permittivity and conductivity values of 60 and 1.79 S/m, respectively, at a frequency of 1.6 GHz within the head model [47], and [49]. The transmitting antenna was positioned 17 cm away from the center of the Ella model's head.

S11 measurements, representing the input port voltage reflection coefficient, were conducted in an anechoic chamber. These measurements were taken in two scenarios: one in free space and the other in the presence of a human head. A VNA produced by Anritsu EMEA Ltd., specifically the Anritsu MS2028C Master, was employed for this purpose.

Fig. 5.6 depicts the remarkable consistency between measured and simulated S11 values, both in the absence and presence of a human head. Moreover, the data indicates a slight enhancement in matching and bandwidth when the antenna is placed in front of a human head. Additionally, the operational bandwidth exceeding 10% cantered at 1.6 GHz positions this antenna as highly suitable for brain imaging experiments. Previous research [32] has demonstrated that higher frequencies suffer from significant signal attenuation, while lower frequencies compromise resolution, hence emphasizing the significance of the chosen frequency band.

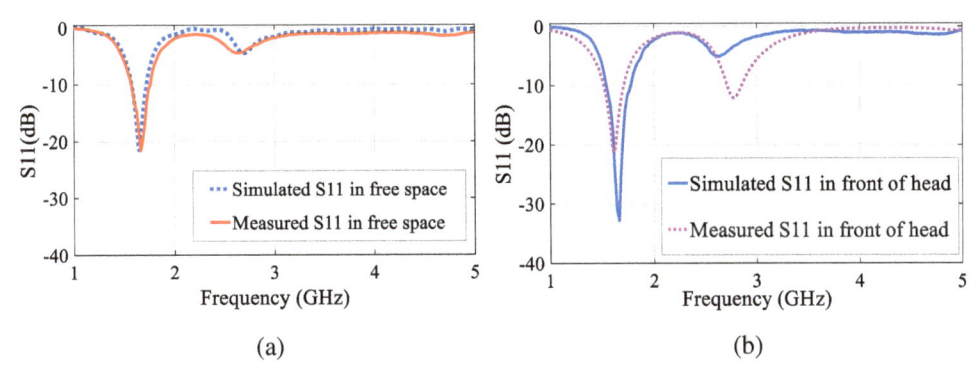

Fig. 5.6 Comparative analysis of simulated and measured reflection coefficients (S11) for the patch antenna: (A) when deployed in open space and (B) when positioned in front of a human head.

To furnish the requisite initial data, various procedural steps are necessary. Initially, both simulations and measurements were conducted for two distinct scenarios: one with a normal brain condition and the other with a cerebral hemorrhage within the head. To this end, for the simulation, a healthy head model, referred to earlier as the Ella model, and the other with a spherical simulated hemorrhagic stroke within the head model, have been used. Furthermore, simulations were executed for the antenna in four distinct positions relative to the Ella model. It is worth noting that instead of rotating the Ella model around its longitudinal axis, we achieved these four different positions, namely 0, 5, 40, and 45°, by rotating the microstrip patch antenna itself. For the frequency-domain experiments conducted within the confines of the anechoic chamber, experiments were performed for two similar scenarios: head phantom with inclusion (mimicking the blood) and head phantom without inclusion. Moreover, the subsequent transmitting positions were generated: 0 and 5°, 90 and 95°, 180 and 185°, 270 and 275°. In order to analyze signal variations across different frequencies, we recorded complex S21 values spanning the entire frequency spectrum spanning from 1 to 2 GHz, with frequency increments of 5 MHz.

5.2.4 Description of signal preprocessing techniques

Signal preprocessing methods are typically applied to mitigate artifacts stemming from both direct and first-layer reflected fields. Failure to effectively remove these artifacts may result in the masking of stroke detection. To eliminate the artifact, we employ two distinct approaches: first, subtracting data from a model representing a healthy head and corresponding data from a head model exhibiting stroke characteristics; second, performing rotational subtraction among data acquired from different transmitter positions.

5.2.4.1 Techniques for artifact removal: Optimal approach to artifact elimination

In the context of artifact mitigation, a dual set of empirical experiments is conducted with the aim of the imaging procedure. Initially, the "absence of target" scenario entails the use of a phantom devoid of any target. Subsequently, the "target presence" scenario involves a replication of the procedure employing a phantom containing a cylindrical inclusion with millimetric dimensions designed to simulate a hemorrhagic brain stroke.

For the simulation, artifact removal has been accomplished through the subtraction of the electric field computed on a round array of points with a radius of 110 mm and a sampling increment of 6° in azimuth angle, situated immediately beyond the confines of the head, for two distinct conditions: Ella in the presence of stroke symptoms and Ella without any stroke manifestations.

In Eq. (5.3), the presence of the inclusion is discerned in the generated image by subtracting the recorded S21 parameter obtained from the "no target" scenario from that of the "target" scenario ($S21_{np,tx_m}^{known,target} - S21_{np,tx_m}^{known,notarget}$). To establish a baseline, an 'Ideal' image is generated for the purpose of illustrating the technology concept.

It is imperative to underscore that, in practical medical imaging scenarios, the application of this artifact removal method is not feasible. The primary intention behind employing this method is to demonstrate the robust feasibility of detecting brain hemorrhages under idealized conditions. Furthermore, one of the key objectives of this study is to develop an algorithm capable of closely approximating the ideal outcome. By employing various artifact removal algorithms, the resulting images may exhibit variability. Consequently, it is impractical to evaluate the algorithm against imaging methodologies where the ideal response is neither calculated nor known, such as real human head measurements involving brain stroke cases. Consequently, in clinical trials, this artifact removal method does not offer practical utility or effectiveness. Hence, another alternative will be the Rotation Subtraction (RS) Artifact Removal Method.

5.2.4.2 RS artifact removal method

In the technique known as the RS method [50], the removal of artifacts is accomplished by conducting a subtraction operation between two datasets acquired by making slight rotational adjustments to the placement of the transmitter relative to the object. With reference to the notation introduced in Section 5.2.3, the following equation can be employed:

$$S21_{np,tx_{Diff}} = S21_{np,tx_1} - S21_{np,tx_2} \qquad (5.4)$$

Here, tx_1 and tx_2 denote the two nearest transmitter locations. The artifact removal technique involving rotational subtraction can be practical for both simulation and experimental experiments.

5.2.4.3 Quantitative image analysis metrics

The evaluation of image quality has been conducted through image quantification. As an integral component of this research, the computation of specific parameters becomes essential for quantifying the detection capabilities of the imaging system, contrasting the efficacy of the proposed artifact removal methods, and establishing a quantifiable measurement framework for image comparisons. Various metrics are employed to quantify the system's ability to detect strokes.

Even after the application of artifact removal procedures, residual clutter may persist within the images. Therefore, it is pertinent to introduce a parameter to systematically assess and compare the detection performance when employing various artifact removal algorithms. These metrics encompass the Area Difference (ArD) index, Polyshape Construction, Centroid Difference, Signal-to-Noise Ratio, Signal-to-Clutter Ratio (S/C), and the Structural Similarity Index Metric. However, here we presented the signal-to-clutter ratio (S/C). In this context, S/C is delineated as the quotient of the maximum intensity assessed within the region containing the lesion, divided by the maximum intensity measured outside the lesion region [51]. The S/C ratio is computed individually for each image, taking into account both artifact removal methods.

5.3 Experimental validation
5.3.1 Imaging results
5.3.1.1 Simulated imaging: A computational approach

The simulated images, generated through both subtraction and RS artifact removal methods, are depicted in Figs. 5.7 and 5.8. Specifically, Fig. 5.9 displays the images (normalized to their respective maximum values) derived from Eq. (5.3) following the artifact subtraction process that has been applied for four distinct transmitter locations (0, 5, 40, and 45°). The corresponding signal-to-clutter ratios (S/C) are presented in Table 5.3. It is noteworthy that all images presented in this section and subsequent subsections underwent normalization and adjustment, with intensity values below 0.5 being set to zero. Notably, the S/C values were consistently computed prior to the image adjustment.

Each of the images showcased in Fig. 5.7 is the result of subtracting the signals acquired from the phantom prior to and following the insertion of the target (subtraction method). Hence, the images involve the subtraction of electric fields recorded for Ella with a stroke, computed on a spherical arrangement of points situated immediately outside the head, from those calculated for Ella without a stroke, using the same grid of points.

It is important to note that the placement of the transmitter remained constant during the subtraction process. The four images correspond to the four distinct placements of the transmitter employed in the simulation. For clarity and consistency, all images have been subjected to normalization, where their intensity values have been scaled relative to the maximum value, and any intensity values below 0.5 have been adjusted to 0. The x and y axes in these images are measured in meters, while the intensity is represented in arbitrary units.

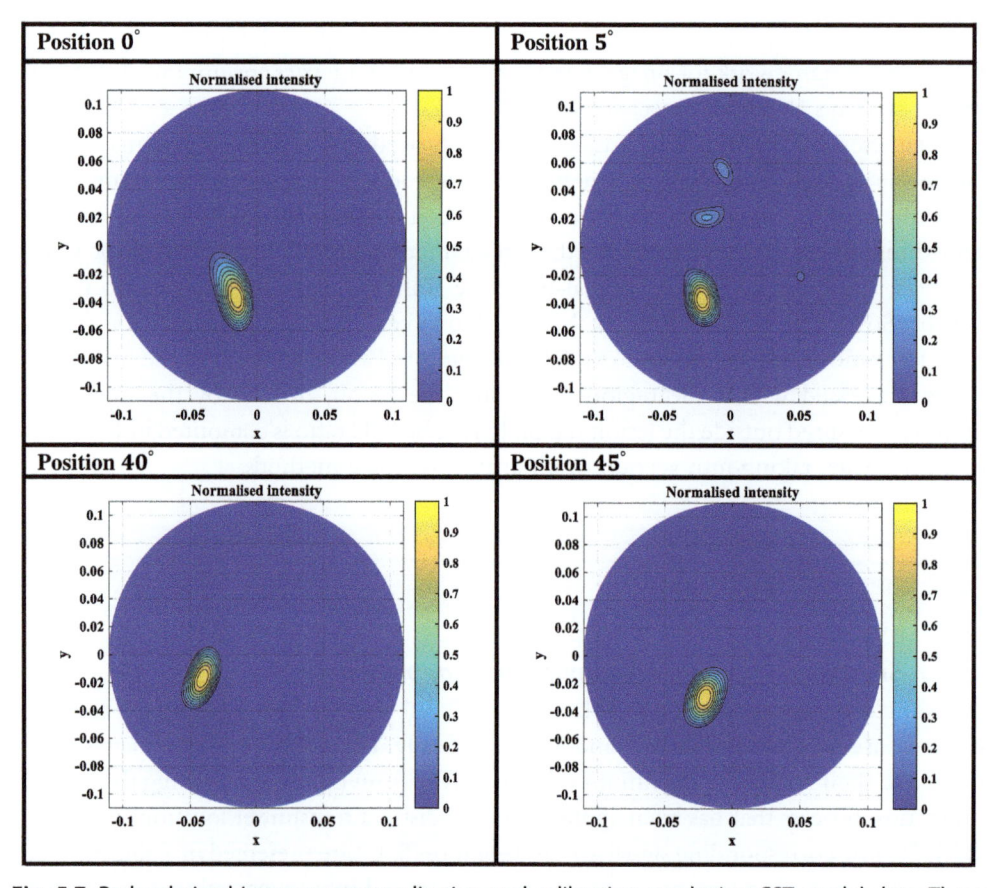

Fig. 5.7 Radar-derived image postnormalization and calibration employing CST model data. These have undergone artifact removal using the subtraction method [14].

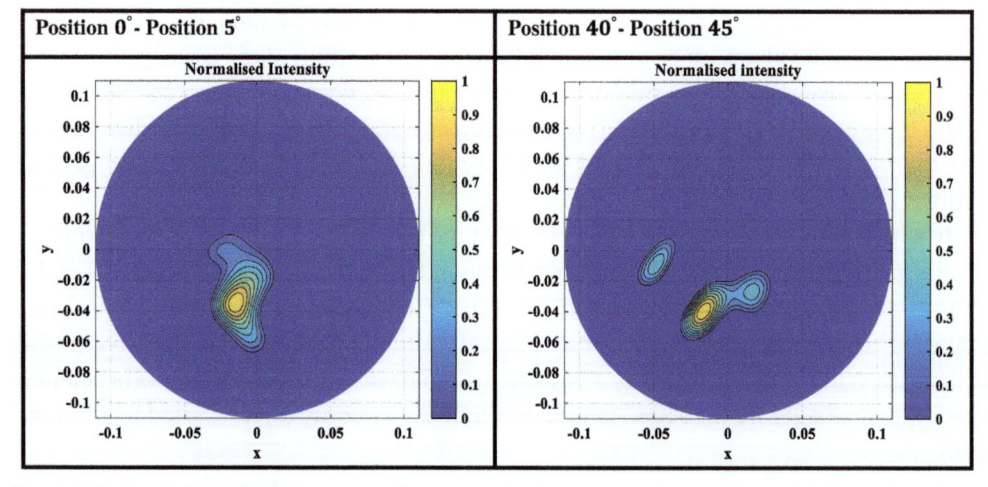

Fig. 5.8 Radar-derived depiction postcalibration and adjustment utilizing CST model data. These have undergone artifact removal using the rotation subtraction method [14].

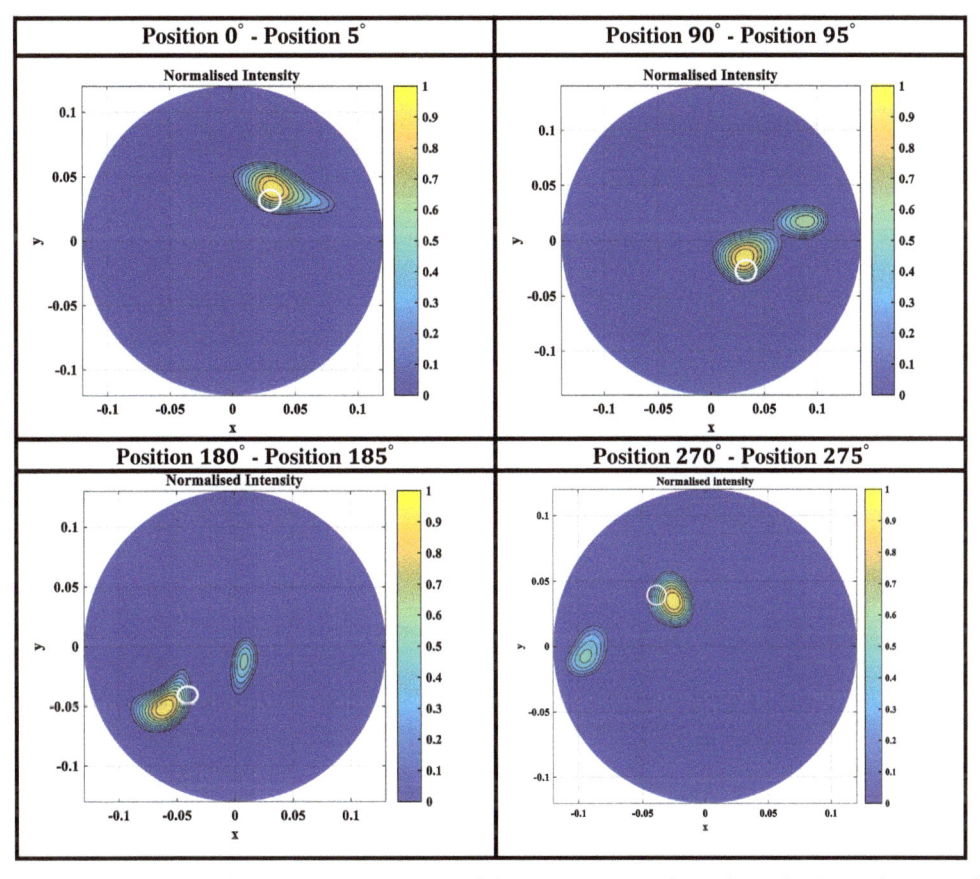

Application of multibistatic frequency-domain measurements 103

Fig. 5.9 Postprocessed images were generated by removing artifacts through the technique of rotation subtraction, where four pairs of datasets were obtained by slightly adjusting the position of the transmitting antenna around the phantom with the inclusion. The images have been normalized to their maximum value, with intensity values below 0.5 set to 0. The axes are labeled in meters, and the intensity is represented in arbitrary units. The white circles indicate the true position of the inclusion, simulating a hemorrhagic stroke within the head phantom.

Table 5.3 Intracerebral S/C Ratio (linear scale) at 1.6 GHz (computed via simulation and subtraction).

Positions	Within-brain S/C (linear) subtraction
Position 0°	2.50
Position 5°	1.91
Position 40°	1.93
Position 45°	2.49

Table. 5.4 Intracerebral signal-to-clutter ratio (linear scale) at 1.6 GHz (computed via simulation and rotational subtraction) [14].

Positions	Within-brain S/C (linear) rotation subtraction
Position 0°–position 5°	1.53
Position 40°–position 45°	1.60

Table. 5.5 Signal-to-clutter ratio (linear scale) at 1.6 GHz (computed via measurements and rotational subtraction) [14].

Positions	S/C (linear) Rotation Subtraction
Position 0°–position 5°	1.85
Position 90°–position 95°	1.48
Position 180°–position 185°	1.63
Position 270°–position 275°	1.50

In Fig. 5.8, depictions of the cranial model featuring a cerebral hemorrhage are presented, employing the rotational subtraction artifact removal procedure on synthetic data (simulation) by means of the transmitting sets of 0, 5° (on the left), and 40, 45° (on the right). The corresponding S/C values can be found in Table 5.4.

The RS method involves subtracting two sets of data acquired by making slight rotational adjustments to the placement of the transmitter in the vicinity of Ella exhibiting stroke symptoms. For clarity and consistency, all images have been subjected to normalization, where their intensity values have been scaled relative to the maximum value, and any intensity values below 0.5 have been adjusted to 0. The x and y axes in these images are measured in meters, while the intensity is represented in arbitrary units.

5.3.1.2 Imaging with phantom models

Fig. 5.9 illustrates the microwave renderings of the phantom acquired via Eq. (5.3) subsequent to the application of the RS artifact removal technique for four distinct doublets of transmitting positions (0° and 5°; 90° and 95°; 180° and 185°; 270° and 275°), each analyzed independently. The corresponding signal-to-clutter ratios (S/C) are provided in Table 5.5.

5.4 Discussion

The current chapter has performed preliminary numerical and experimental outcomes on MWI systems for brain imaging, which can demonstrate the promise of this approach in delivering credible results. Specifically, it exhibits the capability to detect a target (simulating cerebral hemorrhage) positioned at various locations. Simulation and experimental studies were conducted to evaluate the efficacy of the suggested approach in distinguishing cerebral hemorrhage. The simulated and fabricated in-house WB antennas (as shown in Fig. 5.5) applied an HP-based MWI approach for diagnosing cerebral hemorrhage within the multilayered human head phantom.

The examination validates the efficacy of the radar algorithms delineated in Section 5.2.2 to effectively identify and locate a target resembling cerebral hemorrhage within its proximate region. Both simulations and empirical experiments were performed with the custom-made MWI system presented in Figs. 5.1 and 5.2. From the provided outcomes in Sect. 5.3.1, detection through both simulation (employing artifact removal techniques such as subtraction and rotational subtraction) and empirical experiments (the artifact removal method based on rotational subtraction) is achieved at different head models and phantom orientations.

In this chapter, the proposed technique applied HP, with the aim of successful detection owing to variations in dielectric characteristics among the brain hemorrhagic stroke and surrounding healthy tissues. The outcomes presented in this chapter usher in a new era for the creation and employment of a low-complexity MWI scanner for the detection of brain hemorrhagic stroke, where the antennas function in free-space.

References

[1] D. Ireland, M. Bialkowski, Microwave head imaging for stroke detection, Prog. Electromagn. Res. M 21 (2012).
[2] S.Y. Semenov, D.R. Corfield, Microwave tomography for brain imaging: feasibility assessment for stroke detection, Int. J. Antennas Propag. 2008 (2008).
[3] J.A. Tobon Vasquez, et al., First experimental assessment of a microwave imaging prototype for cerebrovascular diseases monitoring, in: *Proceedings of the* 2018 20th International Conference on Electromagnetics in Advanced Applications, ICEAA 2018, 2018.
[4] B.J. Mohammed, A.M. Abbosh, S. Mustafa, D. Ireland, Microwave system for head imaging, IEEE Trans. Instrum. Meas. 63 (1) (2014).
[5] S. Semenov, Microwave tomography: review of the progress towards clinical applications, Philos. Trans. R. Soc. A Math. Phys. Eng. Sci. 367 (1900) 2009.
[6] S. Semenov, T. Huynh, T. Williams, B. Nicholson, A. Vasilenko, Dielectric properties of brain tissue at 1 GHz in acute ischemic stroke: experimental study on swine, Bioelectromagnetics 38 (2) (2017).
[7] A.T. Mobashsher, B.J. Mohammed, S. Mustafa, A. Abbosh, Ultra wideband antenna for portable brain stroke diagnostic system, in: 2013 IEEE MTT-S International Microwave Workshop Series on RF and Wireless Technologies for Biomedical and Healthcare Applications, IMWS-BIO 2013 - Proceedings, 2013.
[8] I. Merunka, O. Fiser, D. Vrba, J. Vrba, Numerical analysis of microwave tomography system for brain stroke detection, in: 2018 28th International Conference Radioelektronika, RADIO-ELEKTRONIKA 2018, 2018.
[9] V.L. Coli, et al., Detection of simulated brain strokes using microwave tomography, IEEE J. Electromagn. RF Microwaves Med. Biol. 3 (4) (2019).
[10] M. Klemm, J.A. Leendertz, D. Gibbins, I.J. Craddock, A. Preece, R. Benjamin, Microwave radar-based differential breast cancer imaging: imaging in homogeneous breast phantoms and low contrast scenarios, IEEE Trans. Antennas Propag. 58 (7) (2010).

[11] F. Wang, Assembly conformal antenna array for wearable microwave breast imaging application, in: IET Conference Publications, vol. 2017, 2017. no. CP732.
[12] R. Scapaticci, J. Tobon, G. Bellizzi, F. Vipiana, L. Crocco, Design and numerical characterization of a low-complexity microwave device for brain stroke monitoring, IEEE Trans. Antennas Propag. 66 (12) (2018).
[13] S. Ahsan, M. Koutsoupidou, E. Razzicchia, I. Sotiriou, P. Kosmas, Advances towards the development of a brain microwave imaging scanner, in: 13th European Conference on Antennas and Propagation, EuCAP 2019, 2019.
[14] B. Sohani, et al., Detection of haemorrhagic stroke in simulation and realistic 3-D human head phantom using microwave imaging, Biomed. Signal Process. Control 61 (2020).
[15] B. Sohani, et al., Developing artefact removal algorithms to process data from a microwave imaging device for haemorrhagic stroke detection, Sensors 20 (19) (2020).
[16] B. Sohani, G. Tiberi, N. Ghavami, M. Ghavami, S. Dudley, A. Rahmani, Microwave imaging for stroke detection: validation on head-mimicking phantom, in: Progress in Electromagnetics Research Symposium, vol. 2019-June, 2019.
[17] B. Khalesi, B. Sohani, N. Ghavami, M. Ghavami, S. Dudley, G. Tiberi, A phantom investigation to quantify huygens principle based microwave imaging for bone lesion detection, Electronics 8 (12) (2019).
[18] B. Khalesi, B. Sohani, N. Ghavami, M. Ghavami, S. Dudley, G. Tiberi, Free-space operating microwave imaging device for bone lesion detection: a phantom investigation, IEEE Antennas Wirel. Propag. Lett. 19 (12) (2020).
[19] J. Puttock, B. Sohani, B. Khalesi, G. Tiberi, S. Dudley-McEvoy, M. Ghavami, UWB microwave imaging for inclusions detection: Methodology for comparing artefact removal algorithms, in: Lecture Notes of the Institute for Computer Sciences, 330, Social-Informatics and Telecommunications Engineering, LNICST, 2020.
[20] G. Tiberi, B. Khalesi, B. Sohani, S. Dudley, M. Ghavami, N. Ghavami, Phase-weighted UWB imaging through Huygens principle, in: Progress in Electromagnetics Research Symposium, vol. 2019-June, 2019.
[21] B. Sohani, A.D. Abdallah, G. Tiberi, N. Ghavami, M. Ghavami, S. Dudley, An analytically based approach for evaluating the impact of the noise on the microwave imaging detection, in: Progress in Electromagnetics Research Symposium, vol. 2021-November, 2021.
[22] D.B. Arciniegas, N.D. Zasler, R.D. Vanderploeg, M.S. Jaffee, T.A. Garcia, Management of Adults with Traumatic Brain Injury, 2013.
[23] W.J. Powers, et al., 2018 guidelines for the early Management of Patients with Acute Ischemic Stroke: a guideline for healthcare professionals from the American Heart Association/American Stroke Association, Stroke 49 (3) (2018).
[24] L. Chen, L. Xia, H. Li, S. Zhang, S. Lan, An improved head imaging algorithm based on Huygens principle, in: ISAP 2018–2018 International Symposium on Antennas and Propagation, 2019.
[25] L. Sani, et al., Novel microwave apparatus for breast lesions detection: preliminary clinical results, Biomed. Signal Process. Control 52 (2019).
[26] N. Ghavami, P.P. Smith, G. Tiberi, D. Edwards, I. Craddock, Non-iterative beamforming based on Huygens principle for multistatic ultrawide band radar: application to breast imaging, IET Microwaves, Antennas Propag. 9 (12) (2015).
[27] A. Vispa, et al., UWB device for breast microwave imaging: phantom and clinical validations, Meas. J. Int. Meas. Confed. 146 (2019).
[28] N. Ghavami, G. Tiberi, M. Ghavami, S. Dudley, M. Lane, Huygens principle based UWB microwave imaging method for skin cancer detection, in: 2016 10th International Symposium on Communication Systems, Networks and Digital Signal Processing, CSNDSP, 2016, p. 2016.
[29] WHO, Reducing risks, promoting healthy life, in: World Heal. Rep. 2002, Press kit, 2002.
[30] M. Hopfer, R. Planas, A. Hamidipour, T. Henriksson, S. Semenov, Electromagnetic tomography for detection, differentiation, and monitoring of brain stroke: a virtual data and human head phantom study, IEEE Antennas Propag. Mag. 59 (5) (2017).
[31] R. Scapaticci, L. Di Donato, I. Catapano, L. Crocco, Feasibility study on microwave imaging for brain stroke monitoring, Prog. Electromagn. Res. B 40 (2012).

[32] N. Ghavami, G. Tiberi, D.J. Edwards, A. Monorchio, UWB microwave imaging of objects with canonical shape, IEEE Trans. Antennas Propag. 60 (1) (2012).
[33] S. Semenov, et al., Electromagnetic tomography for brain imaging: Initial assessment for stroke detection, in: IEEE Biomedical Circuits and Systems Conference: Engineering for Healthy Minds and Able Bodies, BioCAS 2015 - Proceedings, 2015.
[34] P. Enders, Huygens' principle as universal model of propagation, Lat. Am. J. Phys. Educ. 3 (1) (2009).
[35] G. Tiberi, N. Ghavami, D.J. Edwards, A. Monorchio, Ultrawideband microwave imaging of cylindrical objects with inclusions, IET Microwaves, Antennas Propag. 5 (12) (2011).
[36] R.P. Porter, A.J. Devaney, Holography and the inverse source problem, J. Opt. Soc. Am. 72 (3) (1982).
[37] A.J. Devaney, R.P. Porter, Holography and the inverse source problem part II: inhomogeneous media, J. Opt. Soc. Am. A 2 (11) (1985).
[38] Y. Xu, L.V. Wang, Time reversal and its application to tomography with diffracting sources, Phys. Rev. Lett. 92 (3) (2004).
[39] S. Gabriel, R.W. Lau, C. Gabriel, The dielectric properties of biological tissues: II. Measurements in the frequency range 10 Hz to 20 GHz, Phys. Med. Biol. 41 (11) (1996).
[40] M. Lazebnik, E.L. Madsen, G.R. Frank, S.C. Hagness, Tissue-mimicking phantom materials for narrowband and ultrawideband microwave applications, Phys. Med. Biol. 50 (18) (2005).
[41] M. Sperandio, M. Guermandi, R. Guerrieri, A four-shell diffusion phantom of the head for electrical impedance tomography, IEEE Trans. Biomed. Eng. 59 (2) (2012).
[42] M. Akter, et al., Detection of hemorrhagic Hypointense foci in the brain on susceptibility-weighted imaging. Clinical and phantom studies, Acad. Radiol. 14 (9) (2007).
[43] A.T. Mobashsher, A.M. Abbosh, Y. Wang, Microwave system to detect traumatic brain injuries using compact unidirectional antenna and wideband transceiver with verification on realistic head phantom, IEEE Trans. Microw. Theory Tech. 62 (9) (2014).
[44] A.T. Mobashsher, P.T. Nguyen, A. Abbosh, Detection and localization of brain strokes in realistic 3-D human head phantom, in: 2013 IEEE MTT-S International Microwave Workshop Series on RF and Wireless Technologies for Biomedical and Healthcare Applications, IMWS-BIO 2013 - Proceedings, 2013.
[45] S. Symeonidis, W.G. Whittow, C. Panagamuwa, Design and characterization of a three material anatomical bone phantom for implanted antenna applications, in: IET Conference Publications, vol. 2017, 2017. no. CP732.
[46] M.J. O'Donnell, et al., Risk factors for ischaemic and intracerebral haemorrhagic stroke in 22 countries (the INTERSTROKE study): a case-control study, Lancet 376 (9735) (2010).
[47] M. Aldhaeebi, I. Elshafiey, New antenna design for hyperthermia treatment of human head, in: Proceedings - UKSim-AMSS 16th International Conference on Computer Modelling and Simulation, UKSim 2014, 2014.
[48] S.-H. Nawel, B.T. Fethi, Compact triangular microstrip antenna with fractal ground, Int. J. Ind. Electron. Electr. Eng. 33 (6) (2016).
[49] "No Title." [Online]. Available: https://itis.swiss/virtual-population/tissue-properties/database/dielectric-properties/.
[50] M. Klemm, I.J. Craddock, J.A. Leendertz, A. Preece, R. Benjamin, Improved delay-and-sum beamforming algorithm for breast Cancer detection, Int. J. Antennas Propag. 2008 (2008).
[51] E.C. Fear, X. Li, S.C. Hagness, M.A. Stuchly, Confocal microwave imaging for breast cancer detection: localization of tumors in three dimensions, IEEE Trans. Biomed. Eng. 49 (8) (2002).

CHAPTER 6

Sleep posture analysis: state-of-the-art and opportunities of wearable technologies from clinical, sensing and intelligent perception perspectives

Omar Elnaggar[a], Paolo Paoletti[a], Andrew Hopkinson[b], and Frans Coenen[c]
[a]School of Engineering, University of Liverpool, Liverpool, United Kingdom
[b]School of Psychology, University of Liverpool, Liverpool, United Kingdom
[c]School of Electrical Engineering, Electronics and Computer Science, University of Liverpool, Liverpool, United Kingdom

6.1 Introduction

Musculoskeletal conditions are a significant challenge for a large portion of the global population, causing individual health issues and imposing economic and social burdens [1,2]. Although various factors play a role in the onset and progression of these conditions, their risk factors remain partially understood. Sleep is one key risk factor that has gained recognition for its potential adverse impact on musculoskeletal health. Understanding the relationship between sleep and musculoskeletal conditions can yield valuable insights that benefit both areas, paving the way for targeted interventions and therapeutic approaches. This chapter provides a comprehensive review from two perspectives. Firstly, the chapter discusses the clinical literature at the intersection between human sleep behavior and musculoskeletal health complications, encompassing the implications of sleep and the clinical practices for the assessment, management and treatment of sleep-related musculoskeletal conditions and sleep disorders. Secondly, the chapter then provides a review of the technical literature within the domain of sleep posture analysis from two complementary angles: sensor technologies and data processing algorithms. Across both perspectives, the chapter highlights the unmet clinical needs and the most critical opportunities for technological improvement in responding to these needs.

6.2 Health complications: A sleep behavior perspective

This section presents a clinical background and introduces terminology and concepts related to sleep and musculoskeletal health. It focuses on the relationship between sleep and various health complications, with a particular emphasis on musculoskeletal pathology. It will elucidate how certain sleep patterns indicate musculoskeletal pathologies and how musculoskeletal patterns and habits can impact sleep and drive other health problems. The discussion extends to clinical practices for assessing sleep disorders and sleep-related musculoskeletal pathologies, as well as the options clinicians have for condition management and treatment. As recommended by the National Sleep Foundation, adults should aim for 7–9 h of sleep per night for optimal health [3]. Contrary to the widespread belief that sleep solely aids in recovery and restoration after daytime fatigue, there is empirical evidence suggesting broader implications [4]. While sleep is not intrinsically harmful or unhealthy, it is nonetheless a complex phenomenon with interrelated processes that may lead to risk factors. Therefore, it is important to study human sleep behavior from a biomarker perspective to trace the development of sleep-related morbidities and identify underlying health conditions. *Human sleep behavior* refers to the patterns and habits individuals exhibit while sleeping, including aspects like sleep staging, sleep episodes and duration, physiological processes, biomotor behavioral patterns, and psychosocial changes [5,6]. The bidirectional relationship between sleep disorders and musculoskeletal conditions will be revealed, with examples showing how sleep disorders manifest in physical sleep behavior and how certain musculoskeletal habits can lead to sleep-related pathologies.

6.2.1 The musculoskeletal system: A biomarker of and risk factor for sleep-related pathologies

The abnormalities in the human sleep behavior are indicators of sleep disorders. These disorders can be symptomatic or sign of developing morbidity. The etiology of sleep disorders is influenced by the physical behavior that involves the musculoskeletal system, which is viewed as a biomarker of underlying sleep disorders and a risk factor for sleep-related health complications [7]. According to the International Classification of Sleep Disorders [8], sleep disorders follow a six-level taxonomy, including insomnia, sleep-related breathing disorders, central disorders of hypersomnolence, circadian rhythm sleep–wake disorders, parasomnias, and sleep-related movement disorders. The etiology of sleep disorders can be internal or external [9–12], with internal causes including physical pain, genetic predisposition, psychological factors, and abnormalities with the central nervous system. External causes include environmental factors, pharmacological effects of medications, and substance abuse.

The musculoskeletal system supports the body's posture and movement through a unique integration of bones, joints, muscles, tendons, and ligaments [13]. It is a vital system that has direct interactions with various other body systems, including cardiovascular, respiratory, and neurologic systems. Understanding the associations between sleep disorders and the musculoskeletal system is crucial for understanding and treating sleep-related musculoskeletal pathologies.

The term "*risk factor*" refers to a characteristic or hazard that increases an individual's chance of developing a disorder [14]. Sleep habits and patterns, such as posture and in-bed

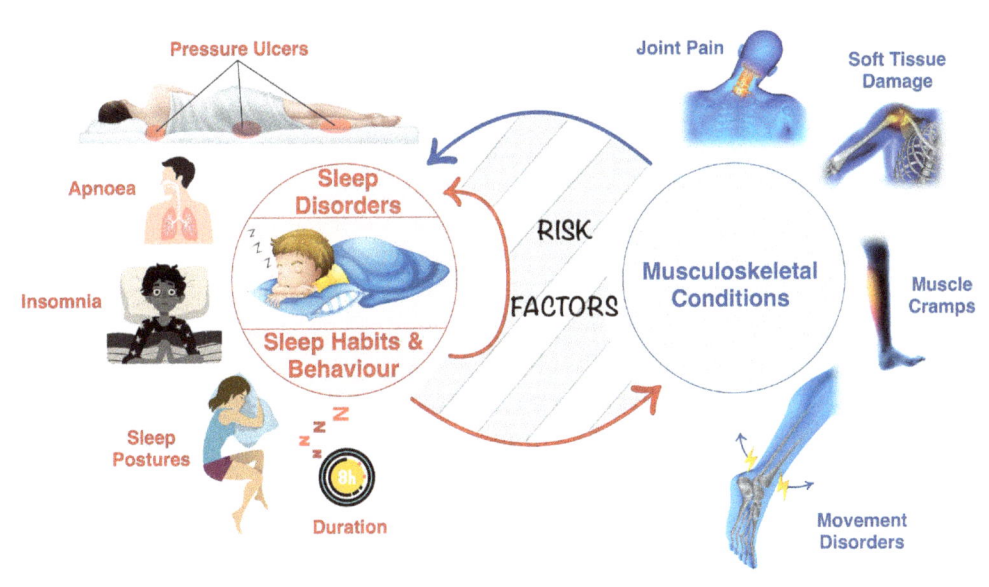

Fig. 6.1 The bidirectional relationship between sleep disorders and musculoskeletal conditions. *(No permission required.)*

body movement, can be considered risk factors for health complications. Similarly, musculoskeletal conditions can also be risk factors for sleep disorders. The bidirectional relationship between sleep disorders and musculoskeletal conditions is illustrated in Fig. 6.1. There are two types of sleep behavior: *movement* and *stable state behaviors* [15].

Movement behavior comprises a pattern or sequence of movement states spanning the duration of sleep, which can be useful for different purposes, such as differentiation between sleep and wake episodes, evaluating sleep quality and duration, and diagnosing circadian rhythm disorders [16]. Abnormal movements during sleep vary in complexity. Simple behaviors include single, repetitive, or rhythmic movements affecting specific body parts or larger muscle groups [17]. Complex behaviors, such as parasomnias, can involve bizarre actions during various sleep states and may pose risks to the sleeper or those around them [18].

Stable state sleep behavior corresponds to periods of no movement [19], which are independent of the sleep stage and provide insights into sleep postures, such as the supine and lateral positions. The sleep posture behavior has significant implications for the health [20,21], and can exacerbate conditions, such as *obstructive sleep apnoea* due to the gravitational pull on the upper airway [22,23]. Moreover, prolonged pressure on certain body parts during sleep can cause pressure ulcers, leading to severe consequences in some cases [24].

Over the past decade, specialized studies have linked postural cues to musculoskeletal morbidities, for example, spinal health. Poor spinal posture during sleep increases biomechanical stresses along the spine, which triggers neck pain episodes and stiffness [25,26]. Studies on patients with neck pain investigated factors such as pillow type, neck muscle activity, and asymmetrical lateral sleep postures [27]. Additionally, stable state sleep behaviors can provide sensible explanations for musculoskeletal joint pain, which cannot be understood through the conventional joint overuse theory. For example, unilateral shoulder pain, which often affects the right shoulder (dominant side), is a strong example of this [28].

Sleep posture is not the sole cause of musculoskeletal pain. The prolonged duration in certain provocative sleep postures can aggravate musculoskeletal pain, potentially causing pressure sores, tissue damage, and inflammation [26,28]. Prolonged joint immobilization can lead to muscular contractions, which can develop into chronic pain episodes [29]. Thus, changes in sleep posture overnight play a crucial role in preventing these complications.

6.2.2 Clinical assessment of sleep disorders

The understanding of sleep disorders and their associated health complications is crucial. Equally important is the grasp of the methods healthcare professionals utilize to diagnose these disorders. This review delves into the various clinical practices adopted for sleep disorder assessment, highlighting their benefits and challenges.

Sleep assessment methods can be broadly categorized based on their focus. Some methods, for instance, are tailored to scrutinize sleep at the behavioral level, which encompasses aspects such as movements and responsiveness. Others delve deeper, examining the quality, duration, and brain activity patterns of sleep [30]. Moreover, specialized diagnostic tools target specific disorders like respiratory sleep disorders [31]. The choice of the most suitable method depends on factors such as the clinical need being addressed and the availability of specialized equipment or trained personnel.

The hierarchy of clinical sleep assessments typically starts with patient-reported sleep diaries and questionnaires, which offer a rapid and inexpensive preliminary evaluation of a patient's sleep [32]. Sleep diaries offer an advantage over questionnaires due to the extended period of self-monitoring, which helps capture the variability in sleep behavior across different days [33]. However, both methods lack the capability to precisely gauge certain aspects of human sleep behavior, such as movement and posture states and their duration due to the absence of direct behavioral observation.

When further diagnosis is deemed necessary, the clinical gold standard for sleep disorder diagnosis is *polysomnography*, an in-clinic medical procedure that involves simultaneous recording of several parameters linked to sleep staging and physiology. Polysomnography uses electrodes in contact with the skin to record a wide range of measurements [34], including electroencephalograms to measure brain activity and distinguish sleep stages, electrocardiograms to assess cardiovascular health, and electromyography to monitor electrical muscle activity of muscles. Some polysomnography systems integrate further measurements for specific analyses, such as a thoracic sensor for sleep posture tracking to study posture-dependent breathing disorders [35]. While polysomnongraphy offers comprehensive insights on sleep, it faces challenges such as costly overnight hospitalization, discomfort from electrodes and sensors attached to the body, and rudimentary insights in relation to, for example, sleep posture analysis. Not to mention, its operation demands the expertise of a trained sleep technologist [36].

An alternative method, *videosomnography*, involves video recordings, capturing the patient's behavior in their natural sleep setting [37]. It is particularly effective for disorders like sleepwalking, not adequately addressed by polysomnography. Yet, videosomnography is not without downsides. The ethical and privacy implications associated with video surveillance often act as a deterrent to its widespread adoption [30,38].

A relatively recent entrant in the sleep assessment landscape is *actigraphy*. This non-invasive method employs a wearable sensor, drawing the attention of sleep specialists due to its convenience and lesser privacy concerns. Actigraphy has shown promise in assessing a range of sleep disorders and in monitoring the efficacy of medical interventions [39,40]. Actigraphy has shown strong correlations with polysomnography in some clinical studies, but its validity remains questionable in other settings [41]. However, despite advances in sensor precision and algorithm accuracy, the clinical use of actigraphic devices remains limited, with further validation and standardization of proprietary algorithms required before a smooth integration into healthcare can be realized [42,43]. Regulation concerns include potential harmful consequences from device misuse, measurement inaccuracy, algorithm uncertainty, failure modes, and misinterpretation of device-generated results [44,45]. These risks may necessitate specialized training of healthcare professionals on wearable sleep technologies to increase their awareness of the effective use and limitations of these devices.

In summary, while numerous methods for sleep disorder assessment exist, each comes with its unique set of advantages and challenges. As technology progresses, the hope is for the development of more accurate, convenient, and patient-friendly tools to improve sleep disorder diagnosis and management.

6.2.3 Management and treatment practices for sleep disorders

Understanding sleep disorders, and their subsequent management and treatment, is paramount for optimal patient care. Once a healthcare practitioner diagnoses a sleep-related disorder, various strategies, encompassing management and treatment, are employed to address it effectively.

Management of sleep disorders is a comprehensive process enabling patients to actively cope with an underlying sleep disorder, with the aim of managing symptoms and mitigating its impact on their quality of life [46]. Clinicians recommend several management techniques for sleep disorders, one of which is improving sleep hygiene. Sleep hygiene encompasses daily routines, behaviors, and environmental factors that promote healthy sleep [47]. Research indicates that improved sleep hygiene can alleviate symptoms in patients with sleep-related behavioral disorders, such as restless leg syndrome and periodic limb movement disorder [48,49].

The treatment of sleep disorders comprises a multitude of pharmacological and non-pharmacological clinical interventions aimed at addressing the underlying cause of a sleep disorder and potentially reversing its progression. For instance, medications can target specific biochemical pathways, such as increasing dopamine levels to alleviate restless leg syndrome [50]. Others relax muscles to reduce the characteristic twitches of the periodic limb movement disorder [51]. However, it is worth noting that while many of these medications are effective, they often come with side effects that can further disrupt sleep or pose other health risks [50].

Beyond medications, non-pharmacological treatments are also available. A common example is continuous positive airway pressure, which is effective for obstructive sleep apnea by keeping the airway open during sleep [52]. However, this treatment does not cure apnea, as breathing difficulties may return if treatment is halted. Additionally, there is an emphasis on addressing psychiatric disturbances, which, if marginalized and left untreated, can aggravate sleep disorders. One prominent option is cognitive-behavioral therapy, which combines cognitive and behavioral components to treat sleep disorders like insomnia, restless leg syndrome, and periodic limb movement disorder [53]. However, this therapy has limitations, such as the need for patient commitment and its unsuitability for patients with complex mental health needs [54].

Physical therapy, or physiotherapy, is another effective non-pharmacological treatment for sleep-related musculoskeletal pathologies, such as sleep pain and nocturnal leg cramps [55,56]. Physiotherapy methods typically involve self- or clinician-administered exercises or passive massage of affected muscles. However, like other treatments, physiotherapy has its challenges, such as high costs or the need for further clinical validation [57].

In cases where the aforementioned treatments fail to achieve the desired outcomes, surgical interventions might be considered. Examples include gastrocnemius release surgery, which aims to relieve tension in the calf muscle, causing pain episodes during sleep and early morning [58]. Other surgeries target conditions like obstructive sleep apnoea by focusing on weight loss or tissue removal [59]. However, while surgical intervention can be justified for some conditions, it should be approached with caution due to potential risks during and after the surgery.

6.2.4 Clinical needs and challenges in sleep posture analysis

The pursuit of understanding sleep-related behavioral and musculoskeletal pathologies has indeed advanced, yet a distinct gap persists between clinical needs and challenges. This section discusses these challenges in relation to the clinical assessment, management, and treatment of sleep-related conditions, while highlighting areas where improvements in clinical practices and patient outcomes can be further enhanced.

Medical screening for sleep disorders faces several inefficiencies. Patient-reported tools, such as diaries and questionnaires, are subjective and sensitive to factors such as bias and forgetfulness [25]. These tools often overlook crucial information, like the duration spent in each sleep posture or the intensity of abnormal movements during sleep. Observation-based assessments, such as polysomnography and videosomnography, provide a more objective and evidence-based evaluation of sleep-related disorders, but they still have major limitations. These limitations include the need for overnight hospitalization, sleeping in unfamiliar environments, heavy use of intrusive electrodes, trained personnel, and laborious manual assessments [60]. Even wearable actigraphic devices are far from being reliable clinical tools in sleep medicine due to several challenges. Notably, the *American Academy of Sleep Medicine*'s recommendations on the use of actigraphy in clinical practice do not exceed the "conditional" strength category [61], citing limited confidence in the outcomes of actigraphy-based diagnosis [62]. Additionally, there are challenges tied to the lack of accuracy and reliability of actigraphy-generated results, difficulty in interpreting device outcomes, and potential misuse of these devices.

The management and treatment of sleep-related pathologies also face hurdles. Many individuals remain unaware of their sleep disorders, and this lack of awareness leads to delayed treatments, which can be exacerbated by the shortage of sleep specialists. Post-diagnosis, the multifactorial nature of sleep pathologies can make treatment selection challenging. Clinicians are increasingly questioning the cost-to-benefit ratio of current treatments [25,28] and are constantly looking for new, cheaper medical interventions, such as postural modifications, wearable night splints, and vibrational devices [63,64]. Furthermore, evaluating the effectiveness of these treatments becomes problematic due to the reliance on subjective measures, such as patient-reported outcomes. This can result in patients switching between different therapies that did not work for them, leading to a lack of patient commitment to the treatment protocol.

Further technological advancement would be essential to address the aforementioned unmet needs and challenges. More broadly, these advancements could also support clinicians in understanding the causes of sleep-related conditions, facilitating the early detection of their risk factors, and devising optimal treatments.

While current clinical assessments are effective in diagnosing certain sleep-related conditions, they fall short in sleep posture sensing as they typically consider only four standard sleep postures (supine, prone, left and right lateral positions). This lack of information about the position of the upper or lower limbs relative to the trunk makes it difficult to provide insight into the underlying etiology. Therefore, the posture sensing capability still needs refinement to provide clinicians with access to more granular measurements that would, in turn, contribute to a better understanding of how postural cues correlate with sleep-related musculoskeletal conditions.

Moreover, sleep technologists manually assess postural immobility and duration to avoid errors inherent to automatic algorithms in sleep medicine [65]. This leads to inefficiency loops in providing care to patients, leaving many without diagnosis. It is, therefore, important to develop advanced algorithms, such as automatic posture recognition and posture duration estimation, to automate this laborious task while maintaining satisfactory reliability of automatic determination of sleep posture duration.

There are methodological considerations fundamental to technological interventions in sleep medicine. At the top of these considerations is the human interpretability of device-reported outcomes, which is important to reassure the clinicians about the technology and gain their trust in using it. Moreover, the safety and usability are crucial factors to ensure the device is reliable and easy to use. The major drawbacks of existing clinical assessments in sleep medicine also qualify as considerations for improvement. Examples of these drawbacks include the sensor intrusiveness of polysomnography and the privacy violations of videosomnography.

6.3 Sleep posture analysis: Current state of research

Sleep posture analysis is a vital area of research with significant implications for sleep-related musculoskeletal conditions. The field encompasses various subtopics, including human motion analysis, sensor technologies, algorithmic trends, and intelligent perception.

The human body undergoes various movements and postural adjustments during sleep, which can be analyzed digitally as a sequence of body postures [66]. This analysis involves two main research directions: motion quantification and classification [67]. Motion quantification is concerned with the estimation of body- or motion-specific parameters, whereas classification focuses on obtaining high-level interpretations or descriptions of the recorded human motion. Sleep posture analysis can be a quantification problem, a classification problem, or both, depending on the output definition. Clinical practice typically involves classification, examining four standard sleep postures.

After gaining an understanding of sleep posture analysis through the lens of human motion analysis, the following section embarks on an exploration of the sensor technology options available for capturing and assessing human sleep postures. The discussion will encompass the distinctive sensor categories, their sensing principles, and the general advantages and disadvantages associated with each option.

6.3.1 Human sleep posture sensing technologies

Sleep posture analysis is crucial for understanding and managing sleep-related disorders. Various sensor technologies have been developed for this purpose, broadly categorized into contact-based and contactless sensors [68].

6.3.1.1 Contactless sensor technologies

Contactless sensor technologies represent a category of devices that can capture and analyze data without the need for direct contact with the human body. In the context of sleep posture analysis, contactless sensor technologies offer a non-intrusive way to monitor a person's sleep posture throughout the night. These technologies can be broadly categorized into two groups: wireless sensors and vision sensors.

Wireless sensors operate at different frequencies and include radio frequency identification (RFID), WiFi, ultra-wideband (UWB), and millimeter wave (mmWave) technologies. RFID technology involves passive tag devices attached to the beddings or mattress that communicate with an RFID reader device [69,70]. This communication helps in identifying the posture of the person sleeping. WiFi-based sleep posture sensing takes advantage of the reflection of radiofrequency signals upon striking objects and obstacles, producing a unique reflected signal signature indicative of the posture [71,72]. UWB technology provides higher spatial scanning resolution compared to WiFi systems, capturing finer-grain postural variations [73]. mmWave technology shares the same working principle as UWB and WiFi signals but has a much wider bandwidth, allowing for higher data transfer rates, although it has relatively weaker penetrability [74]. Wireless sensors are non-intrusive and can be deployed in the bedroom without the need for a dedicated sleep laboratory, but they have limited angular and/or spatial resolution [71] and are susceptible to noise from environmental changes and radio signal interference [72].

Vision sensors, on the other hand, are popular for sleep posture monitoring in both academic and clinical settings and can be classified into marker-based and markerless vision systems. Marker-based systems track the positions of on-body retroreflective markers but are not suitable for sleep posture monitoring due to several reasons, including severe marker occlusion, high costs, and lack of portability. Markerless vision sensors do not require the placement of markers on the human body and include visible light imaging, depth imaging, infrared imaging, and thermal imaging. Visible light imaging captures full-color images of the sleeping person and their surroundings [75]. Depth imaging constructs a depth map of the camera's surroundings [76,77]. Infrared imaging detects the infrared spectrum present in the naturally emitted thermal radiation in the scene [78]. Thermal imaging captures the thermal state of different objects in the scene [79]. Vision sensors have a large field of view and no physical intrusiveness, but they raise ethical concerns surrounding personal privacy and data usage, and their reliability degrades under occlusion by blankets and certain environmental factors.

6.3.1.2 Contact-based sensor technologies

Contact-based sleep posture sensors require physical contact with the body or bed and are divided into bed-embedded and wearable sensors.

Bed-embedded sensors are further classified based on their location, either in the mattress or attached to the bed frame. Various types of pressure-sensitive mattresses exist, such as piezoresistive, piezoelectric, and triboelectric mattresses [80–85]. These mattresses gauge spatial weight distribution, equilibrium air pressures, or cardiac activity to infer sleep postures [86–89]. Load cells attached to bed frames measure vertical reaction forces acting on the bed legs to classify sleep postures [90,91]. Although bed-embedded sensors are non-invasive and convenient, they have limitations such as indirect pose inference methods, high fabrication costs, and potential failure to capture slight posture variations.

Wearable sensors, specifically magneto-inertial sensors, measure physical quantities correlated with sleep postures. These sensors include accelerometers, gyroscopes, and magnetometers [92,93]. Actigraphy, using accelerometers, measures Earth's gravitational acceleration in sensor space to discriminate between different sleep postures [94,95]. Integrating accelerometers with gyroscopes forms an inertial measurement unit (IMU) that provides information on both tilt and rotational movements of body parts [96]. The magneto-inertial measurement unit (M-IMU) adds a magnetometer to the IMU, providing a richer pool of information for sleep posture classification [97]. Smartphones, with built-in magneto-inertial sensors, have also been used for sleep posture classification [98–102]. Sensor placement on the human body is crucial for collecting accurate information about sleep postures [103–105]. While wearable inertial sensors offer direct observability of the body, low computational cost, social acceptability, and cost-effectiveness, they also have downsides such as physical intrusiveness, placement inconsistency, and susceptibility to environmental factors [15,106,107].

6.3.1.3 The sensor technology debate: Which one tops the list?

The suitability of sensor technologies for sleep posture analysis is a critical consideration in sleep medicine research. The selection of appropriate sensor technology is influenced by several criteria, including research needs and constraints, data privacy, usability, affordability, and clinical relevance of the sensor technology. These criteria play a crucial role in determining the sensor technology most appropriate for fulfilling the needs of clinical practice.

The central need is the advanced sensing of sleep postures, moving beyond the four standard postures—supine, prone, left and right lateral positions—to a higher granularity that includes limb positions relative to the trunk. This is essential for diagnosing orthopedic conditions related to limb position or contracture, which cannot be concluded from the trunk position alone.

Besides, there are additional criteria critically related to the implemetability of the sensor technology. Data privacy is a paramount consideration due to the sensitive nature of sleep data. The protection of privacy and confidentiality of patients with sleep disorders influences the adoption of sensor technology. Usability is another vital factor, affecting user satisfaction and adoption. It encompasses the level of physical intrusiveness of the device and the ease of setup and use. Affordability is a key selection criterion as it determines the accessibility of healthcare devices to a larger portion of the patient population, including low-income individuals and marginalized communities. Lastly, the meaningfulness of quantitative measurements is crucial for developing trust in the sensor technology among healthcare professionals and supporting clinicians in the diagnosis and monitoring of medical conditions.

In light of the aforementioned criteria, several studies have underscored the impracticality of using vision sensors due to the associated privacy concerns and computational challenges [75,79,108]. Similarly, contactless wireless sensor technologies also score poorly against these criteria as they are generally capable of classifying no more than four standard postures, a limitation primarily attributed to the effective reflectance area of the body [71,73]. This major limitation hinders the ability to capture slight variations in body posture, such as limb positions. The approach of utilizing contact-based bed-embedded sensors is also compromised due to the ambiguity in sleep posture recognition and the indirect means of sensing sleep posture [80,82,83]. It has been observed that similar data patterns can emerge from different positions, and the spatial distribution of body weight can be influenced by variations in body sizes and weights. Additionally, the fabrication and installation of bed-embedded sensors can be costly, and the deployment of these systems in patient homes is challenging.

Among the considered options, wearable inertial sensors perhaps hold the most promise for sleep posture analysis, albeit with some limitations that need to be addressed. These sensors offer several advantages, including the direct measurement of body posture, high resolution and bandwidth, and cost-effectiveness. Wearable inertial sensors are affixed onto body parts, such as limbs, allowing them to capture slight variations in quasistatic sleep posture as well as in-bed dynamic movements. The MEMS technology driving these sensors is well-established, rendering them significantly cost-effective for utilization in the healthcare sector. Moreover, many lay individuals have grown accustomed to employing wearable devices, making their adoption and operation feasible without the presence of specialist technical staff.

However, there are challenges associated with wearable inertial sensors, such as potential discomfort and physical intrusiveness [97], measurement errors [107,109], sensor misalignment [106,110], and soft tissue artifacts [111,112]. These challenges can affect the comfort of the user, the accuracy of the data, and the performance of the employed algorithms. For example, sensor misalignment, which is the orientation offset between the sensor and the attached body part, can alter the inertial data distribution each time the sensor is worn. Soft tissue artifacts, which arise due to motion, vibration, or deformation of the underlying soft tissues, can cause the sensors to record data that is not reflective of the actual physical movement or posture of the body.

Despite these challenges, wearable inertial sensors present opportunities for improvement and innovation in the development of wearable sleep technology. Their advantageous position compared to other sleep sensor technologies makes them a promising choice for sleep posture monitoring in sleep medicine.

6.3.2 Algorithmic trends in wearable sensor-based sleep posture analysis

Sleep posture analysis is procedurally similar to human motion analysis, involving two main research directions: motion quantification and classification. Posture quantification involves measuring and quantifying parameters related to sleep posture, such as joint angles, duration spent in different postures, and in-bed activity level. Understanding these characteristics and patterns can help medical consultants draw important conclusions about the severity of abnormal body movements during sleep [113]. Posture classification involves categorizing sleep posture-related parameters into discrete states or classes, such as classifying sleep postures and detecting temporal postural changes. This is particularly useful in studying specific sleep disorders, as it enables clinicians to identify the role of provocative sleep postures and their durations in developing spinal pain [26].

Most literature on sleep posture analysis using wearable sensors focuses on classification-based approaches. No prior research has attempted to quantify sleep posture as a continuous variable via wearable sensors, although vision sensors have been employed for this purpose [114]. Even in the less common works that involved quantifying parameters like the torso's inclination angle [99] or extremity joint angles [115,116], some classification was still necessary to categorize sleep posture.

6.3.2.1 Sensor data classification pipeline

In the context of wearable sensors for sleep posture analysis, the classification of sensor data is a critical task that involves several stages to transform raw sensor data into a trained model that can be used for labelling the data. The classification pipeline typically involves data preprocessing, feature extraction, model selection, model training, model evaluation, and model deployment [117]. Understanding each stage of the classification pipeline is crucial for comprehending and gaining insights into published works on wearable sensor data processing for sleep posture analysis.

Data preprocessing: This stage involves cleaning up the data, handling missing data, converting it to a standard or normalized format, removing outliers, or encoding categorical variables [118].

Feature extraction: This involves extracting the most relevant features from the preprocessed data, which can then be passed as inputs to a learning algorithm [119]. There are four main types of extractable features: time-domain features, frequency-domain features, time-frequency features, and pseudo features [119,120].

Model selection: This stage involves selecting the most appropriate machine learning model for the task. There are generally two known pipelines to building a machine learning system: modular learning approach and end-to-end learning approach [121]. There are five common categories of classifiers used in sleep posture analysis: rule-based classifiers, decision tree classifiers, neural network classifiers, nearest neighbor classifiers, and statistical classifiers [119,122].

Model training: This involves adjusting the internal model parameters so it can more accurately classify the data. The training procedure varies depending on the underlying algorithm and model architecture [122,123].

Model evaluation: This involves assessing the performance of the trained model on a testing dataset to determine how well the model generalizes to unseen data [124]. Several metrics can be used for this purpose, such as accuracy, precision, recall, and F1 score [125].

Model deployment: This involves making the model available for use in production, either through web services, mobile applications or otherwise. In research settings, there is typically less emphasis on this stage, but it is crucial for the usability and scalability of the model in the real world.

6.3.2.2 Hierarchical sensor information fusion

Magneto-inertial sensors provide valuable insights into sleep posture and movements, such as torso tilt angle and in-bed body rollovers, despite their limitations and caveats. To compensate for individual sensor weaknesses, obtain more accurate and reliable measurements, and compute more advanced features, it is common practice to package these sensors together in multi-sensor devices like IMUs and M-IMUs, and perform multi-sensor information fusion [126]. This approach is also extended to the deployment of multiple wearable sensors forming a body sensor network (BSN) that clinicians often welcome, as it enables low-cost and non-invasive monitoring of vital signs and physiology, overcoming many shortcomings of single-sensor systems or systems with multiple standalone sensors [34,115,127].

Sensor data can either be *uni-modal* or *multi-modal*. Uni-modal data refers to data originating from a single type of sensor or data source, whereas multi-modal data refers to data collected from multiple different types of sensors or data sources. Information fusion can occur at different stages of the classification pipeline, namely at the data, feature, or decision levels [126–128]. Data-level fusion strategies combine data from multiple sources at the data level, producing a single stream of data or features for further processing or direct input into the classification model. This can involve concatenating raw or preprocessed sensor data into a single data vector, data compression to speed up transmission and reduce computational burden, or feature extraction techniques based on statistical measures, biomechanical, and behavioral features [97,98,129–131].

Feature-level fusion strategies combine multiple features extracted from one or more data sources at the feature level, producing a new feature set for the classification model. This can involve simple concatenation of extracted features into an extended feature vector, feature selection algorithms to obtain a subset of features that improve classification accuracy, or a two-stage feature extraction process where basic features are used to compute more advanced features [116,132–135].

Decision-level fusion involves selecting or generating a single hypothesis from a set of hypotheses generated by individual decisions from multiple independent sensor data streams or decision-making nodes like classifiers [136]. Inference methods, such as Bayesian inference, fuzzy logic, and the mixture of experts framework, are commonly used in decision fusion to draw conclusions from partially abstracted information from preliminary data- or feature-level processing [96,97,115,137,138].

6.4 Monitoring sleep postures using wearable sensors

Monitoring sleep postures is fundamental for comprehending the effects of various sleeping postures on overall health and well-being. This is one of the two clinical risk factors underpinning the stable state sleep behavior. The review presented here provides a thorough examination of the significant works that have aimed to address the challenge of sleep posture monitoring. It covers a broad spectrum of study elements, including the study's objectives, the types of wearable sensors used, their placement on the body, the number of participants, the duration of the sensor data collected, the features extracted from the sensor data, the algorithms used for posture classification, the performance metrics reported, and any notable findings.

The existing literature on sleep posture classification can be organized in several ways. This review categorizes the works based on the number of sleep postures considered. Organizing the literature in this fashion aids in clarifying how the complexity of the sleep posture classification problem increases with the number of postures included. Moreover, this categorization helps in comprehending the effectiveness of algorithms at varying levels of complexity, thereby providing crucial insights into the challenges that need addressing.

6.4.1 The standard four sleep postures

The literature predominantly considers four standard sleep postures: supine, prone, and right and left lateral positions. These postures are prevalent in both technical research and clinical studies. The literature on this topic can be classified into three distinct subcategories based on the posture learning methodology underpinning the classification process.

The first subcategory comprises early attempts at classifying sleep postures using either raw or lightly preprocessed sensor data. For instance, Kishimoto et al. [139] used a single accelerometer attached to the chest and employed a three-stage classification method, achieving 100% accuracy for all participants. Similarly, Zhang and Yang [103] used a single accelerometer and a linear discriminant analysis (LDA) classifier, achieving 99% posture recognition accuracy.

The second subcategory of studies involves extracting features from the sensor data to describe the patterns. Sun et al. [140] used a smartwatch-based system and compared four classifiers, achieving the highest accuracy of 91.8% with the random forest classifier. Chang et al. [131] proposed a two-stage approach using actigraphy-based orientation and respiratory information and achieved an average accuracy of 98%. Jeng et al. [94] used two accelerometers for intelligent sleep posture monitoring and achieved an accuracy of 72%–84% using an ensemble of SVM binary classifiers and the random forest classifier. Jeon et al. [132] used three wearable sensors and a two-stage dynamic state transition framework, achieving an F1 score of 87% in a pilot experiment but only 79% in a more realistic on-site experiment. Abdulsadig et al. [141] used a neck-located accelerometer sensor and two classifiers, achieving 99% accuracy and F1 score with the Extra Trees classifier. Eyobu et al. [104] used a single device equipped with an accelerometer and gyroscope and a deep long short-term memory (LSTM) neural network classifier, achieving 99% classification accuracy.

The third subcategory leverages human expert knowledge of sleep posture definitions. Behar et al. [98] used a smartphone with a built-in accelerometer, a microphone, and an oximeter to classify users as either *obstructive sleep apnoea* (OSA) patients or non-OSA users. Ferrer-Lluis et al. [99] used a smartphone accelerometer sensor and an oximeter to explore the relationship between sleep postures and oxygen desaturation events. They found that smartphone vibrations helped participants reduce the average time spent in the supine posture from 45.6% to only 2%. In a separate study, Ferrer-Lluis et al. [100] used a video-based polysomnography system for ground-truth sleep posture monitoring and achieved an average accuracy of up to 95.9% when compared to reference polysomnography data.

The literature demonstrates the feasibility of learning a few sleep postures using sensor data, extracted features and expert knowledge. Several studies have achieved high classification accuracies using various sensor placements, classifiers, and methodologies. However, some limitations include the lack of interpretability of extracted features in deeper network layers, computationally expensive training, and the requirement of large datasets for reliable performance. Additionally, some studies [94] found that certain postures, such as the prone posture, were harder to correctly classify, and the reliability of some systems remained questionable. Therefore, further research is needed to address these limitations and develop more reliable and efficient systems for sleep posture classification.

6.4.2 Beyond the standard four sleep postures

While most research focuses on the standard four sleep postures—supine, prone, right lateral, and left lateral—some studies have attempted to increase the granularity of sleep posture classification by considering minor variations of the standard postures, such as Fowler's position and torso postures with varying arm and leg positions. This increased granularity has the potential to provide clinicians with more valuable insights into sleep behavior.

Bernal Monroy et al. [96] integrated three wearable devices into two socks and a T-shirt to classify six sleep postures and automatically determine the priority of in-bed postural changes to prevent pressure ulcers in care homes. The study employed the k-nearest neighbor, decision tree, and SVM classifiers, with the SVM classifier performing the best during pilot experiments, achieving an average F1 score exceeding 99%.

Fallmann et al. [130] used three accelerometers attached to the ankles and chest to classify two sets of sleep postures consisting of six and eight postures, respectively. The authors employed a distance-based sleep posture classification algorithm called the generalized matrix learning vector quantization. The personalized classifier achieved an average classification accuracy of 99.8% on the set of eight postures in the pilot study, while the multi-subject classifier achieved 83.6% accuracy. However, fusing variations of the left and right lateral postures improved the multi-subject classifier's performance, resulting in 98.3% accuracy on the reduced set of six postures. In the real sleep study, the multi-subject classifier achieved an average accuracy of 98% for the two participants, while the personalized classifier had a lower accuracy, scoring 58% for one participant.

Kwansicki et al. [97] used three wearable devices equipped with accelerometers, gyroscopes, and magnetometers to monitor sleep posture and quality. The study included two sets of sleep postures: the four standard postures and eight minor variations of the standard postures. The k-nearest neighbor classifier achieved an overall classification accuracy of 99.5% for the set of four postures and 92.5% for the set of eight postures. The lowest participant accuracy was reported to be 84.3%. The study also investigated the estimation of sleep stages based on the activity level present in the actigraphy data. However, the authors identified short battery life and bulky sensor size as limitations of their work.

While the aforementioned studies have achieved remarkable accuracies in sleep posture classification, it is important to note that these results were obtained using a significant amount of training data, which is a practical barrier to the widespread application of wearable sensors for sleep posture monitoring. The requirement for large datasets not only increases the time and cost associated with data collection but also raises privacy concerns. Therefore, there has been a pressing need for novel approaches that can achieve high classification accuracies with a minimal amount of training data.

Recently proposed was a novel approach to augmenting human sleep postures using a one-shot learning method [115], which significantly boosted the classification of 12 sleep postures by up to 50% even with single-observations of each posture. The authors utilized four bespoke miniature wearable sensor modules to measure four extremity joints' orientations that formed a unique posture representation that is more comprehensible to non-technical end users, such as clinicians. Additionally, new metric-based and data visualization approaches were utilized to extract insights on postural analysis, the added value of data augmentation, and the interpretation of the classification performance. The proposed framework attained promising overall accuracy as high as 100% on synthetic data and 92.7% on real data, on par with state-of-the-art data-hungry algorithms available in the literature.

6.5 Temporal analysis of in-bed postural activity using wearable sensors

The use of wearable sensors for sleep posture analysis offers the potential to understand the relationship between physical sleep behavior and musculoskeletal health. While in-bed postures themselves do not pose potential risks, it is the extended periods spent in "*provocative postures*" that can exert strain on various body regions and physiological systems, adversely affecting overall well-being. Despite its significance, there has been limited research focused on the estimation of posture-wise durations, necessitating the consideration of related studies on active-idle state classification, sleep–wake state classification, and sleep stage classification. The review herein categorizes literature according to the classification approach underpinning the research methodology, rule-based classification, linear regression-based classification, supervised classification, and hybrid approaches.

Rule-based classification approaches involve applying rules or conditions to specific sensor measurements or features. For example, Ref. [140] reported a rule-based classification approach for respiratory rate estimation using smartwatch actigraphy. Another study investigated sleep stage classification using three accelerometers attached to the wrists and chest [97]. However, these approaches have limitations, such as the need for participant-specific calibration and the potential for overestimation of sleep time. Other studies, such as Refs. [131,142], adopted two consecutive rules for classification to distinguish between different micromovements, achieving improved classification performance near 80% in accuracy.

Linear regression-based classification methods prominently relied conditioning an extracted feature called the "activity count" to make classifications. Palotti et al. [143] compared several methods within this category in the domain of wake–sleep state classification. Despite achieving a category-wide average F1 score of 80.4%, these methods tended to overestimate the "sleep" state. The use of rescoring rules, as proposed by Webster et al. [144], can enhance the specificity and accuracy of the classification.

Supervised classification approaches involved training machine learning models on labeled examples to classify new and unseen data. Khademi et al. [145] found that personalized models performed significantly better than generalized models in estimating sleep quality parameters. Banfi et al. [146] proposed a lightweight CNN architecture, lightCCNA, which outperformed baseline models with an average F1 score of 90.9%. While deep learning models have relatively higher performance, Palotti et al. [143] discouraged augmenting them with rescoring rules as they resulted in decreased accuracy and F1 score.

Hybrid approaches combine rule-based classification and supervised classification and aim at harnessing the interpretability of rule-based classifiers and the predictive power of supervised classifiers. Domingues et al. [147] demonstrated the efficacy of an advanced hierarchical synergistic approach in addressing the challenge of overestimating sleep in wake–sleep state classification. The proposed approach achieved an average geometric mean of 78.5% in distinguishing between wake and sleep states, outperforming traditional methods reported in clinical research. Chang et al. [30] proposed a hybrid approach for detecting body rollovers, achieving an average accuracy of 92%. More recently, Elnaggar et al. [148] proposed a novel hybrid framework for the temporal segmentation of sleep posture. The framework combines a Bayesian inference method with a rule-based changepoint detection logic in its decision-making core. The method achieved superior performance compared to other related approached within the literature, yielding consistently over 96% in the correlation between predicted and ground-truth posture durations.

6.6 Conclusion

The role of sleep in musculoskeletal health is an area of critical importance, given the substantial burden that musculoskeletal conditions impose on both individual and societal levels. As the chapter has highlighted, sustained provocative sleep postures can initiate or exacerbate musculoskeletal conditions, contributing to a vicious cycle that also detrimentally impacts sleep hygiene and quality. Although current clinical assessments provide some insight into sleep physiology and its related disorders, they present considerable limitations, particularly in the area of sleep posture analysis. These limitations include being physically intrusive, privacy-invading, and requiring trained personnel, all of which hinder the development of optimal treatments and accurate prognoses. In light of these challenges, the rise of sensor technologies, and particularly wearable devices, presents a promising avenue for automating and democratizing sleep posture analysis beyond in-the-clinic environments. The potential of wearable sensors to measure or classify sleep postures has been proven by several groups, but further research and innovation to overcome or work around the difficulty of obtaining training data for sleep postures is required before their wider adoption by the healthcare sector is possible.

Overall, the chapter has provided a systematic and critical review of the state-of-the-art in sleep posture sensor technologies and data processing algorithms, arguing that wearable devices are best suited to address the unmet clinical needs identified. Despite the limitations of current sensor technologies, including wearable devices, the chapter has highlighted key limitations that could merit opportunities of future research and development from both sensing and intelligent perception standpoints. These opportunities encompass the need for further research into hierarchical sensor information fusion, among other intelligent perception trends, to enhance the accuracy and usability of sleep posture analysis. Furthermore, the chapter has emphasized the limitations of existing sensor technologies and approaches, and in guiding the development of more effective solutions.

References

[1] S. Bevan, Economic impact of musculoskeletal disorders (MSDs) on work in Europe, Best Pract. Res.: Clin. Rheumatol. 29 (3) (2015), https://doi.org/10.1016/j.berh.2015.08.002.

[2] S.B. Rosenfeld, K. Schroeder, S.I. Watkins-Castillo, The economic burden of musculoskeletal disease in children and adolescents in the United States, J. Pediatr. Orthop. 38 (4) (2018), https://doi.org/10.1097/BPO.0000000000001131.

[3] M. Hirshkowitz, K. Whiton, S.M. Albert, C. Alessi, O. Bruni, L. DonCarlos, N. Hazen, J. Herman, P.J. Adams Hillard, E.S. Katz, L. Kheirandish-Gozal, D.N. Neubauer, A.E. O'Donnell, M. Ohayon, J. Peever, R. Rawding, R.C. Sachdeva, B. Setters, M.V. Vitiello, J.C. Ware, National Sleep Foundation's updated sleep duration recommendations: final report, Sleep Health 1 (4) (2015), https://doi.org/10.1016/j.sleh.2015.10.004.

[4] V.V. Vyazovskiy, Sleep, recovery, and metaregulation: explaining the benefits of sleep, Nat. Sci. Sleep 7 (2015), https://doi.org/10.2147/NSS.S54036.

[5] M.W. Mahowald, C.H. Schenck, Insights from studying human sleep disorders, Nature 437 (7063) (2005), https://doi.org/10.1038/nature04287.

[6] R.E. Dahl, D.S. Lewin, Pathways to adolescent health: sleep regulation and behavior, J. Adolesc. Health 31 (6 Suppl) (2002), https://doi.org/10.1016/S1054-139X(02)00506-2.

[7] V. Ibáñez, J. Silva, O. Cauli, A survey on sleep assessment methods, PeerJ 2018 (5) (2018), https://doi.org/10.7717/peerj.4849.

[8] M.J. Sateia, International classification of sleep disorders-third edition highlights and modifications, Chest 146 (5) (2014), https://doi.org/10.1378/chest.14-0970.

[9] B. Karna, A. Sankari, G. Tatikonda, Sleep Disorder, in: In *StatPearls [Internet]*, StatPearls Publishing, Treasure Island (FL), 2022. https://www.ncbi.nlm.nih.gov/books/NBK560720/.

[10] T.L. Sletten, S.M.W. Rajaratnam, M.J. Wright, G. Zhu, S. Naismith, N.G. Martin, I. Hickie, Genetic and environmental contributions to sleep-wake behavior in 12-year-old twins, Sleep 36 (11) (2013), https://doi.org/10.5665/sleep.3136.

[11] F.H. Fadhel, Exploring the relationship of sleep quality with drug use and substance abuse among university students: a cross-cultural study. *Middle East current*, Psychiatry 27 (1) (2020), https://doi.org/10.1186/s43045-020-00072-7.

[12] G.D.M. Potter, D.J. Skene, J. Arendt, J.E. Cade, P.J. Grant, L.J. Hardie, Circadian rhythm and sleep disruption: causes, metabolic consequences, and countermeasures, Endocr. Rev. 37 (6) (2016), https://doi.org/10.1210/er.2016-1083.

[13] J.C. Paz, M.P. West, Acute Care Handbook for Physical Therapists, fourth ed., 2013, https://doi.org/10.1016/C2011-0-05707-1.

[14] E.E. Werner, R.S. Smith, Overcoming the odds: High risk children from birth to adulthood, in: Overcoming the Odds: High Risk Children from Birth to Adulthood, 1992.

[15] S. Fallmann, L. Chen, Computational sleep behavior analysis: a survey, IEEE Access 7 (2019) 142421–142440, https://doi.org/10.1109/ACCESS.2019.2944801.

[16] C.E. Kuo, Y.C. Liu, D.W. Chang, C.P. Young, F.Z. Shaw, S.F. Liang, Development and evaluation of a wearable device for sleep quality assessment, IEEE Trans. Biomed. Eng. 64 (7) (2017), https://doi.org/10.1109/TBME.2016.2612938.

[17] M. Bergmann, A. Stefani, E. Brandauer, E. Holzknecht, H. Hackner, B. Högl, Hypnagogic foot tremor, alternating leg muscle activation or high frequency leg movements: clinical and phenomenological considerations in two cousins, Sleep Med. 54 (2019), https://doi.org/10.1016/j.sleep.2018.10.024.

[18] B.V. Vaughn, A.Y. Avidan, A.F. Eichler, Approach to Abnormal Movements and Behaviors during Sleep, 2018. UpToDate. Updated June 6.

[19] L.E. Bilston, S.C. Gandevia, Biomechanical properties of the human upper airway and their effect on its behavior during breathing and in obstructive sleep apnea, J. Appl. Physiol. 116 (3) (2014), https://doi.org/10.1152/japplphysiol.00539.2013.

[20] B. Haex, Bed and Back: ergonomic aspects of sleeping, in: Back and Bed: Ergonomic Aspects of Sleeping, vol. 1, issue 1, 2004.

[21] S. Gordon, K. Grimmer, P. Trott, Self-reported versus recorded sleep position: an observational study, Internet J. Allied Health Sci. Pract. (2004). https://doi.org/10.46743/1540-580x/2004.1034.

[22] A. Menon, M. Kumar, Influence of body position on severity of obstructive sleep apnea: a systematic review, ISRN Otolaryngol. 2013 (2013), https://doi.org/10.1155/2013/670381.

[23] A. Bidarian-Moniri, M. Nilsson, L. Rasmusson, J. Attia, H. Ejnell, The effect of the prone sleeping position on obstructive sleep apnea, Acta Otolaryngol. 135 (1) (2015), https://doi.org/10.3109/00016489.2014.962183.

[24] E. Jaul, Assessment and management of pressure ulcers in the elderly, Drugs Aging 27 (4) (2010) 311–325.

[25] D. Cary, K. Briffa, L. McKenna, Identifying relationships between sleep posture and non-specific spinal symptoms in adults: a scoping review, BMJ Open 9 (6) (2019) 1–10, https://doi.org/10.1136/bmjopen-2018-027633.

[26] D. Cary, A. Jacques, K. Briffa, Examining relationships between sleep posture, waking spinal symptoms and quality of sleep: a cross sectional study, PLoS One 16 (11) (2021), https://doi.org/10.1371/journal.pone.0260582.

[27] W.H. Lee, M.S. Ko, Effect of sleep posture on neck muscle activity, J. Phys. Ther. Sci. 29 (6) (2017), https://doi.org/10.1589/jpts.29.1021.

[28] J. Zenian, Sleep position and shoulder pain, Med. Hypotheses 74 (4) (2010), https://doi.org/10.1016/j.mehy.2009.11.013.

[29] L. Parisi, F. Pierelli, G. Amabile, G. Valente, E. Calandriello, F. Fattaposta, P. Rossi, M. Serrao, Muscular cramps: proposals for a new classification, Acta Neurol. Scand. 107 (3) (2003) 176–186, https://doi.org/10.1034/j.1600-0404.2003.01289.x.

[30] A. Sadeh, Iii. Sleep assessment methods, Monogr. Soc. Res. Child Dev. 80 (1) (2015) 33–48, https://doi.org/10.1111/mono.12143.

[31] Riha, & L., R., Diagnostic approaches to respiratory sleep disorders, J. Thorac. Dis. 7 (8) (2015).

[32] C.E. Carney, D.J. Buysse, S. Ancoli-Israel, J.D. Edinger, A.D. Krystal, K.L. Lichstein, C.M. Morin, The consensus sleep diary: standardizing prospective sleep self-monitoring, Sleep 35 (2) (2012), https://doi.org/10.5665/sleep.1642.

[33] V. Ibáñez, J. Silva, O. Cauli, A survey on sleep questionnaires and diaries, Sleep Med. 42 (2018) 90–96, https://doi.org/10.1016/j.sleep.2017.08.026.

[34] L.C. Markun, A. Sampat, Clinician-focused overview and developments in polysomnography, Curr. Sleep Med. Rep. 6 (4) (2020) 309–321, https://doi.org/10.1007/s40675-020-00197-5.

[35] A. Tiotiu, O. Mairesse, G. Hoffmann, D. Todea, A. Noseda, Body position and breathing abnormalities during sleep: a systematic study, Pneumologia 60 (4) (2011) 216–221. https://europepmc.org/article/med/22420172.

[36] F. Mendonça, S.S. Mostafa, F. Morgado-Dias, A.G. Ravelo-Garcia, T. Penzel, A review of approaches for sleep quality analysis, IEEE Access 7 (2019) 24527–24546, https://doi.org/10.1109/ACCESS.2019.2900345.

[37] O.S. Ipsiroglu, Y.H.A. Hung, F. Chan, M.L. Ross, D. Veer, S. Soo, G. Ho, M. Berger, G. McAllister, H. Garn, G. Kloesch, A.V. Barbosa, S. Stockler, W. McKellin, E. Vatikiotis-Bateson, Diagnosis by behavioral observation home-videosomnography—a rigorous ethnographic approach to sleep of children with neurodevelopmental conditions, Front. Psych. 6 (MAR) (2015), https://doi.org/10.3389/fpsyt.2015.00039.

[38] A.J. Schwichtenberg, J. Choe, A. Kellerman, E.A. Abel, E.J. Delp, Pediatric videosomnography: can signal/video processing distinguish sleep and wake states? Front. Pediatr. 6 (2018), https://doi.org/10.3389/fped.2018.00158.

[39] R. Allen, C. Chen, A. Soaita, C. Wohlberg, L. Knapp, B.T. Peterson, D. García-Borreguero, J. Miceli, A randomized, double-blind, 6-week, dose-ranging study of pregabalin in patients with restless legs syndrome, Sleep Med. 11 (6) (2010), https://doi.org/10.1016/j.sleep.2010.03.003.

[40] V. Natale, G. Plazzi, M. Martoni, Actigraphy in the assessment of insomnia: a quantitative approach, Sleep 32 (6) (2009), https://doi.org/10.1093/sleep/32.6.767.

[41] A. Sadeh, The role and validity of actigraphy in sleep medicine: an update, Sleep Med. Rev. 15 (4) (2011), https://doi.org/10.1016/j.smrv.2010.10.001.

[42] D.J. Miller, M. Lastella, A.T. Scanlan, C. Bellenger, S.L. Halson, G.D. Roach, C. Sargent, A validation study of the WHOOP strap against polysomnography to assess sleep, J. Sports Sci. 38 (22) (2020), https://doi.org/10.1080/02640414.2020.1797448.

[43] K. Boyne, D.D. Sherry, P.R. Gallagher, M. Olsen, L.J. Brooks, Accuracy of computer algorithms and the human eye in scoring actigraphy, Sleep Breath. 17 (1) (2013), https://doi.org/10.1007/s11325-012-0709-z.

[44] C.P. Bonafide, D.T. Jamison, E.E. Foglia, The emerging market of smartphone-integrated infant physiologic monitors, JAMA 317 (4) (2017) 353–354.

[45] L. Piwek, D.A. Ellis, S. Andrews, A. Joinson, The rise of consumer health wearables: promises and barriers, PLoS Med. 13 (2) (2016), https://doi.org/10.1371/journal.pmed.1001953.

[46] W.R. Miller, S. Lasiter, R.B. Ellis, J.M. Buelow, Chronic disease self-management: a hybrid concept analysis, Nurs. Outlook 63 (2) (2015) 154–161.

[47] E.J. Stepanski, J.K. Wyatt, Use of sleep hygiene in the treatment of insomnia, Sleep Med. Rev. 7 (3) (2003), https://doi.org/10.1053/smrv.2001.0246.

[48] A. Sönmez, Y. Aksoy Derya, Effects of sleep hygiene training given to pregnant women with restless leg syndrome on their sleep quality, Sleep Breath. 22 (2) (2018) 527–535, https://doi.org/10.1007/s11325-018-1619-5.

[49] W.R. Pigeon, M. Yurcheshen, Behavioral sleep medicine interventions for restless legs syndrome and periodic limb movement disorder, Sleep Med. Clin. 4 (4) (2009), https://doi.org/10.1016/j.jsmc.2009.07.008.

[50] K. Suzuki, M. Miyamoto, K. Hirata, Sleep disorders in the elderly: diagnosis and management, J. Gen. Family Med. 18 (2) (2017), https://doi.org/10.1002/jgf2.27.

[51] O. Hoxha, T. Jairam, T. Kendzerska, P. Rajendram, R. Zhou, P. Ravindran, S. Osman, M. Banayoty, Y. Qian, B.J. Murray, M.I. Boulos, Association of periodic limb movements with medication classes, Neurology 98 (15) (2022) e1585, https://doi.org/10.1212/WNL.0000000000200012.

[52] R.C. Basner, Continuous positive airway pressure for obstructive sleep apnea, N. Engl. J. Med. 356 (17) (2007) 1751–1758.

[53] K.A. Babson, M.T. Feldner, C.L. Badour, Cognitive behavioral therapy for sleep disorders, Psychiatr. Clin. 33 (3) (2010) 629–640.

[54] J. Holmes, All you need is cognitive behaviour therapy? Br. Med. J. 324 (7332) (2002), https://doi.org/10.1136/bmj.324.7352.1522.

[55] A.W. Andrews, R. Pine, Physical therapy for nocturnal lower limb cramping: a case report, Physiother. Theory Pract. 35 (2) (2019), https://doi.org/10.1080/09593985.2018.1441932.

[56] J. Eadie, A.T. Van De Water, C. Lonsdale, M.A. Tully, W. Van Mechelen, C.A. Boreham, L. Daly, S.M. McDonough, D.A. Hurley, Physiotherapy for sleep disturbance in people with chronic low back pain: results of a feasibility randomized controlled trial, Arch. Phys. Med. Rehabil. 94 (11) (2013), https://doi.org/10.1016/j.apmr.2013.04.017.

[57] M. Tramontano, S. De Angelis, G. Galeoto, M.C. Cucinotta, D. Lisi, R.M. Botta, D'ippolito, M., Morone, G., & Buzzi, M. G., Physical therapy exercises for sleep disorders in a rehabilitation setting for neurological patients: a systematic review and meta-analysis, Brain Sci. 11 (9) (2021), https://doi.org/10.3390/brainsci11091176.

[58] Z. Arshad, A. Aslam, M.A. Razzaq, M. Bhatia, Gastrocnemius release in the Management of Chronic Plantar Fasciitis: a systematic review, Foot Ankle Int. 43 (4) (2022), https://doi.org/10.1177/10711007211052290.

[59] H. Ashrafian, T. Toma, S.P. Rowland, L. Harling, A. Tan, E. Efthimiou, A. Darzi, T. Athanasiou, Bariatric surgery or non-surgical weight loss for obstructive sleep Apnoea? A systematic review and comparison of Meta-analyses, Obes. Surg. 25 (7) (2015), https://doi.org/10.1007/s11695-014-1533-2.

[60] J.L. Hossain, C.M. Shapiro, The prevalence, cost implications, and management of sleep disorders: an overview, Sleep Breath. 6 (2) (2002), https://doi.org/10.1007/s11325-002-0085-1.

[61] M. Dijkers, Introducing GRADE: a systematic approach to rating evidence in systematic reviews and to guideline development, in: E-Newsletter: Center on Knowledge Translation for Disability and Rehabilitation Research, vol. 1(5), 2013.

[62] M.T. Smith, C.S. McCrae, J. Cheung, J.L. Martin, C.G. Harrod, J.L. Heald, K.A. Carden, Use of Actigraphy for the evaluation of sleep disorders and circadian rhythm sleep-wake disorders: an American Academy of sleep medicine clinical practice guideline, J. Clin. Sleep Med. 14 (7) (2018), https://doi.org/10.5664/jcsm.7230.

[63] W.C. Chen, L.A. Lee, N.H. Chen, T.J. Fang, C.G. Huang, W.N. Cheng, H.Y. Li, Treatment of snoring with positional therapy in patients with positional obstructive sleep apnea syndrome, Sci. Rep. 5 (2015), https://doi.org/10.1038/srep18188.

[64] J.P. Van Maanen, N. De Vries, Long-term effectiveness and compliance of positional therapy with the sleep position trainer in the treatment of positional obstructive sleep apnea syndrome, Sleep 37 (7) (2014), https://doi.org/10.5665/sleep.3840.

[65] M. Tripathi, Technical notes for digital polysomnography recording in sleep medicine practice, Ann. Indian Acad. Neurol. 11 (2) (2008), https://doi.org/10.4103/0972-2327.41887.

[66] C. Park, S.D. Noh, A. Srivastava, Data science for motion and time analysis with modern motion sensor data, Oper. Res. 70 (6) (2022), https://doi.org/10.1287/opre.2021.2216.

[67] I.H. Lopez-Nava, M.M. Angelica, Wearable inertial sensors for human motion analysis: a review, IEEE Sensors J. 16 (22) (2016) 7821–7834, https://doi.org/10.1109/JSEN.2016.2609392.

[68] X. Li, Y. Gong, X. Jin, P. Shang, Sleep posture recognition based on machine learning: a systematic review, Pervasive Mob. Comput. 90 (101752) (2023), https://doi.org/10.1016/j.pmcj.2023.101752.

[69] X. Hu, K. Naya, P. Li, T. Miyazaki, K. Wang, Y. Sun, Non-invasive sleeping posture recognition and body movement detection based on RFID, in: 2018 IEEE International Conference on Internet of Things (iThings) and IEEE Green Computing and Communications (GreenCom) and IEEE Cyber, Physical and Social Computing (CPSCom) and IEEE Smart Data (SmartData), 2018, pp. 1817–1820. https://doi.org/10.1109/Cybermatics_2018.2018.00302.

[70] P.-J. Chen, T.-H. Hu, M.-S. Wang, Raspberry pi-based sleep posture recognition system using AIoT technique, Healthcare 10 (3) (2022), https://doi.org/10.3390/healthcare10030513.

[71] S. Yue, Y. Yang, H. Wang, H. Rahul, D. Katabi, BodyCompass: monitoring sleep posture with wireless signals, Proc. ACM Interact. Mob. Wearable Ubiquitous Technol. 4 (2) (2020), https://doi.org/10.1145/3397311.

[72] J. Liu, Y. Chen, Y. Wang, X. Chen, J. Cheng, J. Yang, Monitoring vital signs and postures during sleep using WiFi signals, IEEE Internet Things J. 5 (3) (2018) 2071–2084, https://doi.org/10.1109/JIOT.2018.2822818.

[73] D.K.-H. Lai, L.-W. Zha, T.Y.-N. Leung, A.Y.-C. Tam, B.P.-H. So, H.-J. Lim, D.S.K. Cheung, D.W.-C. Wong, J.C.-W. Cheung, Dual ultra-wideband (UWB) radar-based sleep posture recognition system: towards ubiquitous sleep monitoring, Eng. Regen. 4 (1) (2023) 36–43, https://doi.org/10.1016/j.engreg.2022.11.003.

[74] E.M. Sitar, S. Sur, A millimeter-wave wireless sensing approach for sleep posture classification, in: Proceedings of the 20th ACM Conference on Embedded Networked Sensor Systems, Association for Computing Machinery, 2023, pp. 794–796. https://doi.org/10.1145/3560905.3568088.

[75] S. Liu, S. Ostadabbas, A vision-based system for in-bed posture tracking, in: Proceedings — 2017 IEEE International Conference on Computer Vision Workshops, ICCVW 2017, vols. 2018-Janua, 2017. https://doi.org/10.1109/ICCVW.2017.163.

[76] A.Y.C. Tam, B.P.H. So, T.T.C. Chan, A.K.Y. Cheung, D.W.C. Wong, J.C.W. Cheung, A blanket accommodative sleep posture classification system using an infrared depth camera: a deep learning approach with synthetic augmentation of blanket conditions, Sensors 21 (16) (2021), https://doi.org/10.3390/s21165553.

[77] W. Ren, O. Ma, H. Ji, X. Liu, Human posture recognition using a hybrid of fuzzy logic and machine learning approaches, IEEE Access 8 (2020), https://doi.org/10.1109/ACCESS.2020.3011697.

[78] S. Liu, Y. Yin, S. Ostadabbas, In-bed pose estimation: deep learning with shallow dataset, IEEE J. Transl. Eng. Health Med. 7 (2019), https://doi.org/10.1109/JTEHM.2019.2892970.

[79] Z. Chen, Y. Wang, Remote recognition of in-bed postures using a thermopile Array sensor with machine learning, IEEE Sensors J. 21 (9) (2021), https://doi.org/10.1109/JSEN.2021.3059681.

[80] K. Tang, A. Kumar, M. Nadeem, I. Maaz, CNN-based smart sleep posture recognition system, IoT 2 (1) (2021), https://doi.org/10.3390/iot2010007.

[81] Q. Hu, X. Tang, W. Tang, A real-time patient-specific sleeping posture recognition system using pressure sensitive conductive sheet and transfer learning, IEEE Sensors J. 21 (5) (2021), https://doi.org/10.1109/JSEN.2020.3043416.

[82] R.S. Hsiao, T.X. Chen, M.A. Bitew, C.H. Kao, T.Y. Li, Sleeping posture recognition using fuzzy c-means algorithm, Biomed. Eng. Online 17 (2018), https://doi.org/10.1186/s12938-018-0584-3.

[83] W. Viriyavit, V. Sornlertlamvanich, Bed position classification by a neural network and Bayesian network using noninvasive sensors for fall prevention, J. Sens. 2020 (2020), https://doi.org/10.1155/2020/5689860.

[84] Z. Zhou, S. Padgett, Z. Cai, G. Conta, Y. Wu, Q. He, S. Zhang, C. Sun, J. Liu, E. Fan, K. Meng, Z. Lin, C. Uy, J. Yang, J. Chen, Single-layered ultra-soft washable smart textiles for all-around ballistocardiograph, respiration, and posture monitoring during sleep, Biosens. Bioelectron. 155 (2020), https://doi.org/10.1016/j.bios.2020.112064.

[85] Y. Chao, T. Liu, L.-M. Shen, Method of recognizing sleep postures based on air pressure sensor and convolutional neural network: for an air spring mattress, Eng. Appl. Artif. Intell. 121 (2023) 106009, https://doi.org/10.1016/j.engappai.2023.106009.

[86] E. Hoque, R.F. Dickerson, J.A. Stankovic, Monitoring body positions and movements during sleep using WISPs, in: Wireless Health 2010, Association for Computing Machinery, 2010, pp. 44–53, https://doi.org/10.1145/1921081.1921088.

[87] S. Khare, A. Chawala, Effect of change in body position on resting electrocardiogram in young healthy adults, Niger. J. Cardiol. 13 (2) (2016), https://doi.org/10.4103/0189-7969.187711.

[88] S. Peng, Y. Li, R. Cui, K. Xu, Y. Wu, M. Huang, C. Dai, T. Tamur, S. Mukhopadhyay, C. Chen, W. Chen, Sleep postures monitoring based on capacitively coupled electrodes and deep recurrent neural networks, Biomed. Eng. Online 21 (1) (2022) 75, https://doi.org/10.1186/s12938-022-01031-5.

[89] M. Liu, S. Ye, A novel body posture recognition system on bed, in: 2018 IEEE 3rd International Conference on Signal and Image Processing (ICSIP), 2018, pp. 38–42, https://doi.org/10.1109/SIPROCESS.2018.8600465.

[90] Z.T. Beattie, C.C. Hagen, T.L. Hayes, Classification of lying position using load cells under the bed, in: Proceedings of the Annual International Conference of the IEEE Engineering in Medicine and Biology Society, EMBS, 2011, https://doi.org/10.1109/IEMBS.2011.6090068.

[91] G. Wong, S. Gabison, E. Dolatabadi, G. Evans, T. Kajaks, P. Holliday, H. Alshaer, G. Fernie, T. Dutta, Toward mitigating pressure injuries: detecting patient orientation from vertical bed reaction forces, J. Rehabil. Assist. Technol. Eng. 7 (2020), https://doi.org/10.1177/2055668320912168.

[92] C. Jussi, P. Davidson, K.-J. Martti, L. Helena, Inertial sensors and their applications, in: Handbook of Signal Processing Systems, Springer International Publishing, 2019, pp. 51–85, https://doi.org/10.1007/978-3-319-91734-4_2.

[93] N. El-Sheimy, A. Youssef, Inertial sensors technologies for navigation applications: state of the art and future trends, SatNav 1 (1) (2020) 2, https://doi.org/10.1186/s43020-019-0001-5.

[94] P.-Y. Jeng, L.-C. Wang, C.-J. Hu, D. Wu, A wrist sensor sleep posture monitoring system: an automatic labeling approach, Sensors 21 (1) (2021), https://doi.org/10.3390/s21010258.

[95] J. Razjouyan, H. Lee, S. Parthasarathy, J. Mohler, A. Sharafkhaneh, B. Najafi, Improving sleep quality assessment using wearable sensors by including information from postural/sleep position changes and body acceleration: a comparison of chest-worn sensors, wrist Actigraphy, and polysomnography, J. Clin. Sleep Med. 13 (11) (2017), https://doi.org/10.5664/jcsm.6802.

[96] E. Bernal Monroy, A. Polo Rodríguez, M. Espinilla Estevez, J. Medina Quero, Fuzzy monitoring of in-bed postural changes for the prevention of pressure ulcers using inertial sensors attached to clothing, J. Biomed. Inform. 107 (103476) (2020) 1–12, https://doi.org/10.1016/j.jbi.2020.103476.

[97] R.M. Kwasnicki, G.W.V. Cross, L. Geoghegan, Z. Zhang, P. Reilly, A. Darzi, G.Z. Yang, R. Emery, A lightweight sensing platform for monitoring sleep quality and posture: a simulated validation study, Eur. J. Med. Res. 23 (28) (2018) 1–9, https://doi.org/10.1186/s40001-018-0326-9.

[98] J. Behar, A. Roebuck, M. Shahid, J. Daly, A. Hallack, N. Palmius, J. Stradling, G.D. Clifford, SleepAp: an automated obstructive sleep apnoea screening application for smartphones, IEEE J. Biomed. Health Inform. 19 (1) (2015), https://doi.org/10.1109/JBHI.2014.2307913.

[99] I. Ferrer-Lluis, Y. Castillo-Escario, J.M. Montserrat, R. Jané, Enhanced monitoring of sleep position in sleep apnea patients: smartphone triaxial accelerometry compared with video-validated position from polysomnography, Sensors 21 (11) (2021), https://doi.org/10.3390/s21113689.

[100] I. Ferrer-Lluis, Y. Castillo-Escario, J.M. Montserrat, R. Jané, Sleeppos app: an automated smartphone application for angle based high resolution sleep position monitoring and treatment, Sensors 21 (13) (2021), https://doi.org/10.3390/s21134531.

[101] E. Ramanujam, T. Perumal, S. Padmavathi, Human activity recognition with smartphone and wearable sensors using deep learning techniques: a review, IEEE Sensors J. 21 (12) (2021), https://doi.org/10.1109/JSEN.2021.3069927.

[102] W.S. Lima, E. Souto, K. El-Khatib, R. Jalali, J. Gama, Human activity recognition using inertial sensors in a smartphone: an overview, Sensors 19 (14) (2019), https://doi.org/10.3390/s19143213.

[103] Z. Zhang, G.Z. Yang, Monitoring cardio-respiratory and posture movements during sleep: what can be achieved by a single motion sensor, in: IEEE 12th International Conference on Wearable and Implantable Body Sensor Networks (BSN), 2015, pp. 1–6, https://doi.org/10.1109/BSN.2015.7299409.

[104] O.S. Eyobu, Y.W. Kim, D. Cha, D.S. Han, A real-time sleeping position recognition system using IMU sensor motion data, in: IEEE International Conference on Consumer Electronics (ICCE), vols. 2018-Janua, 2018, pp. 1–2, https://doi.org/10.1109/ICCE.2018.8326209.

[105] P. Alinia, A. Samadani, M. Milosevic, H. Ghasemzadeh, S. Parvaneh, Pervasive lying posture tracking, Sensors 20 (20) (2020) 1–22. https://doi.org/10.3390/s20205953.

[106] B. Fan, Q. Li, T. Tan, P. Kang, P.B. Shull, Effects of IMU sensor-to-segment misalignment and orientation error on 3-D knee joint angle estimation, IEEE Sensors J. 22 (3) (2022) 2543–2552, https://doi.org/10.1109/JSEN.2021.3137305.

[107] U. Qureshi, F. Golnaraghi, An algorithm for the in-field calibration of a MEMS IMU, IEEE Sensors J. 17 (22) (2017) 7479–7486, https://doi.org/10.1109/JSEN.2017.2751572.

[108] F. Cabitza, R. Rasoini, G.F. Gensini, Unintended consequences of machine learning in medicine, JAMA J. Am. Med. Assoc. 318 (6) (2017), https://doi.org/10.1001/jama.2017.7797.

[109] O.J. Woodman, An Introduction to Inertial Navigation (Report No. UCAM-CL-TR-696), University of Cambridge, 2007. https://www.cl.cam.ac.uk/techreports/UCAM-CL-TR-696.pdf.

[110] Z. Wang, D. Wu, R. Gravina, G. Fortino, Y. Jiang, K. Tang, Kernel fusion based extreme learning machine for cross-location activity recognition, Inf. Fusion 37 (2017) 1–9, https://doi.org/10.1016/j.inffus.2017.01.004.

[111] A. Forner-Cordero, M. Mateu-Arce, I. Forner-Cordero, E. Alcántara, J.C. Moreno, J.L. Pons, Study of the motion artefacts of skin-mounted inertial sensors under different attachment conditions, Physiol. Meas. 29 (4) (2008), https://doi.org/10.1088/0967-3334/29/4/N01.

[112] A. Leardini, A. Chiari, U. Della Croce, A. Cappozzo, Human movement analysis using stereophotogrammetry part 3. Soft tissue artifact assessment and compensation, Gait Posture 21 (2) (2005) 212–225, https://doi.org/10.1016/j.gaitpost.2004.05.002.

[113] A. Zampogna, A. Manoni, F. Asci, C. Liguori, F. Irrera, A. Suppa, Shedding light on nocturnal movements in parkinson's disease: evidence from wearable technologies, Sensors 20 (18) (2020), https://doi.org/10.3390/s20185171.

[114] F. Achilles, A.E. Ichim, H. Coskun, F. Tombari, S. Noachtar, N. Navab, Patient MoCap: human pose estimation under blanket occlusion for hospital monitoring applications, in: Lecture Notes in Computer Science (including subseries Lecture Notes in Artificial Intelligence and Lecture Notes in Bioinformatics, vol. 9900 LNCS, 2016. https://doi.org/10.1007/978-3-319-46720-7_57.

[115] O. Elnaggar, F. Coenen, A. Hopkinson, L. Mason, P. Paoletti, Information Fusion, 95, 2023, pp. 215–236, https://doi.org/10.1016/j.inffus.2023.02.003.

[116] O. Elnaggar, F. Coenen, P. Paoletti, In-Bed Human Pose Classification Using Sparse Inertial Signals, Springer International Publishing, 2020, pp. 331–344.

[117] A. Paleyes, R.G. Urma, N.D. Lawrence, Challenges in deploying machine learning: a survey of case studies, ACM Comput. Surv. 55 (6) (2022), https://doi.org/10.1145/3533378.

[118] Z. Abedjan, X. Chu, D. Deng, R.C. Fernandez, I.F. Ilyas, M. Ouzzani, P. Papotti, M. Stonebraker, N. Tang, Detecting data errors: where are we and what needs to be done? in: Proceedings of the VLDB Endowment, vol. 9, issue 12, 2016. https://doi.org/10.14778/2994509.2994518.

[119] T.R. Bennett, J. Wu, N. Kehtarnavaz, R. Jafari, Inertial measurement unit-based wearable computers for assisted living applications: a signal processing perspective, IEEE Signal Process. Mag. 33 (2) (2016), https://doi.org/10.1109/MSP.2015.2499314.

[120] S. Krishnan, Y. Athavale, Trends in biomedical signal feature extraction, in: Biomedical Signal Processing and Control, vol. 43, 2018. https://doi.org/10.1016/j.bspc.2018.02.008.

[121] C. Janiesch, P. Zschech, K. Heinrich, Machine learning and deep learning, Electron. Mark. 31 (3) (2021), https://doi.org/10.1007/s12525-021-00475-2.

[122] C.M. Bishop, N.M. Nasrabadi, Pattern Recognition and Machine Learning, vol. 4, issue 4, Springer, 2006.

[123] Q. Wang, Y. Ma, K. Zhao, Y. Tian, A comprehensive survey of loss functions in machine learning, Ann. Data Sci. 9 (2) (2022), https://doi.org/10.1007/s40745-020-00253-5.

[124] I. Goodfellow, Y. Bengio, A. Courville, Deep Learning, MIT Press, 2016.

[125] H. Mohammad, M.N. Sulaiman, A review on evaluation metrics for data classification evaluations, Int. J. Data Min. Knowl. Manag. 5 (2) (2015), https://doi.org/10.5121/ijdkp.2015.5201.

[126] E.F. Nakamura, A.A.F. Loureiro, A.C. Frery, Information fusion for wireless sensor networks: methods, models, and classifications, ACM Comput. Surv. 39 (3) (2007), https://doi.org/10.1145/1267070.1267073.

[127] R. Gravina, P. Alinia, H. Ghasemzadeh, G. Fortino, Multi-sensor fusion in body sensor networks: state-of-the-art and research challenges, Inf. Fusion 35 (2017) 68–80, https://doi.org/10.1016/j.inffus.2016.09.005.

[128] Q. Li, R. Gravina, Y. Li, S.H. Alsamhi, F. Sun, G. Fortino, Multi-user activity recognition: challenges and opportunities, Inf. Fusion 63 (2020) 121–135, https://doi.org/10.1016/j.inffus.2020.06.004.

[129] M. Pesenti, G. Invernizzi, J. Mazzella, M. Bocciolone, A. Pedrocchi, M. Gandolla, IMU-based human activity recognition and payload classification for low-back exoskeletons, Sci. Rep. 13 (1) (2023), https://doi.org/10.1038/s41598-023-28195-x.

[130] S. Fallmann, R. Van Veen, L. Chen, D. Walker, F. Chen, C. Pan, Wearable accelerometer based extended sleep position recognition, in: IEEE 19th International Conference on e-Health Networking, Applications and Services (Healthcom), 2017, pp. 1–6. https://doi.org/10.1109/HealthCom.2017.8210806.

[131] L. Chang, J. Lu, J. Wang, X. Chen, D. Fang, Z. Tang, P. Nurmi, Z. Wang, SLEEPGUARD: capturing rich sleep information using smartwatch sensing data, Proc. ACM Interact. Mob. Wearable Ubiquitous Technol. 2 (3) (2018) 1–34, https://doi.org/10.1145/3264908.

[132] S. Jeon, T. Park, A. Paul, Y.S. Lee, S.H. Son, A wearable sleep position tracking system based on dynamic state transition framework, IEEE Access 7 (2019) 135742–135756, https://doi.org/10.1109/ACCESS.2019.2942608.

[133] R. Muthukrishnan, R. Rohini, LASSO: a feature selection technique in predictive modeling for machine learning, in: 2016 IEEE International Conference on Advances in Computer Applications, ICACA 2016, 2017. https://doi.org/10.1109/ICACA.2016.7887916.

[134] A. Leone, G. Rescio, A. Caroppo, P. Siciliano, A. Manni, Human postures recognition by accelerometer sensor and ML architecture integrated in embedded platforms: benchmarking and performance evaluation, Sensors 23 (2) (2023), https://doi.org/10.3390/s23021039.

[135] K. Nakazaki, S. Kitamura, Y. Motomura, A. Hida, Y. Kamei, N. Miura, K. Mishima, Validity of an algorithm for determining sleep/wake states using a new actigraph, J. Physiol. Anthropol. 33 (31) (2014), https://doi.org/10.1186/1880-6805-33-31.

[136] A. Bulling, U. Blanke, B. Schiele, A tutorial on human activity recognition using body-worn inertial sensors, ACM Comput. Surv. 46 (3) (2014), https://doi.org/10.1145/2499621.

[137] C.A. Reyes-García, A.A. Torres-García, Fuzzy logic and fuzzy systems, in: Biosignal Processing and Classification Using Computational Learning and Intelligence: Principles, Algorithms, and Applications, 2021, https://doi.org/10.1016/B978-0-12-820125-1.00020-8.

[138] M. Airaksinen, O. Räsänen, E. Ilén, T. Häyrinen, A. Kivi, V. Marchi, A. Gallen, S. Blom, A. Varhe, N. Kaartinen, L. Haataja, S. Vanhatalo, Automatic posture and movement tracking of infants with wearable movement sensors, Sci. Rep. 10 (169) (2020) 1–12, https://doi.org/10.1038/s41598-019-56862-5.

[139] Y. Kishimoto, A. Akahori, K. Oguri, Estimation of sleeping posture for M-health by a wearable tri-axis accelerometer, in: Proceedings of the 3rd IEEE-EMBS International Summer School and Symposium on Medical Devices and Biosensors, ISSS-MDBS 2006, 2006, pp. 45–48. https://doi.org/10.1109/ISSMDBS.2006.360093.

[140] X. Sun, L. Qiu, Y. Wu, Y. Tang, G. Cao, SleepMonitor: monitoring respiratory rate and body position during sleep using smartwatch, Proc. ACM Interact. Mob. Wearable Ubiquitous Technol. 1 (3) (2017) 1–22, https://doi.org/10.1145/3130969.

[141] R.S. Abdulsadig, S. Singh, Z. Patel, E. Rodriguez-Villegas, Sleep posture detection using an accelerometer placed on the neck, in: Proceedings of the Annual International Conference of the IEEE Engineering in Medicine and Biology Society, vols. 2022-July, EMBS, 2022. https://doi.org/10.1109/EMBC48229.2022.9871300.

[142] M. Borazio, E. Berlin, N. Kucukyildiz, P. Scholl, K. Van Laerhoven, Towards benchmarked sleep detection with wrist-worn sensing units, in: Proceedings—2014 IEEE International Conference on Healthcare Informatics, ICHI 2014, 2014, pp. 125–134, https://doi.org/10.1109/ICHI.2014.24.

[143] J. Palotti, R. Mall, M. Aupetit, M. Rueschman, M. Singh, A. Sathyanarayana, S. Taheri, L. Fernandez-Luque, Benchmark on a large cohort for sleep-wake classification with machine learning techniques, NPJ Digit. Med. 2 (50) (2019), https://doi.org/10.1038/s41746-019-0126-9.

[144] J.B. Webster, D.F. Kripke, S. Messin, D.J. Mullaney, G. Wyborney, An activity-based sleep monitor system for ambulatory use, Sleep 5 (4) (1982) 389–399, https://doi.org/10.1093/sleep/5.4.389.

[145] A. Khademi, Y. El-Manzalawy, L. Master, O.M. Buxton, V.G. Honavar, Personalized sleep parameters estimation from actigraphy: a machine learning approach, Nat. Sci. Sleep 11 (2019), https://doi.org/10.2147/NSS.S220716.

[146] T. Banfi, N. Valigi, M. di Galante, P. d'Ascanio, G. Ciuti, U. Faraguna, Efficient embedded sleep wake classification for open-source actigraphy, Sci. Rep. 11 (345) (2021), https://doi.org/10.1038/s41598-020-79294-y.

[147] A. Domingues, T. Paiva, J.M. Sanches, Sleep and wakefulness state detection in nocturnal actigraphy based on movement information, IEEE Trans. Biomed. Eng. 61 (2) (2014) 426–434, https://doi.org/10.1109/TBME.2013.2280538.

[148] O. Elnaggar, R. Arelhi, F. Coenen, A. Hopkinson, L. Mason, P. Paoletti, arXiv Preprint arXiv:2301.03469, 2023.

CHAPTER 7

Comparative evaluation of deep learning techniques for multistage Alzheimer's prediction from magnetic resonance images

Pushpendra Gupta[a], Pradeep Nahak[a], Vidyapati Kumar[a], Dilip Kumar Pratihar[a], and Kalyanmoy Deb[b]

[a]Department of Mechanical Engineering, Indian Institute of Technology Kharagpur, Kharagpur, West Bengal, India
[b]Electrical and Computer Engineering, Michigan State University, East Lansing, MI, United States

7.1 Introduction

Alzheimer's disease (AD) stands as a neurodegenerative ailment causing irreversible and severe damage to brain cells, resulting in a gradual decline in memory and cognitive functions [1]. As the primary cause of dementia, AD accounts for a substantial portion, approximately 60%–80%, of all dementia cases [2]. Its impact resonates profoundly, affecting not only patients but also their families, posing a significant societal and financial burden. This disease has emerged as a substantial public health challenge, significantly affecting individuals, families, and healthcare systems globally. According to the World Health Organization, nearly 55 million individuals worldwide are affected by Alzheimer's dementia, with more than 60% of these cases prevalent in low- and middle-income countries [3]. Without medical advancements to prevent, decelerate, or cure AD, the annual influx of new cases might surpass 10 million [4]. Projections indicate a substantial surge in the number of individuals living with AD, estimated to surpass 78 million worldwide by 2030 [5]. This escalation underscores the pressing need for advancements in managing and addressing the challenges posed by AD on a global scale.

The consequent damage to brain tissue results in steadily declining cognitive abilities, changes in behavior and personality, and inability to carry out daily activities. The initial stage of AD is marked by mild forgetfulness and difficulty retaining new information. As the disease progresses through moderate and severe stages, language breakdown, disorientation, mood swings, and loss of bodily functions manifest [6]. Currently, there are no treatments available to reverse or stall the neurodegeneration caused by AD. However, early diagnosis before the appearance of symptoms can aid in initiating therapies to improve quality of life and delay further deterioration [7]. This imminent crisis underscores the urgency and significance of research efforts aimed at the early prediction and diagnosis of AD to prevent permanent memory loss and to develop treatments that can be used in the future. However, diagnosing AD is challenging, as the symptoms are often subtle and variable in the early stages. Moreover, there is no definitive biomarker or test that can confirm the presence of AD. Therefore, there is a need for reliable and accurate methods to predict AD using noninvasive and accessible data sources.

Early detection of AD is of paramount importance, as it not only facilitates early intervention and potential treatments but also plays a pivotal role in mitigating the irreversible memory loss associated with the disease. Magnetic resonance imaging (MRI) [8] data is one type of medical imaging data that can offer useful insights into the structural and functional changes in the brain that are connected to AD. MRI data have shown promise for detecting early pathological changes in AD [9,10]. The shrinkage of AD-affected brain areas, including the hippocampus and temporal lobes, can be captured using MRI. The hallmark pathological characteristics of AD are the accumulation of amyloid beta plaques and neurofibrillary tangles composed of tau protein in the brain, leading to neuronal dysfunction and loss [11]. MRI can easily reveal these changes and detect AD in its early stage [12]. The characteristic structural changes noted in MRI scans include hippocampus and temporal lobe atrophy, dilation of ventricles and sulci, and reduced cortical thickness [13]. Manual analysis of MRI data is laborious and susceptible to inaccuracies, demanding significant time investment. Therefore, automated techniques that can extract relevant features and classify MRI images into different stages of AD are needed. DL techniques can enable the automated analysis of MRI images to identify patterns predictive of AD onset and progression [14]. DL can learn from enormous amounts of data and complete challenging tasks. DL has already achieved outstanding achievements in fields like speech recognition, natural language processing, and computer vision [15]. DL can also be applied to medical imaging data, such as MRI, to perform tasks such as segmentation, detection, classification, and prediction.

This chapter focuses on the early prediction of AD using augmented medical image data with DL techniques. The dataset used for this study consists of MRI images of AD patients and healthy subjects. The images are classified into four classes: mild demented (MD), moderate demented (MoD), nondemented (ND), and very mild demented (VMD). These classes represent different stages of the disease, ranging from mild to severe cognitive impairment, thus enabling a comprehensive assessment of the effectiveness of the chosen DL algorithms. Three popular DL algorithms, namely CNN [16], Visual Geometry Group (VGG-16) [17], and Residual Network (ResNet-50) [18], are used to predict the disease. Comparative evaluations of CNN, VGG-16, and ResNet-50 models are undertaken to determine the best-performing technique for multiclass AD prediction using augmented MRI data. Overall, this study demonstrates the potential of DL techniques for AD prediction using medical imaging data and highlights the importance of selecting appropriate algorithms for optimal results.

7.2 Methodology

The primary objective of this study revolves around AD prediction using DL techniques applied to medical image data. The dataset utilized comprises 6400 MRI images, categorized into four classes: MD, MoD, ND, and VMD. The dataset taken from the Kaggle database is elaborated in Section 7.2.1 [19]. Image augmentation techniques [20] are employed, including rotation, flipping, shifting, shearing, zooming, and cropping, to enhance data robustness and diversity. This augmentation process yields a total of 12,800 images, introducing variations crucial for improving model generalization and predictive capabilities. The specifics of various image augmentation methods are elucidated in Section 7.2.2. Three prominent DL models are utilized to classify images into different AD stages: CNN, VGG-16, and ResNet-50. The selection of these models stems from their established prowess in image classification tasks and their adeptness at extracting intricate features from medical imaging data. The CNN model encompasses convolutional, pooling, dropout, and fully connected layers, optimized through stochastic gradient descent and backpropagation. VGG-16 and ResNet-50 represent well-established deep CNN architectures, renowned for their state-of-the-art performance in image classification tasks. Evaluation of model performance on test data employs metrics such as accuracy, precision, recall, and F1 score. The flowchart in Fig. 7.1 shows the steps involved in obtaining the image database, splitting it into training, validation, and testing sets, and comparing different DL models. Further details regarding the dataset, machine learning models, and specific evaluation metrics adopted in this study are expounded upon in subsequent sections, offering a comprehensive understanding of the methodology employed for early AD prediction.

7.2.1 Data set description

Fig. 7.2 shows how the 6400 MRI images are distributed among each class. Three samples from each class are presented in Table 7.1. As evident, there is a significant class imbalance present, which poses an additional challenge for model training and evaluation. The ND class contained the maximum number of images (3200), followed by VMD (2240 images), MD (896 images), and MoD (64 images). The DL models face difficulty in accurately predicting the disease, as they may either favor the majority classes or overfit the minority classes. However, getting a balanced medical dataset across different stages of a disease is often hard due to the limited availability of subjects and image acquisitions [21]. Therefore, it is not feasible to assign equal number of medical images to each category in a real-world medical dataset. Class imbalance can bias machine learning models toward the majority class and lead to poor generalization on under-represented classes [22]. The class imbalance that is observed shows the difficulty of the task that the DL models have to do, as they have to effectively differentiate between these categories despite the large differences in sample sizes.

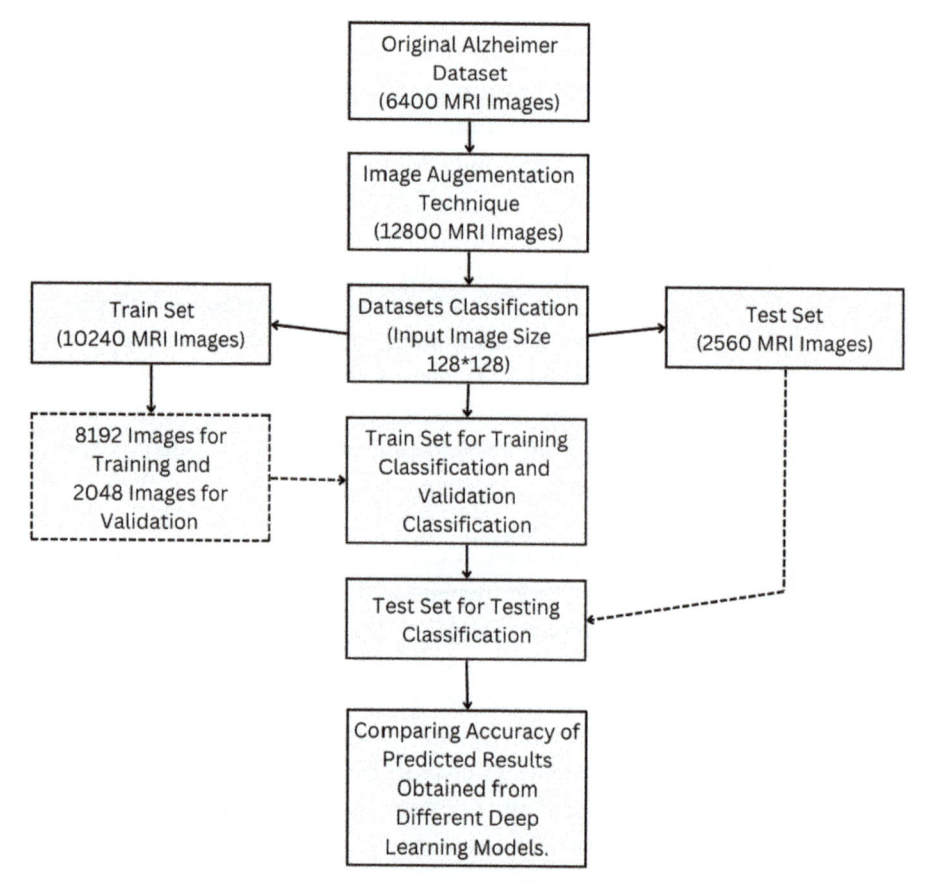

138 Biomedical robots and devices in healthcare

Fig. 7.1 Flowchart illustrates the steps taken from obtaining the image database to comparing different deep learning models.

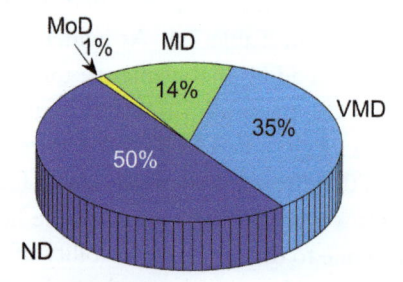

Fig. 7.2 Distribution of Alzheimer's MRI images.

This inherent class imbalance is a crucial test of the strength of the learning models and their ability to generalize well. To mitigate the imbalance and improve model robustness, the number of images was increased to 12,800 using augmentation techniques prior to training. Augmentation helps expose the model to diverse representations of the data and reduces overfitting [23]. Further elaboration on the specifics of the data augmentation

Table 7.1 Brain MRI Samples.

ND brain MRI records

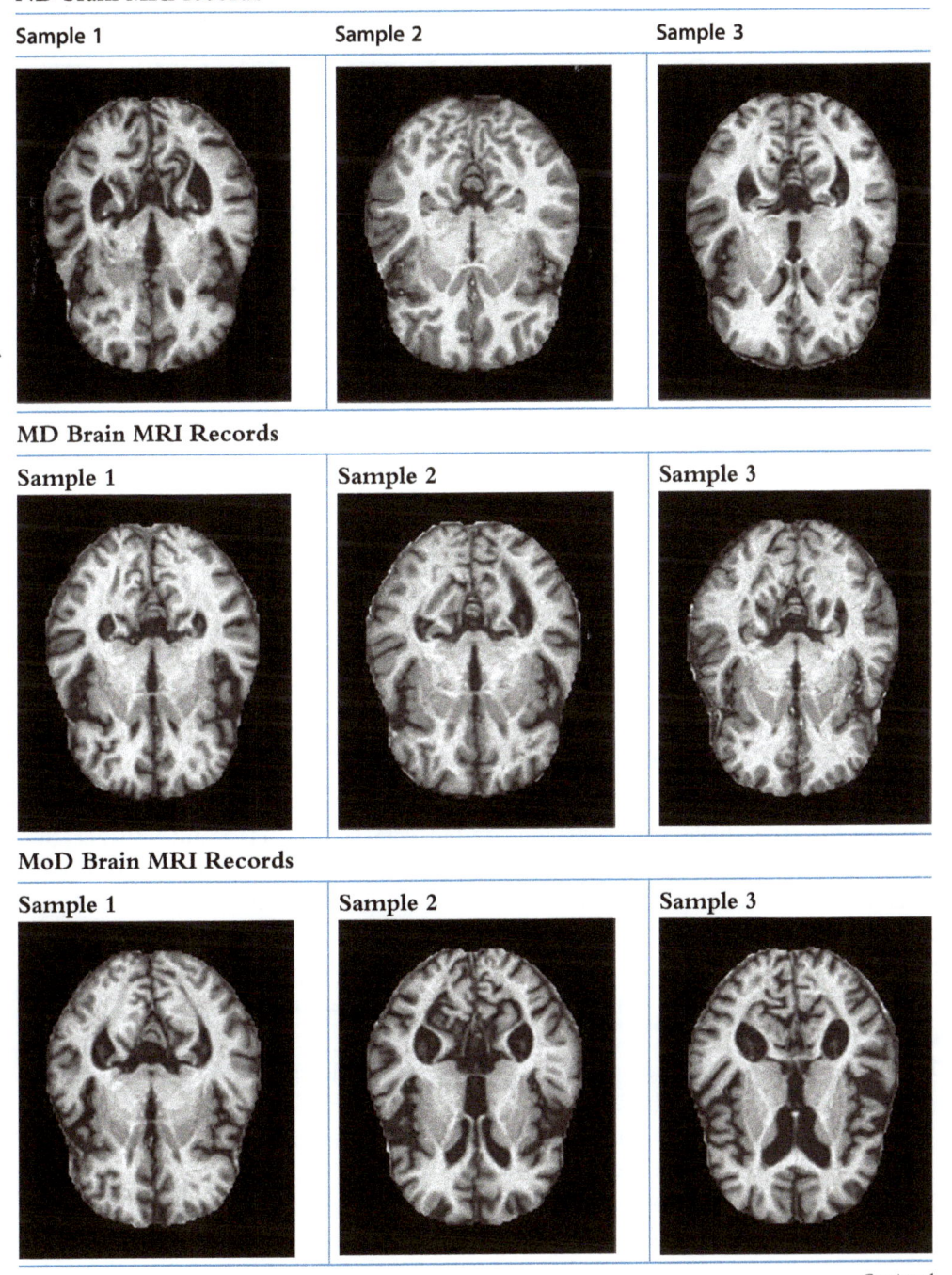

Sample 1	Sample 2	Sample 3

MD Brain MRI Records

Sample 1	Sample 2	Sample 3

MoD Brain MRI Records

Sample 1	Sample 2	Sample 3

Continued

Table 7.1 Brain MRI Samples—cont'd

VMD Brain MRI Records

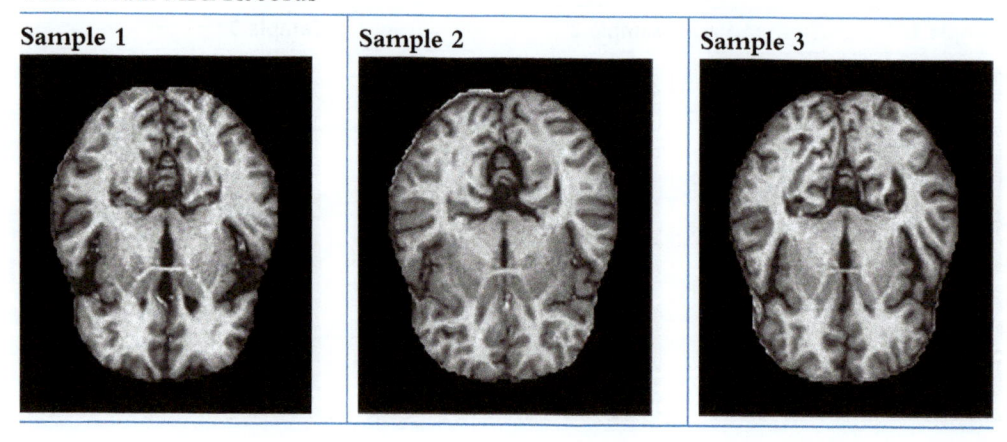

Sample 1	Sample 2	Sample 3

techniques is provided in the subsequent subsection. Despite the imbalance, the variety in data across the four subtle stages of Alzheimer's dementia can allow for granular diagnosis and disease monitoring. Comparative assessment of DL techniques on this dataset can provide insights into optimal models for multiclass classification problems in medical imaging.

7.2.2 Data augmentation

Data augmentation techniques are applied carefully to avoid overfitting. The aim is to overcome the challenges of having limited data in each class and enhance the models' ability to detect important patterns in medical imaging data, regardless of variations and distortions. In the realm of data augmentation, various techniques are judiciously employed to introduce diversity and variability into the dataset, ultimately enhancing the robustness and generalization capacity of the DL models. The following is a concise description of the principal data augmentation techniques utilized in this study:

1. **Rotation:** Rotation augmentation involves rotating images by a specified degree. This technique allows the models to recognize the same features from different orientations, which can be particularly relevant in medical imaging, where the precise orientation of structures may vary.
2. **Flip:** Horizontal and vertical flipping involves mirroring the image. It aids in ensuring that the model is invariant to changes in orientation, which is vital when interpreting medical images with varying perspectives.

3. **Zoom:** Zoom augmentation scales images in and out, introducing variations in the size and perspective of the objects within the image. This assists in improving the model's ability to recognize features regardless of their scale.
4. **Enhances adaptability:** Manipulating the brightness and contrast levels within images serves to simulate different lighting conditions, thereby enhancing the model's adaptability to fluctuations in image quality.
5. **Gaussian Noise:** The introduction of Gaussian noise involves adding random pixel values to the image. This technique helps the model learn to distinguish true features from noise, a crucial skill in real-world medical image analysis.
6. **Shearing:** Shearing introduces slanting distortions in the image, enhancing the model's ability to handle skewed anatomical structures. Rectangular sections of images sheared horizontally and vertically to introduce shape deformations.
7. **Cropping:** Random cropping focuses the model's attention on different regions within the image. This technique enhances the model's capacity to detect relevant features across various image compositions.

7.2.3 Machine learning models

This section discusses the core components of three DL technique that has been used, namely CNN, VGG-16, and ResNet-50. Each of these models plays a pivotal role in the early prediction of AD from medical imaging data.

7.2.3.1 Convolutional neural network

The CNN is a cornerstone within DL, designed specifically for image analysis tasks. Comprised of multiple layers, each serving a distinct purpose in feature extraction and classification, this model recognizes and categorizes visual attributes present in images. Fundamentally, a CNN encompasses various components: an input layer, one or more hidden layers, and an output layer. The hidden layers include convolutional layers, pooling layers, and fully connected layers. These layers execute specialized functions on the input data, sequentially transmitting their outputs to subsequent layers in the network. The convolutional layer employs filters to extract intricate features like edges, shapes, and textures from the input image. These filters, represented as matrices of weights, slide across the image, performing dot product computations with specific image regions. This process captures complex visual patterns within the input data. As the network progresses through these layers, it gains the ability to discern intricate patterns, crucial for medical imaging analysis. The convolutional layers utilize operations to identify crucial features within the input images. This progression aids in recognizing edges, textures, and specific image components relevant to medical imaging data, resulting in a feature map depicting filter activation across the image. The convolutional layers utilize 5×5 kernel filters to extract spatial features from input images, subsequently followed by max-pooling operations to down-sample feature map dimensions. Pooling layers reduce feature map sizes,

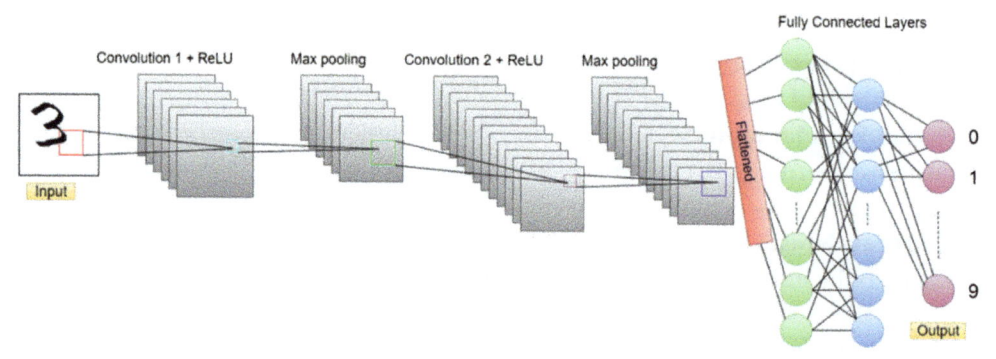

Fig. 7.3 A schematic representation of a CNN architecture [24].

mitigating computational complexity, preventing overfitting, and preserving crucial spatial information. Further in the architecture, fully connected layers integrate high-level features from preceding layers, facilitating the final classification task. Situated at the network's end, these layers map learned features to class labels, crucial for predicting AD within this context. The output layer, typically with neurons equal to the number of classes, leverages a softmax function to generate probability scores for each class. This CNN architecture, as depicted in Fig. 7.3, incorporates two convolutional layers, two pooling layers, and one fully connected layer. The stacked convolutional and pooling layers aid in identifying discriminative features indicative of Alzheimer's stages.

Transfer learning is another approach that can save time and resources by reusing the learned features and avoiding training from scratch. Transfer learning promotes faster convergence and improved performance compared to training networks from scratch [25]. Transfer learning leverages pretrained models developed for general image classification tasks and adapt them to new, specific tasks, such as AD prediction. In our study, two well-established transfer learning architectures are employed: VGG-16 and ResNet-50. These models can extract high-level features that are useful for various image recognition tasks. VGG-16 and ResNet-50 stand as well-established deep CNNs acknowledged for attaining state-of-the-art accuracy in various computer vision tasks [26,27]. These models are initially instantiated with preexisting weights trained on the ImageNet dataset. Subsequently, they underwent fine-tuning via transfer learning techniques specifically applied to the Alzheimer's MRI dataset.

7.2.3.2 VGG-16

The VGG-16 model, proposed by Simonyan and Zisserman [26], is a simple and effective CNN architecture with 16 layers, including 13 convolutional layers and 3 fully connected layers. The convolutional layers use 3×3 filters with a stride of 1 and padding of 1, while the pooling layers use 2×2 max pooling with a stride of 2. The fully

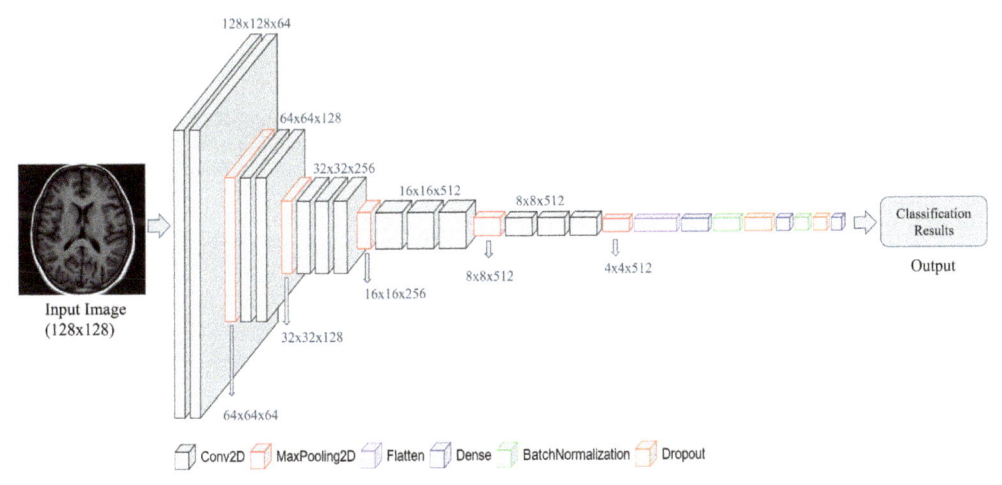

Fig. 7.4 The VGG16 architecture [28].

connected layers have 4096, 4096, and 1000 neurons, respectively. The VGG-16 is known for its ability to capture complex image details, as shown in Fig. 7.4.

It has multiple convolutional layers for spatial feature extraction, followed by fully connected layers for classification. These pretrained models are useful for medical image analysis tasks because they can extract robust features from large datasets. By fine-tuning these models on the AD dataset, we can leverage their pretraining knowledge and adapt their feature extraction skills to the specific challenges of AD prediction. The VGG-16 model is compared with other CNN architectures to gain insights into the optimal DL techniques for multiclass AD prediction from MRI scans.

7.2.3.3 ResNet-50

ResNet-50, introduced by He et al. [27], is a 50-layer CNN architecture that uses residual connections to overcome the vanishing gradient problem in deep networks. These connections act as shortcuts that skip one or more layers and add the input to the output of the skipped layers. This allows the network to learn deeper and more complex features without degrading the performance. The convolutional layers use different filter sizes (1×1, 3×3) with varying channel numbers, while the pooling layers use 2×2 max pooling or average pooling with a stride of 2. The fully connected layers have 2048 and 1000 neurons, respectively. ResNet-50 is shown in Fig. 7.5.

To apply transfer learning with ResNet-50 or VGG-16, the last classification layer of the pretrained model was replaced with a fully connected layer with the number of classes to be predicted. Some or all of the pretrained layers were frozen or fine-tuned by controlling their update during training. This way, the pretrained model was adapted to the specific dataset and task.

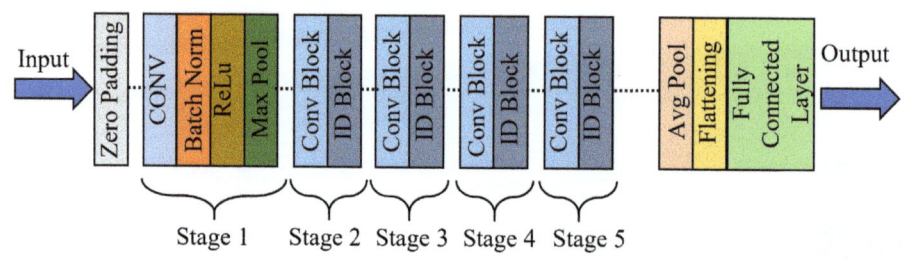

Fig. 7.5 The ResNet50 model architecture.

7.2.4 Evaluation metrics

In the context of evaluating machine learning models, especially for classification tasks such as AD prediction, several metrics are used to assess their performance. Among these, "Accuracy," "Precision," "Recall," "F1 score," and "Support" are fundamental metrics that provide insights into how well a model is performing. These are explained below:

7.2.4.1 Accuracy

Accuracy in the classification model represents the number of correct predictions with respect to the total number of predictions. It is calculated by dividing the number of true positives (TP) and true negatives (TN) by the sum of true positives, true negatives, false positives (FP), and false negatives (FN):

$$\text{Accuracy} = \frac{TP + TN}{TP + TN + FP + FN}$$

Accuracy is a simple and intuitive metric, but it has some limitations. It does not account for the class imbalance problem, where some classes have more samples than others. In such cases, accuracy can be misleading, as it can be inflated by the majority class.

7.2.4.2 Precision

Precision serves as a metric that evaluates the proportion of correctly predicted positive instances within the total predicted positives by the model. It elucidates the model's ability to avoid mislabeling negative samples as positive. A higher precision value indicates the model's confidence and accuracy in positive predictions. Mathematically, precision is calculated as the ratio of TP to the sum of TP and FP, represented by the formula:

$$\text{Precision} = \frac{TP}{TP + FP}$$

Often termed as the positive predictive value, precision gauges the accuracy of a model's positive predictions. Specifically in the domain of AD prediction, precision delineates the proportion of correctly identified cases of AD (true positives) among all the cases that the model predicted as positive (TP and FP). A higher precision value signifies a lower rate of false alarms, indicating the model's proficiency in accurately identifying instances of AD.

7.2.4.3 Recall
The fraction of positive instances that are correctly identified as such among all the actual positives is called recall. It is also known as sensitivity or TP rate. This metric evaluates how effectively the model detects all positive samples, demonstrating its sensitivity in capturing relevant instances of a specific class. Mathematically, recall is calculated using the following formula:

$$\text{Recall} = \frac{\text{TP}}{\text{TP} + \text{FN}}$$

In the context of AD prediction, recall highlights the model's capability to correctly identify cases of AD (True Positives) in relation to all actual Alzheimer's cases (TP and FN). A higher recall value indicates the model's effectiveness in capturing a larger proportion of Alzheimer's cases, emphasizing its comprehensiveness in identifying these instances.

7.2.4.4 F1 score
The F1 score serves as a unified metric that harmonizes both precision (P) and recall (R), offering a comprehensive assessment of a model's performance. It is calculated as the harmonic mean of P and R, aiming to strike a balance between these two metrics. Mathematically, the F1 score is computed using the formula:

$$\text{F1 score} = \frac{2 \times P \times R}{P + R}$$

This metric proves particularly valuable when dealing with class imbalances, as it accounts for FP and FN. A higher F1 score indicates a model that adeptly balances P and R, effectively identifying TP cases while minimizing false alarms. Consequently, it showcases the model's ability to achieve both high P and high R at the same time.

7.2.4.5 Support
Support is an important metric that shows the number of samples in each class in the dataset. It reveals how balanced or imbalanced the dataset is. A class with a low support value means that there are not many samples for that class, which can affect the model's learning ability. For AD prediction, support means the actual number of samples in different classes such as VMD, MD, MoD, and ND. In summary, key metrics have already been discussed to measure the model's accuracy, completeness, and balance in predicting AD versus nondisease cases. However, support provides useful context by showing the data distribution among different classes, which helps to understand other metrics and the model's performance.

7.3 Results and discussion

The original dataset comprised 6400 MRI scans distributed unevenly across MD (896 images), MoD (64 images), ND (3200 images), and VMD (2240 images) classes. Data augmentation techniques are used to increase the number of images to 12,800 and overcome the imbalance across categories. The images, standardized to a size of 128×128, are systematically partitioned into training, validation, and testing sets. Notably, 20% of the data is reserved for testing, with the remaining 80% split into validation and training sets. Thus, the augmented dataset is split into training (8192 images), validation (2048 images), and testing (2560 images) sets. A batch size of 32 and a training duration of 100 epochs are chosen to train the DL models. In this study, three formidable DL models, namely CNN, ResNet-50, and VGG-16, are employed to tackle the task of AD prediction from medical images. These models, known for their efficacy in image analysis, are fine-tuned and trained on the augmented dataset to extract and classify features indicative of AD. The significance of these models' performance lies in their ability to effectively distinguish between cases of AD at different stages and ND individuals, which is vital for early intervention and treatment. Comparative analysis of these models is based on precision, recall, and F1 score and supports critical insights into DL techniques for multiclass classification of Alzheimer's stages. The key findings are discussed in the following section.

Table 7.2 details the training, validation, and testing accuracies, with VGG-16 outperforming the others in all categories, followed by ResNet-50 and CNN. VGG-16 stands out with the highest precision, recall, and F1 score for all classes, indicating its superior accuracy in image classification and its effectiveness in reducing both FP and negatives. While VGG-16 is the preferred model based on these metrics, it is important to consider other factors such as computational resources and training time when

Table 7.2 Performance metrics (precision, recall, F1 score, and support) for various classes achieved by CNN, ResNet-50, and VGG-16 models.

Deep learning model	Class	Precision	Recall	F1 score	Support
CNN	MD	0.85	0.64	0.73	662
	MoD	0.71	0.81	0.76	624
	ND	0.86	0.95	0.90	639
	VMD	0.97	1	0.98	635
ResNet-50	MD	0.86	0.31	0.45	662
	MoD	0.48	0.87	0.62	624
	ND	0.79	0.68	0.73	639
	VMD	1	1	1	635
VGG-16	MD	0.85	0.84	0.85	662
	MoD	0.84	0.82	0.83	624
	ND	0.91	0.94	0.92	639
	VMD	1	1	1	635

choosing a model for practical applications. In scenarios where resources or time are limited, ResNet-50 or CNN may be more suitable choices. The selection process should balance performance with practicality to ensure the chosen model is feasible for the intended use. Accuracy, the primary metric of evaluation, measures the proportion of images correctly classified out of the total number. Further analysis includes confusion matrices for the testing set, which detail the number and percentage of accurate and inaccurate predictions for each class.

Fig. 7.6 presents the confusion matrices for three deep learning models: CNN (top left), ResNet-50 (top right), and VGG-16 (bottom left). Each matrix compares the actual and predicted classes of AD, namely MD, MoD, ND, and VMD. The diagonal entries indicate the correct classifications, while the off-diagonal entries show the misclassifications. The column-normalized column summaries and the row-normalized row summaries provide additional information on the percentage of correct and incorrect classifications for each predicted and true class, respectively. The confusion matrices reveal the superior performance of VGG-16 over CNN and ResNet-50 in this classification task. VGG-16 achieves the highest accuracy for all four classes, with very few errors. It excels in distinguishing the MD class, which is the most challenging category

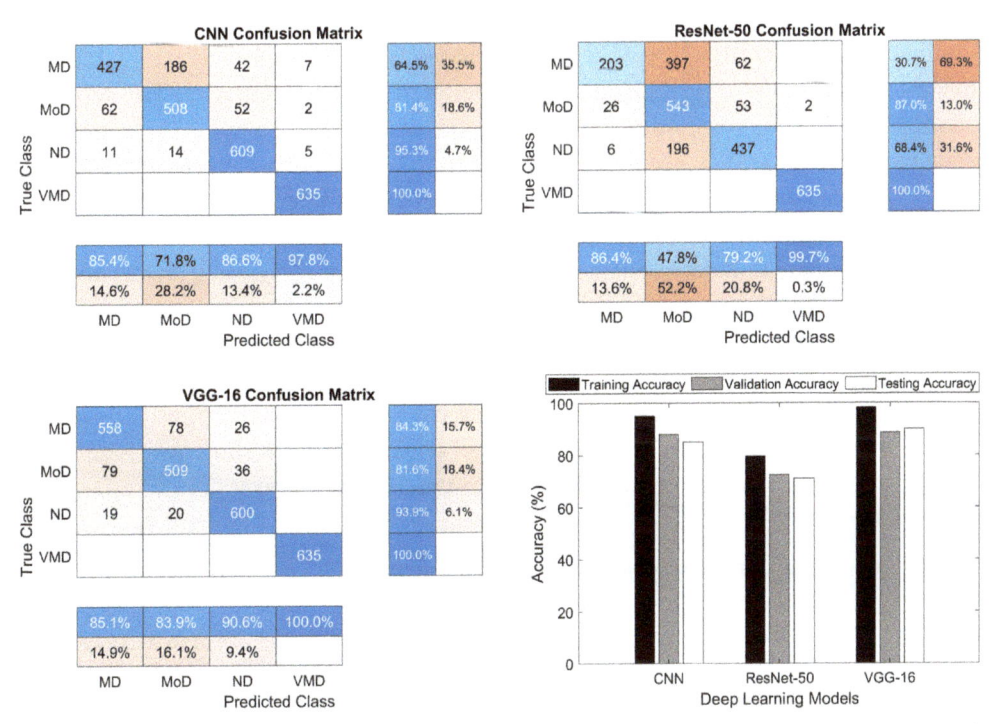

Fig. 7.6 Confusion matrices for CNN, ResNet-50, and VGG-16 models, along with a bar graph comparing their training, validation, and testing accuracy.

for the other two models. The CNN and ResNet-50 models exhibit challenges in accurately predicting the MD class, frequently misclassifying most instances as MoD or ND. However, CNN's accuracy for the MD class is higher than ResNet-50's.

The column-normalized column summaries and the row-normalized row summaries further reveal the performance of these models. For instance, in the CNN confusion matrix, the column summary for the MD class shows that it is correctly predicted 64.5% of the time and incorrectly predicted 35.5% of the time as either MoD, ND, or VMD. The row summary indicates that 85.4% of the actual MD instances are correctly classified, while 14.6% of the instances from other classes are misclassified as MD. Both CNN and ResNet-50 models have a high error rate in classifying MoD, as they often confuse it with MD, ND, or VMD. The row summary shows that 28.2% and 52.2% of the true MoD instances are misclassified by CNN and ResNet-50, respectively. In contrast, VGG-16 has less error, as it most of the time correctly classifies all the MoD instances compared to other models. The column summary for the MD class by ResNet-50 shows a dismal performance, with a 69.3% misclassification rate, indicating that ResNet-50 fails to recognize most of the MD instances. The overall analysis of the confusion matrices confirms that VGG-16 is the most reliable and robust model for this complex classification problem.

Training, validation, and testing accuracy are also given in Fig. 7.6 for different DL techniques in the bottom right as a bar graph. These values are also presented in Table 7.3. They show that VGG-16 is performing much better in all three accuracies. This superior performance of VGG-16 might be attributed to its increased complexity, boasting a higher number of layers that enable the model to learn intricate data patterns. It is essential to recognize that a machine learning model's accuracy can fluctuate depending on the specific dataset and task at hand. Additionally, when assessing model performance, considering other metrics like precision and recall alongside accuracy is crucial for a comprehensive evaluation.

Fig. 7.7A displays the training and validation accuracy for the CNN model, where training accuracy swiftly surpasses 80% within 50 epochs before stabilizing at approximately 90%. The validation accuracy mirrors this pattern but remains consistently lower than the training accuracy. In contrast, the ResNet-50 model, as shown in Fig. 7.7B, achieves a training accuracy of over 75% after 50 epochs, peaking at around 80%. The

Table 7.3 Comparison of training, validation, and testing accuracy for CNN, ResNet-50, and VGG-16 models.

Model	Training accuracy	Validation accuracy	Testing accuracy
CNN	94.89%	87.98%	85.12%
ResNet-50	79.48%	72.41%	71.01%
VGG-16	98.16%	88.57%	89.92%

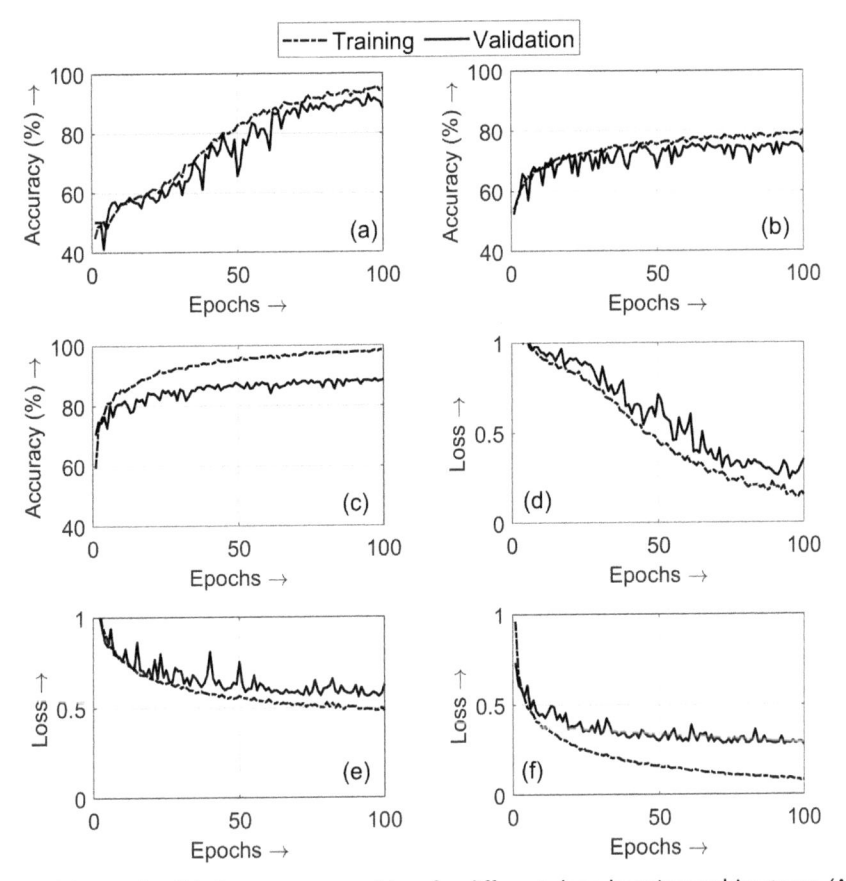

Fig. 7.7 Training and validation accuracy and loss for different deep learning architectures. (A) CNN accuracy, (B) ResNet-50 accuracy, (C) VGG-16 accuracy, (D) CNN loss, (E) ResNet-50 loss, and (F) VGG-16 loss.

VGG-16 model, depicted in Fig. 7.7C, outperforms the other two models with a training accuracy exceeding 95% after 50 epochs and leveling off near 98%. Its validation accuracy also ranks the highest, approaching 90%, which demonstrates VGG-16's superior performance in both training and validation phases compared to CNN and ResNet-50. However, its validation accuracy is also lower than that of its training counterpart, indicating a higher susceptibility to overfitting in this instance. Fig. 7.7D illustrates the training and validation loss for the CNN model, which gradually declines to below 0.5 after 50 epochs and reduces further to under 0.1. The validation loss follows a similar trajectory but is slightly elevated compared to the training loss, indicating effective learning with potential for enhancement. Fig. 7.7E reveals that the ResNet-50 model's training loss diminishes to only 0.6 after 50 epochs and settles around 0.5 after 80 epochs. Its validation loss is comparable to the training loss. Lastly, Fig. 7.7F shows that the VGG-16 model achieves the lowest training and validation loss among the three models. Although the validation loss is higher than the training loss, indicating some overfitting, the small loss percentage suggests that VGG-16 still performs better than the other models. This implies that despite some overfitting, VGG-16 is the most effective model for this dataset.

7.4 Conclusion

This chapter compares the performance of three DL models—CNN, ResNet-50, and VGG-16—for multiclass AD prediction using MRI images. VGG-16 outperforms the other models, achieving a testing accuracy of 89.9% and high precision, recall, and F1 scores for all four classes—nondemented, MD, moderate demented, and VMD. The confusion matrices reveal that VGG-16 accurately classifies most samples, while CNN and ResNet-50 struggle with MD cases. These results confirm the effectiveness of complex deep CNN architectures in capturing subtle imaging patterns indicative of different Alzheimer's stages. The findings also suggest that pretrained networks fine-tuned via transfer learning, such as VGG-16, can surpass shallow CNNs built from scratch. The high accuracy, precision, and recall of VGG-16 demonstrate its reliability for automated medical image analysis and computer-aided diagnosis. However, the performance of DL models may vary depending on the data and task, and VGG-16 shows some signs of overfitting, which can be mitigated by regularization and dropout. This study illustrates the potential of AI techniques for enhancing clinical decision-making in neurological disorders using medical imaging data.

References

[1] T. Zhang, Y. Yang, M. Shokr, C. Mi, X.M. Li, X. Cheng, F. Hui, Deep learning-based sea ice classification with Gaofen-3 fully polarimetric SAR data, Remote Sens. 13 (8) (2021) 1452.
[2] A.L. Fymat, On dementia and other cognitive disorders, Clin. Res. Neurol. 2 (1) (2019) 1–4.
[3] C. Patterson, World Alzheimer Report 2018, The State of the art of Dementia Research: New frontiers, Alzheimer's Disease International, 2018, pp. 1–46.
[4] A. Wimo, G.-C. Ali, M. Guerchet, M. Prince, M. Prina, Y.-T. Wu, World Alzheimer Report 2015, The Global Impact of Dementia: An Analysis of Prevalence, Incidence, Cost and Trends, Alzheimer's Disease International, 2015, pp. 1–82.
[5] Alzheimer's disease international, Dementia statistics, 2021, Available: https://www.alzint.org/about/dementia-facts-figures/dementia-statistics/.
[6] B. Reisberg, S.H. Ferris, M.J. de Leon, T. Crook, The global deterioration scale for assessment of primary degenerative dementia, Am. J. Psychiatry 139 (9) (1982) 1136–1139.
[7] B. Dubois, A. Padovani, P. Scheltens, A. Rossi, G. Dell'Agnello, Timely diagnosis for Alzheimer's disease: a literature review on benefits and challenges, J. Alzheimers Dis. 49 (3) (2016) 617–631.
[8] L. Mittendorff, A. Young, J. Sim, A narrative review of current and emerging MRI safety issues: what every MRI technologist (radiographer) needs to know, J. Med. Radiat. Sci. 69 (2) (2022) 250–260.
[9] P.S. Sisodia, G.K. Ameta, Y. Kumar, N. Chaplot, A review of deep transfer learning approaches for class-wise prediction of Alzheimer's disease using MRI images, Arch. Comput. Methods Eng. 30 (4) (2023) 2409–2429.

[10] A. Khalid, E.M. Senan, K. Al-Wagih, M.M. Ali Al-Azzam, Z.M. Alkhraisha, Automatic analysis of MRI images for early prediction of Alzheimer's disease stages based on hybrid features of CNN and handcrafted features, Diagnostics 13 (9) (2023) 1654.

[11] G. Liu, L. Zhang, Y. Fan, W. Ji, The pathogenesis in Alzheimer's disease: TREM2 as a potential target, J. Integr. Neurosci. 22 (6) (2023) 150.

[12] S.C. Burnham, L. Iaccarino, M.J. Pontecorvo, A.S. Fleisher, M. Lu, E.C. Collins, M.D. Devous Sr., A review of the flortaucipir literature for PET imaging of tau neurofibrillary tangles, Brain Commun. (2023) fcad305.

[13] A. Ayaz, I. Nisar, A. Muhammad, K. Ahmed, P. Chand, F. Jehan, Structural changes in the brain on magnetic resonance imaging in malnourished children: a scoping review of the literature, Pediatr. Neurol. 149 (2023) 151–158.

[14] S. Rathore, M. Habes, M.A. Iftikhar, A. Shacklett, C. Davatzikos, A review on neuroimaging-based classification studies and associated feature extraction methods for Alzheimer's disease and its prodromal stages, NeuroImage 155 (2017) 530–548.

[15] M.M. Yapici, A. Tekerek, N. Topaloğlu, Literature review of deep learning research areas, Gazi Mühendislik Bilimleri Dergisi 5 (3) (2019) 188–215.

[16] Z. Li, F. Liu, W. Yang, S. Peng, J. Zhou, A survey of convolutional neural networks: analysis, applications, and prospects, IEEE Trans. Neural Networks Learn. Syst. 33 (12) (2021) 6999–7019.

[17] S. Tammina, Transfer learning using vgg-16 with deep convolutional neural network for classifying images, Int. J. Sci. Res. Publ. 9 (10) (2019) 143–150.

[18] B. Koonce, B. Koonce, ResNet 50. Convolutional Neural Networks with Swift for Tensorflow: Image Recognition and Dataset Categorization, 2021, pp. 63–72.

[19] S. Kumar, S. Shastri, Alzheimer MRI Preprocessed Dataset, 2022, Retrieved July 15, 2023 from https://www.kaggle.com/datasets/sachinkumar413/alzheimer-mri-dataset. https://doi.org/10.34740/KAGGLE/DSV/3364939.

[20] M. Xu, S. Yoon, A. Fuentes, D.S. Park, A comprehensive survey of image augmentation techniques for deep learning, Pattern Recogn. (2023) 109347.

[21] M.I. Razzak, S. Naz, A. Zaib, Deep Learning for Medical Image Processing: Overview, Challenges and the Future. Classification in BioApps: Automation of Decision Making, 2018, pp. 323–350.

[22] J.M. Johnson, T.M. Khoshgoftaar, Survey on deep learning with class imbalance, J. Big Data 6 (1) (2019) 1–54.

[23] C. Shorten, T.M. Khoshgoftaar, A survey on image data augmentation for deep learning, J. Big Data 6 (1) (2019) 1–48.

[24] A. Al Bataineh, D. Kaur, M. Al-khassaweneh, E. Al-sharoa, Automated CNN architectural design: a simple and efficient methodology for computer vision tasks, Mathematics 11 (5) (2023) 1141.

[25] H.C. Shin, H.R. Roth, M. Gao, L. Lu, Z. Xu, I. Nogues, R.M. Summers, Deep convolutional neural networks for computer-aided detection: CNN architectures, dataset characteristics and transfer learning, IEEE Trans. Med. Imaging 35 (5) (2016) 1285–1298.

[26] K. Simonyan, A. Zisserman, Very deep convolutional networks for large-scale image recognition, arXiv preprint arXiv:1409.1556 (2014).

[27] K. He, X. Zhang, S. Ren, J. Sun, Deep residual learning for image recognition, in: Proceedings of the IEEE Conference on Computer Vision and Pattern Recognition, 2016, pp. 770–778.

[28] A. Gebrehiwot, L. Hashemi-Beni, G. Thompson, P. Kordjamshidi, T.E. Langan, Deep convolutional neural network for flood extent mapping using unmanned aerial vehicles data, Sensors 19 (7) (2019) 1486.

CHAPTER 8

Machine learning brain activation topography for individual skill classification: Need for leave-one-subject-out (LOSO) cross-validation

Takahiro Manabe[a] and Anirban Dutta[b]
[a]University at Buffalo, Amherst, NY, United States
[b]University of Lincoln, United Kingdom

8.1 Background

The fundamentals of laparoscopic surgery (FLS) stands as a pivotal educational curriculum within the realm of surgery training [1]. As an imperative prerequisite for American Board of Surgery certification, it is integral to the Basic and Advanced Laparoscopic Skills Module of the ACS/APDS US Skills Curriculum Project. This module serves as a comprehensive platform for cultivating fundamental surgical skills crucial for the effective execution of laparoscopic procedures. Within this module, learners undertake five psychomotor tasks, namely pegboard transfers, pattern cutting, placement of a ligating loop, and suturing with both extracorporeal and intracorporeal knot tying. Designed to standardize training and assessment methodologies, FLS addresses the cognitive and psychomotor skills indispensable for performing minimally invasive surgery.

We explored the neural underpinnings of FLS skills, delving into the formation of cognitive-perceptual mental models during the initial stages of skill acquisition in a laparoscopic environment. Drawing inspiration from Fitts and Posner's three-stage model for motor skill acquisition, our published study [2] endeavored to unravel the brain-behavior relationship during skill learning through portable brain imaging and machine learning. Here, the brain circuit mechanisms, propelled by motor skill proficiency, involve selective attention and cortical alterations in motor planning and execution. In our investigation [2], we hypothesized that semi-stable brain states [3], embodying selective attention and cortical excitability alterations, can be estimated through the topography of electroencephalogram (EEG). While experts are presumed to possess a preexisting cognitive-perceptual model, novices are anticipated to construct this model upon their initial exposure to FLS tasks. The study leveraged microstate-based analysis of EEG topography, enhancing the traditional common spatial pattern approach [2].

Preliminary results, showcased at the Interservice/Industry Training, Simulation, and Education Conference (I/ITSEC) 2022, demonstrated promising classification accuracy between expert surgeons and novice medical residents [3].

Building upon these findings, our current study presented in this chapter investigates leave-one-subject-out (LOSO) evaluation of the convolutional neural network (CNN)-based approach [2] to identify if individualization is possible. Our CNN approach is motivated by studies demonstrating the classification of cognitive states using an attention-based time-series deep learning framework. By adapting ESNet, a network preserving topography in EEG-based temporal attentive pooling, we provided mechanistic insights into skill learning at a group level [2]. These insights are informed by our own prior studies using functional near-infrared spectroscopy (fNIRS), which identified cortical activation in specific brain regions during FLS tasks [4,5]. However, our studies also found high variability in scalp-recorded EEG signals across individual subjects and recording sessions, a factor often overlooked in EEG-based machine learning studies in many domains [6]. Unlike the common k-fold cross-validation technique used in our prior work [2], this chapter emphasizes the importance of LOSO evaluation for assessing algorithm performance in real-life settings with unseen subjects.

While the holdout method provides a straightforward approach, fivefold cross-validation offers a more robust assessment of a machine learning model's performance [2]. The process of fivefold cross-validation involves segregating a test group from the entire dataset and iteratively dividing the training and test data at a 5:1 ratio for five different combinations. This approach allows for a thorough evaluation of the model's generalization ability, as all data samples are utilized for training, validation, and testing, thus reducing bias and offering a more reliable indication of predictive performance for new data. Despite the advantages of multiple-fold cross-validation, recent discussions have surfaced regarding its application to bio-signal data, particularly in EEG-based machine learning [6]. The authors of the recent paper [6] underscore the significance of "LOSO" cross-validation, particularly in the context of machine learning for EEG (brain waves). Of note, the LOSO evaluation conducted unveiled a crucial insight: k-fold classification results can be misleading when it comes to individual skill classification. Consequently, the paper underscores the necessity of evaluating any EEG-based skill classification method using a LOSO-style cross-validation approach. They highlighted the well-known variability between individual subjects and recording sessions in EEG signals which we also found in our dataset [2]. Surprisingly, most EEG-based machine learning studies do not assess algorithm performance across sessions or subjects, opting instead for training and testing on the entire dataset with established k-fold cross-validation methods.

In summary, this chapter unfolds a comprehensive exploration of the LOSO evaluation of our CNN-based approach [2] to identify if individualization is possible to discern and compare the brain states of experts and novices. The goal is to contribute to a deeper understanding of individual cognitive and perceptual processes involved in laparoscopic surgery skill acquisition.

8.2 Methods

8.2.1 Data collection: Electroencephalography

During the experiment, we employed electroencephalography (EEG) to record brain activity. EEG is a noninvasive method that captures the electrical potentials produced by the brain's electrophysiological activity. These potentials are gathered through electrode channels strategically placed on the human scalp, as illustrated in Fig. 8.1. Given that EEG signals primarily consist of cerebral cortex potentials, they are considered closely linked to an individual's behaviors. For this study, we utilized the wireless LiveAmp system (Brain Vision, USA), depicted by the gray "E" discs in Fig. 8.2, to record 32 channels of EEG signals. The sampling frequency during data collection was set at 500 Hz.

8.2.2 Data preprocessing

All EEG signals obtained underwent a comprehensive preprocessing and epoching process, detailed in Fig. 8.3, utilizing the EEGLAB toolbox within the MATLAB environment (MathWorks Inc., USA). In the initial preprocessing phase, frequency filtering was applied to the EEG signals. Following Klug et al.'s recommendation in our prior work [2], a high-pass filter with a cutoff frequency of 1 Hz was selected. This specific cutoff frequency is known to yield the lowest rejection threshold (RV) for independent components other than EEG, such as electromyograms (EMG), ultimately enhancing the quality of independent component analysis (ICA) decomposition [2].

Subsequently, noise removal procedures were implemented using the *cleanline* and *clean_rawdata* plugins integrated into EEGLAB. The data was then rereferenced to a common average reference, and ICA was employed for artifact removal. ICA, a widely used feature extraction method in EEG preprocessing, was applied using the *runica* function, a mainstream algorithm for ICA signal decomposition. Fig. 8.4 provides visual examples of high-quality, independent components extracted through ICA, typically representing the alpha and beta frequency bands of EEG (1–30 Hz).

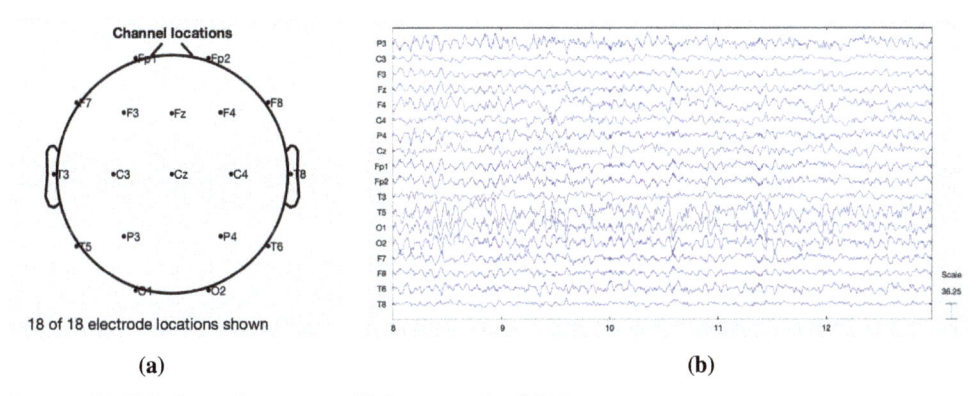

Fig. 8.1 (A) EEG channel montage. (B) An example of EEG.

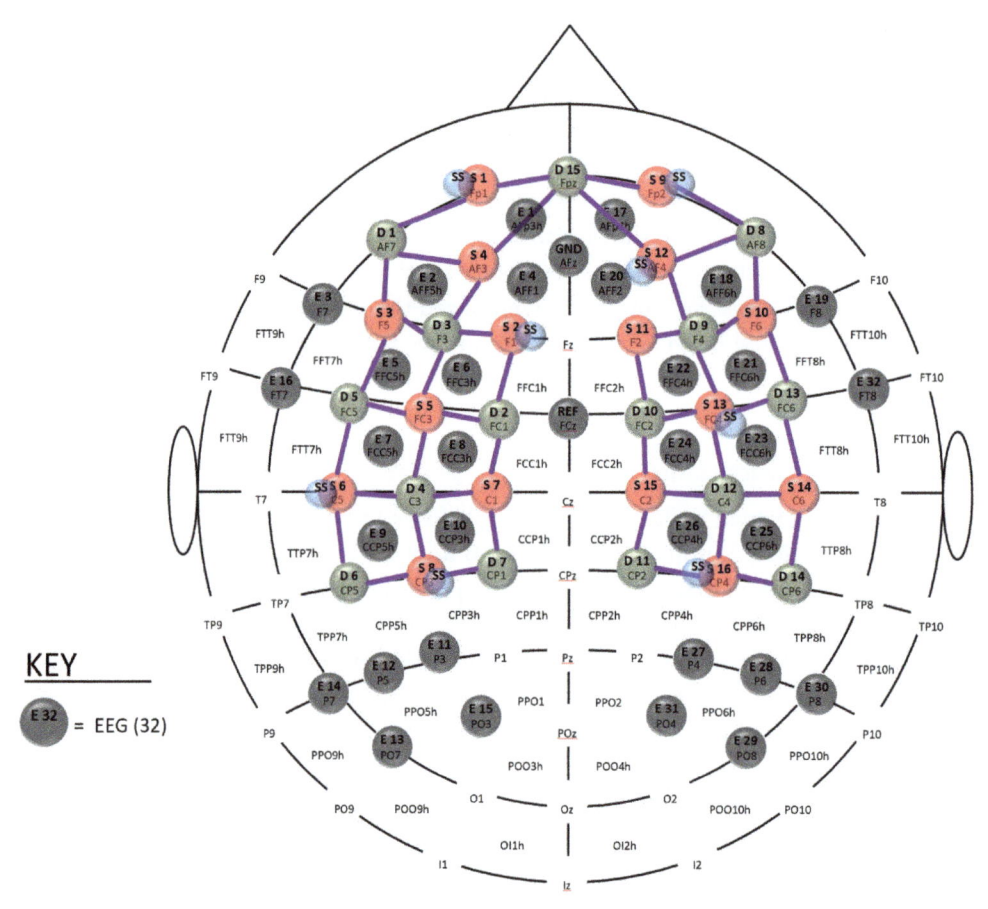

156 Biomedical robots and devices in healthcare

Fig. 8.2 Multimodal sensor montage where the 32 active EEG electrodes are represented with *gray* discs.

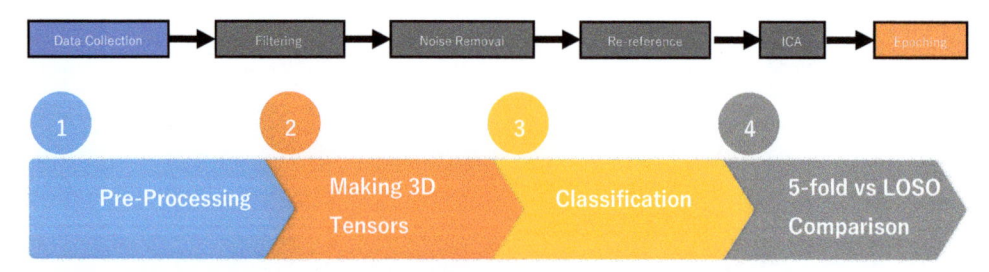

Fig. 8.3 EEG data processing process. Top panel shows the preprocessing steps: after the data measurement, preprocessing was performed using filtering, noise removal, and re-referencing, followed by applying independent component analysis (ICA). Subsequently, the dataset was segmented into 1-s epochs. Bottom panel shows the subsequent CNN analysis steps for comparison of fivefold cross-validation with LOSO cross-validation.

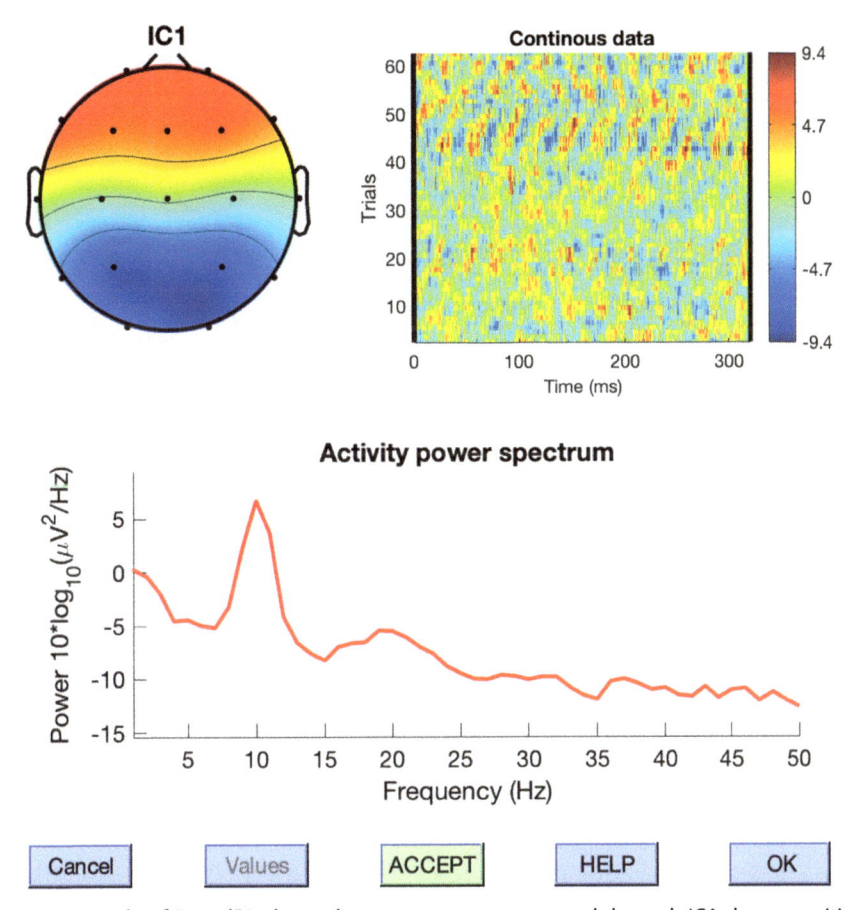

Fig. 8.4 An example of "good" independent components extracted through ICA decomposition with more than 50% brainwave. The top-left figure shows the topography of the decomposed components. The bottom figure represents the power spectrum of the components, highlighting prominent spectral patterns in the frequency range, which is commonly observed in brainwaves (1–30 Hz).

To further enhance the preprocessing pipeline, an automated labeling method was introduced using the ICLabel function, as depicted in Fig. 8.5. This function served to label the components and identify those with a significant number of artifact components. Only components labeled "Brain" with 50% or more confidence were retained. Following these meticulous preprocessing steps, the data was segmented into epochs, each lasting 1 s, with no overlap between epochs. For instance, if an original data segment was precisely 60 s long, it was subdivided into 60 nonoverlapping epochs.

8.2.3 Processing for topography-preserving 3D-CNN

The preprocessing of EEG data is illustrated in Fig. 8.3, capturing unique spatiotemporal patterns exhibited by both experts and novices. Then, transformation into a three-dimensional

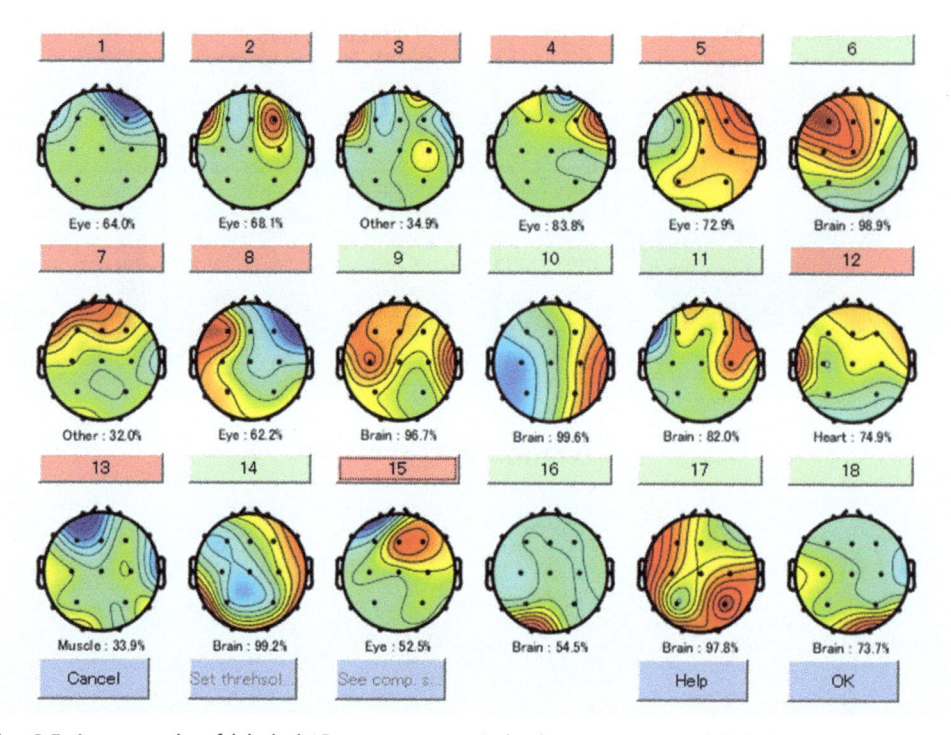

Fig. 8.5 An example of labeled IC components. Only the components labeled as "Brain" with a contribution of 50% or more are kept (*green* labels), while the rest are removed as artifact components (*red* labels).

tensor results in a 3D dataset, where two dimensions represent spatial information, and the third dimension represents time [2]. To achieve this, the EEG time series from each channel is initially downsampled to 120 Hz and then mapped onto a 16 × 16 square grid 2D image using an azimuthal equidistant projection based on the corresponding positions from the scalp EEG montage.

For the FLS task's EEG data analysis, the data 2 s prior to the start trigger is segmented into 3-s segments using a 1-s sliding window, following the method proposed by Kwak et al. [7]. This segmentation process is repeated for all sliding time steps. To interpolate empty locations on the 16 × 16 grid between the projected electrode positions, the griddata() function in Matlab is employed. Notably, the v4 interpolation method is chosen over cubic spline interpolation, as utilized in ESNet, to enhance data quality.

The EEG data is then structured into a 3D tensor, encapsulating spatiotemporal details in the form of height × width × time. Each 3-s EEG time window generates a 3D EEG image (denoted as $X_{eeg} \in R(16 \times 16 \times 360)$) using the ESNet method. With 21 participants (8 experts and 13 novices), each performing the task thrice, this results in 21 participants × 3 repetitions × 180 time windows, yielding a total of 11,340 cuboid tensors.

The ESNet model [7], a 3D CNN, incorporates both spatial and temporal details. It features a specialized temporal attentive pooling (TAP) layer, which efficiently condenses temporal details. Three convolutional layers, each followed by a rectified linear unit (ReLU) activation function, form the core of the model. The channel information is doubled as output in each layer, utilizing short-length kernels and strides for spatial details in all convolutional layers. The TAP layer is vital in pooling spatial and temporal details effectively, enhancing the model's capability. After the three convolutional layers, the TAP layer executes Spatial Attentive Pooling, followed by a fully connected (FC) layer and Softmax activation. This process transforms the original feature, giving more weight to relevant temporal information and efficiently compressing it. Subsequently, the feature undergoes additional processing, passing through an FC layer, ReLU function, Dropout, and Softmax layer. Batch normalization and L2 regularization are strategically implemented to enhance performance and prevent overfitting. Detailed concepts of the TAP layer can be further explored in the original paper by Kwak et al. [7].

8.3 Results

In this chapter, we scrutinized the model accuracy from our prior work [2] by employing two distinct evaluation methods: fivefold cross-validation (see Fig. 8.6) and LOSO cross-validation (see Fig. 8.7). The primary focus of their study was twofold: first, to underscore the importance of LOSO evaluation in EEG-based machine learning, and second, to demonstrate the efficacy of our model [2] in achieving high LOSO accuracy using balanced and clean EEG data. The LOSO approach accounts for the inherent variability in EEG signals across individual subjects and recording sessions, offering a more robust and realistic evaluation of machine learning models in the domain of EEG-based individualization.

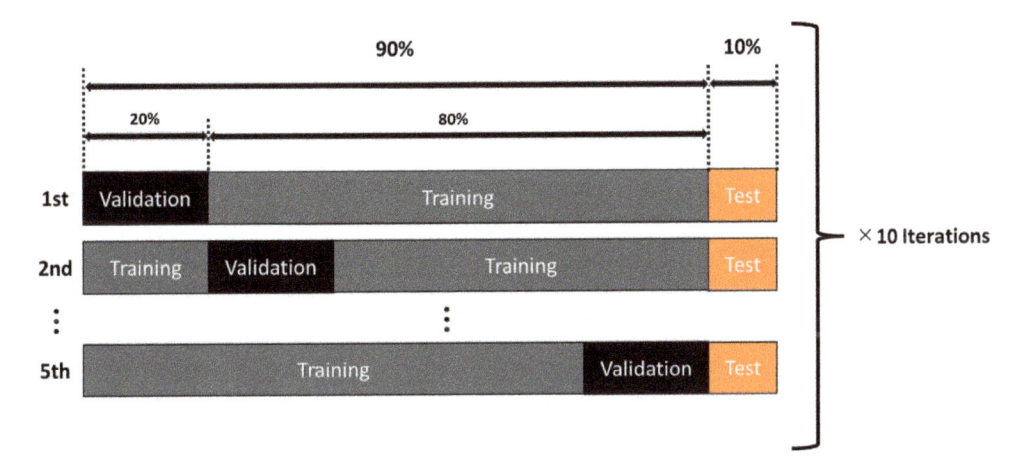

Fig. 8.6 Fivefold cross-validation.

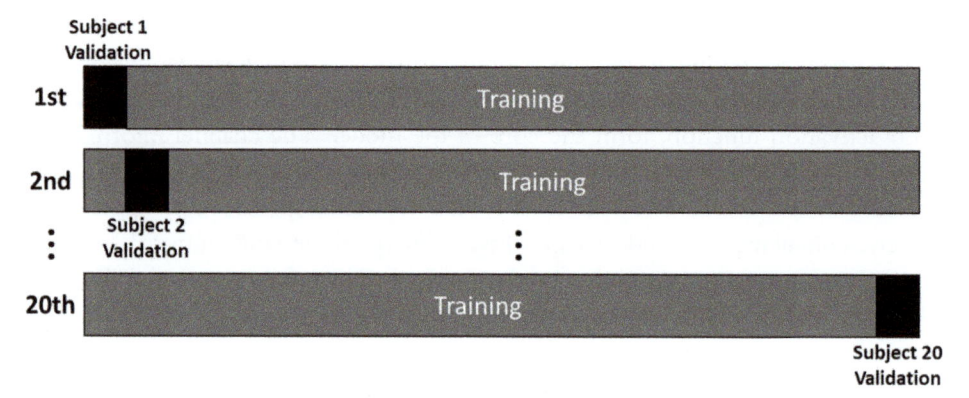

Fig. 8.7 Leave-out-subject-out (LOSO) cross-validation.

8.3.1 Fivefold cross-validation results

Fig. 8.8 provides a visual representation of the model's [2] loss function and accuracy throughout the training and validation processes spanning 200 epochs. The performance of the ESNet model stands out, demonstrating significant learning advancements, albeit with occasional spikes. Notably, the learning curve consistently converges around the midpoint, specifically the 100th epoch, indicating a rapid and effective acquisition of knowledge by the model. Despite the presence of minor fluctuations, the accuracy performance gap between the training and validation phases remains remarkably small. By the conclusion of the 200th epoch, this gap hovers within a modest range of 2.50%. This observation signifies a well-balanced and robust training process, suggesting that the model not only comprehensively learns from the group training data but also generalizes well to unseen data during the validation phase. The stability in the accuracy performance throughout the epochs underscores the model's reliability and consistent predictive

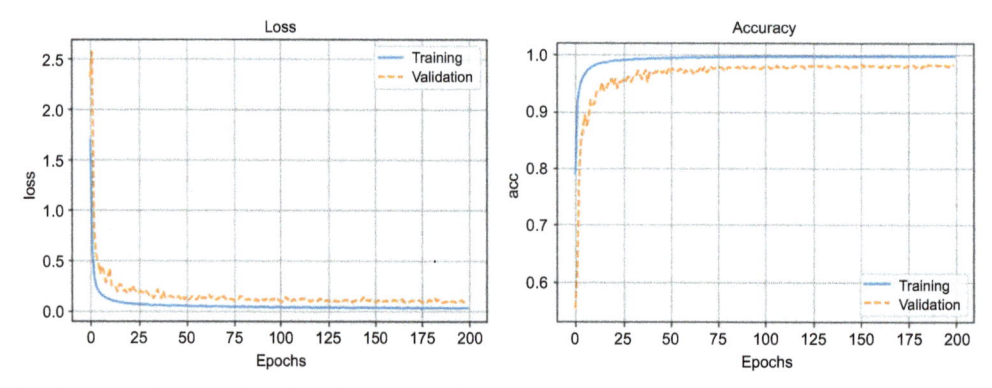

Fig. 8.8 Visualization of the loss function and accuracy of the model [2] during the 200 epochs of training and fivefold cross-validation processes.

capabilities. Overall, the depicted learning curves affirm the ESNet model's proficiency in both rapid learning and maintaining a stable performance across group-level training and validation processes [2].

8.3.2 Leave-one-subject-out cross-validation results

In this analysis, a leave-one-group-out cross-validation, as detailed in the "Methods" section, was executed. This approach involved excluding one participant's epoch from the dataset and employing the removed epochs as validation data. Fig. 8.9 depicts the average results of these validations, irrespective of their classification category. The figures illustrate the loss functions and accuracy of the model over the course of 200 epochs in the one-group-out cross-validation assessment.

The observed patterns indicate successful training of the model, aligning with the outcomes observed in the fivefold cross-validation. However, when it comes to validation, both the loss function and accuracy exhibit random fluctuations across the epochs. Particularly in the case of accuracy, values are scattered in the range of 60%–70%. This variability suggests that, despite effective training, the model's performance during validation may exhibit unpredictability, emphasizing the importance of further investigation into challenges with EEG signal variability [6] and individualization.

To investigate this LOSO issue further, we present two separate classification accuracy curves with LOSO cross-validation process separately for experts and novices, visualized in Figs. 8.10 and 8.11 , respectively. In the case of experts, the model exhibits limited learning, with an accuracy of around 55%, even lower than that of novices. Particularly concerning for experts, the loss function shows an increasing trend with epochs, indicating a potential divergence from learning. The novices' classification curve reveals that the model maintains an accuracy level of approximately 70%, yet there is a lack of discernible improvement over the epochs, suggesting a stagnation in the learning process.

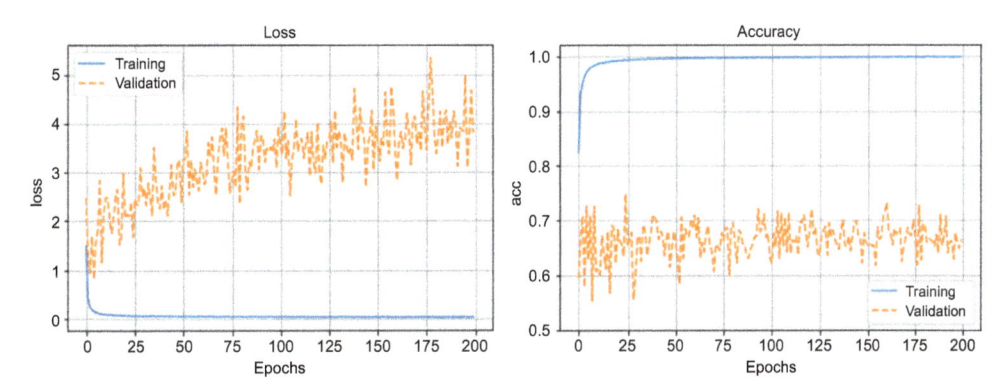

Fig. 8.9 Visualization of the loss function and accuracy of the model [2] during the 200 epochs of training and LOSO cross-validation processes.

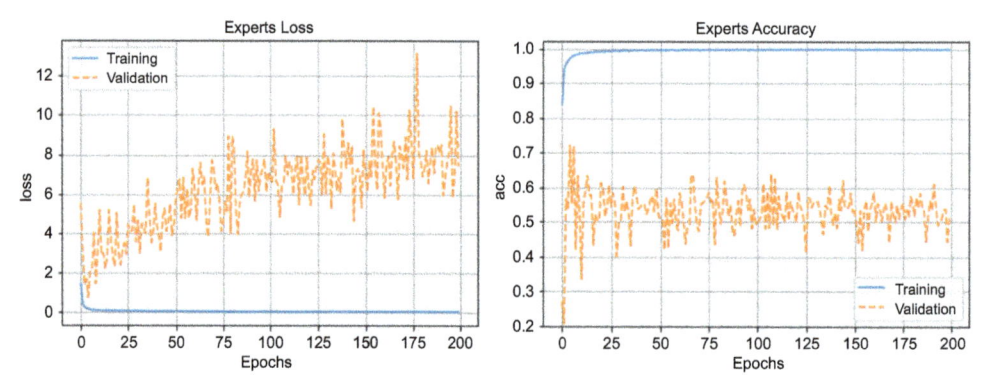

Fig. 8.10 Visualization of the loss function and accuracy of the model [2] during the 200 epochs of training and LOSO cross-validation processes for experts only.

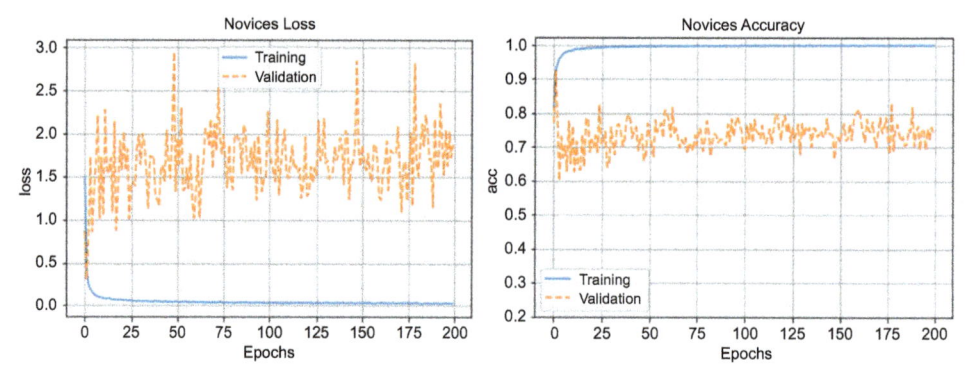

Fig. 8.11 Visualization of the loss function and accuracy of the model [2] during the 200 epochs of training and LOSO cross-validation processes for novices only.

These findings collectively suggest that overall accuracy is not significantly influenced by individual performance. Instead, the key observation is the model's limited capacity to learn essential individual skill-related features from the group data, regardless of whether the subject is in the novices or experts group. This lack of improvement in accuracy over epochs during LOSO cross-validation, coupled with increasing loss in the case of experts, raises concerns about the model's ability to effectively capture and learn meaningful features from the EEG data provided. Further exploration and refinement of the model architecture or training strategy may be necessary to address these limitations and enhance the learning capabilities of the ESNet model for individualization.

8.4 Discussion

The study conducted a crucial evaluation of the LOSO evaluation methodology, emphasizing its necessity in the context of individualized skill classification using scalp-recorded

EEG data. The comparison between k-fold and LOSO evaluations revealed significant insights into the impact of evaluation techniques on the model's performance. Initially, k-fold evaluation demonstrated high accuracy in separating experts versus novices, suggesting a robust learning pattern [2]. However, when the focus shifted to classifying unseen individual subjects, a more realistic scenario, the accuracy dropped with LOSO. This decline implies that, under k-fold, the algorithm tends to learn overall group-specific features rather than individual skill-related features. In conclusion, our study establishes that the k-fold classification result is misleading for individualized skill classification using the scalp-recorded EEG-based ESNet method [7]. Our findings strongly advocate for the adoption of a LOSO-style cross-validation methodology for accurate evaluation of individual skill classification models, ensuring robustness and reliability in real-life scenarios with unseen subjects.

References

[1] FLS Trainer System and Accessories, Fundamentals of Laparoscopic Surgery, 2010, Available at: https://www.flsprogram.org/testing-information/trainer-box/. (Accessed 21 April 2022).

[2] T. Manabe, F.N.U. Rahul, Y. Fu, X. Intes, S.D. Schwaitzberg, S. De, et al., Distinguishing laparoscopic surgery experts from novices using EEG topographic features, Brain Sci. 13 (2023) 1706, https://doi.org/10.3390/brainsci13121706.

[3] T. Manabe, P. Walia, Y. Fu, X. Intes, S. De, S. Schwaitzberg, et al., EEG Topographic Features for Assessing Skill Levels During Laparoscopic Surgical Training, 2022, https://doi.org/10.21203/rs.3.rs-1934633/v1.

[4] P. Walia, Y. Fu, J. Norfleet, S.D. Schwaitzberg, X. Intes, S. De, et al., Error-related brain state analysis using electroencephalography in conjunction with functional near-infrared spectroscopy during a complex surgical motor task, Brain Inform. 9 (2022) 29, https://doi.org/10.1186/s40708-022-00179-z.

[5] P. Walia, Y. Fu, S.D. Schwaitzberg, X. Intes, S. De, A. Dutta, et al., Portable neuroimaging differentiates novices from those with experience for the fundamentals of laparoscopic surgery (FLS) suturing with intracorporeal knot tying task, Surg. Endosc. (2022), https://doi.org/10.1007/s00464-022-09727-4.

[6] S. Kunjan, T.S. Grummett, K.J. Pope, D.M.W. Powers, S.P. Fitzgibbon, T. Bastiampillai, et al., M. Mahmud, M.S. Kaiser, S. Vassanelli, Q. Dai, N. Zhong, The necessity of leave one subject out (LOSO) cross validation for EEG disease diagnosis, in: Brain Informatics Lecture Notes in Computer Science, Springer International Publishing, Cham, 2021, pp. 558–567, https://doi.org/10.1007/978-3-030-86993-9_50.

[7] Y. Kwak, W.-J. Song, S.-E. Kim, FGANet: fNIRS-guided attention network for hybrid EEG-fNIRS brain-computer interfaces, IEEE Trans. Neural Syst. Rehabil. Eng. 30 (2022) 329–339, https://doi.org/10.1109/TNSRE.2022.3149899.

CHAPTER 9

Transfer learning-based disease prognosis in Biomedicine 4.0: Challenges and opportunities

Senthil Kumar Jagatheesaperumal[a] and Sivasankar Ganesan[b]

[a]Department of Electronics and Communication Engineering, Mepco Schlenk Engineering College, Sivakasi, Tamil Nadu, India
[b]Department of Mechanical Engineering, Amrita School of Engineering, Amrita Vishwa Vidyapeetham, Coimbatore, Tamil Nadu, India

9.1 Introduction

As technological advancements continue, the healthcare solution needs novel interfaces for disease prognosis, which faces additional challenges. With the increasing integration of human–computer interfaces into our daily lives, protecting sensitive information in biomedicine for enhancing the healthcare sector has become a critical concern. Successfully tackling these issues necessitates the seamless incorporation of learning techniques, robust decision-making methods, and effective treatment planning, for enhanced patient outcomes mechanisms.

This chapter examines the implications of evolving transfer learning strategies, by shedding light on the critical importance of disease prognosis in this context. Subsequently, it explores the need for efficient analysis of medical data methods that go beyond traditional healthcare systems, as well as the role of learning techniques in ensuring enhanced accuracy in prognostic models based on healthcare data. Furthermore, this article provides potential solutions to mitigate these risks, such as lack of standardization in prognostic models, addressing disease complexity and variability, and incorporating strategies to enhance accuracy in prognostic models.

Further, the article delves into the challenges and opportunities of transfer learning in Biomedicine 4.0. In addition to addressing these challenges, the article presents opportunities in Biomedicine 4.0 for enhancing treatment outcomes. This approach has the potential to develop innovative healthcare solutions, ensuring improved treatment outcomes, and reduced healthcare costs.

The organization of the sections in this chapter is as follows: Section 9.2 delves into the challenges of disease prognosis and the challenges involved in limited data, data complexity, and standardization issues. Section 9.3 provides an overview of using AI/ML in disease prognosis, including efficient analysis of healthcare data and effective forecasting of disease outcomes. In Section 9.4, we examine potential solutions and strategies to address these challenges, highlighting the opportunities that transfer learning offers for disease prognosis. Finally, Section 9.5 concludes the article, emphasizing the need to transfer learning as we innovate and develop the next generation of robust and trustworthy healthcare systems.

9.2 Challenges in disease prognosis

Disease prognosis is the process of predicting the outcome of a specific medical condition for an individual patient. Despite significant advances in medical science in disease prognosis, healthcare professionals and researchers still face several challenges in this area. Major challenges in disease prognosis include limited data availability, disease complexity and variability, and lack of standardization in prognostic models [1]. Fig. 9.1 shows the major impact of disease prognosis in Biomedicine 4.0 for reaching out to various healthcare sector stakeholders.

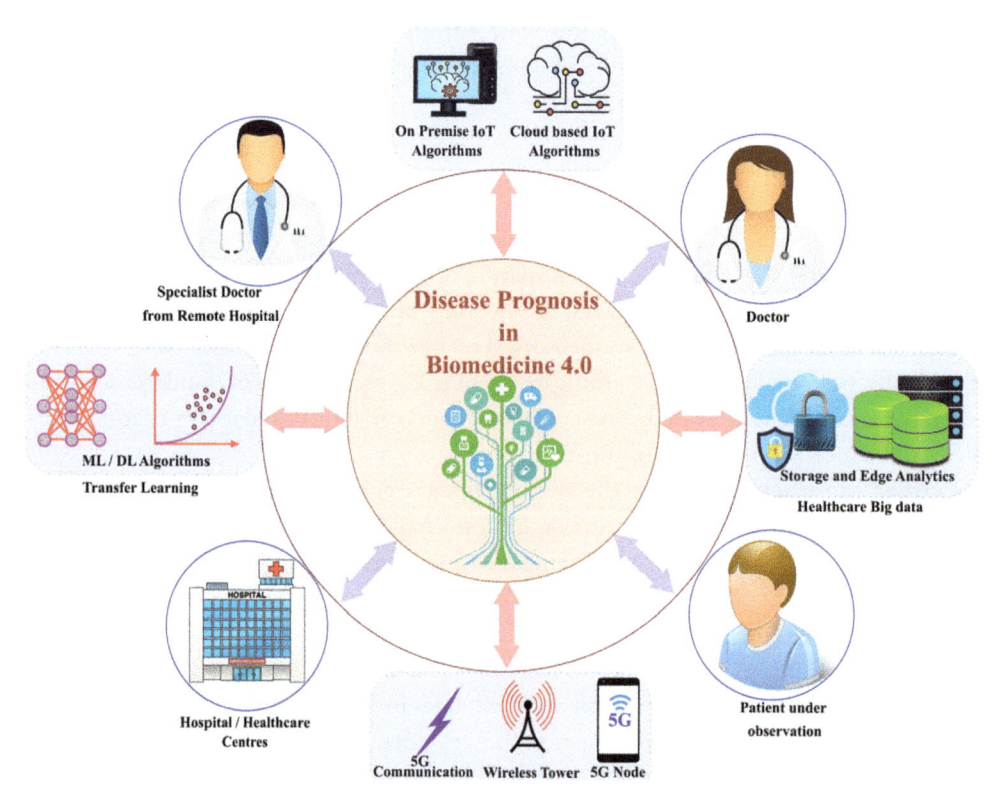

Fig. 9.1 Impact of disease prognosis in Biomedicine 4.0 for the healthcare sector stakeholders.

9.2.1 Limited data availability

Data, such as patient health records, medical imaging, genetic information, and lifestyle factors, are heavily used in disease prognosis. It can be difficult to obtain comprehensive and high-quality data, especially when dealing with rare diseases or patients from diverse backgrounds. The challenge of limited data availability in disease prognosis refers to the difficulty in obtaining a sufficient quantity and quality of data necessary to develop accurate predictive models for estimating the course and outcome of a medical condition [2]. This limitation makes it difficult for healthcare professionals and researchers to make informed decisions about patient care and treatment strategies. Moreover, it has a significant impact on the accuracy of prognosis models.

There are several reasons why data availability on disease prognosis is limited.

- *Small sample size:* Gathering and storing patient data is both costly and time-consuming. Moreover, some diseases are uncommon, affecting only a small number of people. As a result, the patient dataset in that case is quite small. Also, a model trained on a small dataset may not be generalize to new patients. This can result in inaccurate predictions, which can be disastrous for patients.
- *Data privacy:* Patients' medical data is extremely sensitive because it contains personal health information that must be safeguarded to ensure patient privacy. Strict regulations and ethical considerations can limit research access to patient data, impeding the development of comprehensive prognosis models. This can limit access to important datasets.
- *Diversity of patient populations:* Because of genetic, lifestyle, and environmental factors, disease manifestations and outcomes can differ between patient populations. Obtaining data that adequately represents diverse populations, on the other hand, can be difficult, limiting the model's applicability.

There are several approaches that can be taken to address the issue of limited data availability in disease prognosis. One approach is to create new methods for gathering and storing patient data. Another goal is to find new ways to anonymize patient data so that it can be shared without jeopardizing patient privacy.

9.2.2 Disease complexity and variability

The term disease complexity refers to the fact that many diseases are caused by a combination of genetic, environmental, and lifestyle factors. This complicates predicting the course of disease for any given individual. Disease variability is that patients with the same disease can have different symptoms and outcomes. This is due to several factors, such as the patient's unique biology, the severity of the disease, and the treatment the patient receives. The combination of disease complexity and variability makes developing accurate prognosis models difficult [3]. This is because these models must account for a wide range of factors and predict the course of the disease in a variety of patients.

One approach is to create models that can learn from enormous amounts of patient data. These models can detect patterns in data and predict the course of the disease in new patients. Another approach is to create models that can account for the patient's unique biology. These models can predict how a patient will respond to treatment based on genetic information and other biomarkers.

9.2.3 Lack of standardization in prognostic models

A major challenge in disease prognosis is the lack of standardization in prognostic models [4]. This is because different models make predictions using different data, methods, and metrics. This makes comparing the results of different models difficult, and it can lead to confusion and uncertainty among healthcare professionals. There are several reasons why prognostic models lack standardization. First, disease prognosis is still a young field, and there is no single agreed-upon approach to developing and evaluating prognostic models. Second, the data used to train predictive models is frequently heterogeneous and incomplete. This makes developing models that are generalizable to new patients difficult. Third, the metrics used to evaluate prognostic models can differ depending on the application. There are several approaches that can be taken to address the issue of lack of standardization in prognostic models. The first step is to create common data standards for collecting and storing patient data. Another goal is to create standard methods for developing and evaluating prognostic models. Despite the difficulties, quick progress is being made in the field of disease prognosis. The accuracy of prognostic models is likely to improve as more data becomes available and new methods are developed. This will lead to greater standardization in prognostic models, making it easier to compare the results of different models and make informed patient care decisions.

9.3 AI/ML in disease prognosis

In the healthcare industry, AI and ML have been regarded as the most effective and promising analytical tools [10]. It uses algorithms to process and gain insights from data to predict or decision-making that can be applied to disease prognosis [11,12,13,14]. A simple review of the AI/ML-based algorithm used for disease prognosis is listed in Table 9.1.

The analysis of clinical data using the AI/ML algorithm, as shown in Fig. 9.2, enables an understanding of the molecular mechanisms underlying diseases and how risk factors affect their development. This clinical data ranges from clinical symptoms to various sorts of biochemical testing and imaging device outputs. The profile builder creates the patent profile, which is then given to the AI/ML module. AI/ML algorithms efficiently handle and analyze vast and complex profile datasets. These algorithms use pattern recognition to find minor correlations and risk variables that may be difficult for human clinicians to notice. It detects early indications and symptoms of diseases, allowing for early detection

Table 9.1 Disease prognosis through AI/ML models in Biomedicine 4.0.

References	Year	Disease	AI/ML model
[5]	2021	Pancreatic ductal adenocarcinoma	Random forest
[6]	2023	Cryptococcus	CNN
[7]	2022	Sickle cell disease	CNN
[8]	2023	Lung cancer	CNN
[9]	2023	Chronic kidney disease	ANN

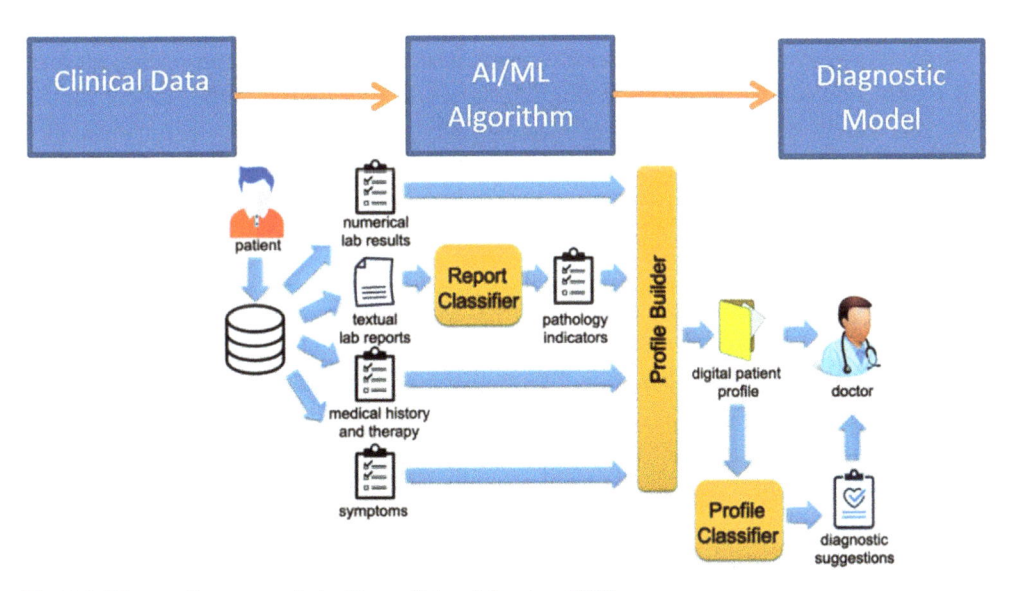

Fig. 9.2 Diagnostic prognosis in Biomedicine 4.0 using AI/ML.

and action. It also creates complex prognostic models that predict disease progression and patient survival rates. These models consider a variety of factors, including medical history, genetic information, lifestyle, and response to previous therapies.

9.3.1 Efficient analysis of medical data

Efficient medical data analysis is important in AI/ML-based disease prognosis to enable timely and accurate forecasts [15]. To achieve effective medical data analysis, multiple methodologies such as data preprocessing, feature selection, network modeling, parallel computing, and cloud computing are required.

- *Data preprocessing:* Thorough preparation is required before feeding data to AI/ML algorithms. Cleaning the data, dealing with missing values, normalizing or scaling numerical characteristics, and encoding categorical variables are all part of this process.

Proper preprocessing ensures that the data are consistent and usable, lowering the likelihood of incorrect predictions.
- *Feature selection:* All medical data details may not be relevant to disease prediction. Feature selection approaches are methods for identifying the most useful and notable features that lead to accurate forecasts. By reducing the number of features, AI/ML algorithms can be trained more effectively, resulting in shorter processing times and enhanced generalization.
- *Network model selection:* Choosing the best AI/ML network model for disease prediction is critical. Some network models may be more efficient than others, particularly when dealing with enormous amounts of medical data. Ensemble approaches such as Random Forest or Gradient Boosting Machines, for example, can be less computationally costly than deep learning models such as convolutional neural networks (CNNs).
- *Parallel computing:* For large datasets and sophisticated models, parallel computing can accelerate analysis. Techniques such as distributing computations across numerous processors or making use of GPUs (graphics processing units) can help to speed up the training and prediction processes.
- *Cloud computing:* Access to scalable computing resources is made easier by using cloud-based platforms for AI/ML analysis. Cloud providers offer powerful machines outfitted with specialized technology (e.g., GPUs) capable of accelerating AI model training and efficiently handling massive medical datasets.

Thus, AI/ML-based algorithms can efficiently manage medical data for disease prognosis.

9.3.2 Forecasting disease outcomes

A critical part of AI/ML in disease prediction is forecasting disease outcomes. It entails forecasting how a disease will progress for an individual patient based on their medical history, present health condition, and other pertinent data. AI/ML algorithms can do better longitudinal patient data analysis, survival analysis, time series analysis, and dynamic risk assessment [16].
- *Longitudinal patient data analysis:* AI/ML algorithms can assess past health records, diagnostic tests, treatment information, and follow-up visits. By analyzing trends and patterns in these data points over time, AI models may estimate how a disease will progress in the future.
- *Survival analysis:* A statistical technique often employed in disease prognosis is survival analysis. Survival analysis can be done using AI/ML algorithms to assess the likelihood of a patient living or experiencing a specific event (e.g., illness progression, relapse, or recovery) during a given time.
- *Time series analysis:* Time series forecasting techniques are used for diseases with changing symptoms or treatment responses over time. Based on historical trends, AI/ML

models can assess time-stamped data and forecast future disease states or health outcomes.
- *Dynamic risk assessment:* AI/ML models can constantly update risk estimates based on fresh data inputs and patient reactions to therapies. This dynamic risk assessment provides real-time insights into illness progression and enables treatment regimens to be adjusted in real-time.

Furthermore, AI/ML algorithms can rapidly integrate and evaluate data from a variety of sources, including electronic health records, medical imaging, genomics, wearable devices, and patient-reported outcomes. Combining several data sources enhances disease prediction accuracy.

9.4 Transfer learning for disease prognosis

In the domain of healthcare, deploying transfer learning harnesses pretrained models and knowledge from diverse medical datasets to enhance disease prognosis accuracy and efficiency. This powerful technique addresses the challenges of limited labeled data and complex feature extraction, enabling personalized medicine and accelerating drug discovery. Through real-world examples, we explore its transformative impact and ethical considerations, empowering researchers, and practitioners in the pursuit of precise and accessible healthcare solutions (Table 9.2).

9.4.1 Understanding transfer learning

Transfer learning is a powerful ML technique that leverages knowledge gained from one task or domain to improve the performance of another related task or domain. Transfer learning addresses challenges such as limited data and complex feature extraction by utilizing pretrained models and knowledge from existing datasets. This approach has transformative applications in various fields, including disease prognosis, enabling more accurate and efficient predictions, accelerating research, and fostering personalized solutions in healthcare. Fig. 9.3 shows the sequence of steps followed for transferring the model weights from the model that learns from the heart disease data to the neurological disorder learning model.

9.4.2 Advantages over traditional ML methods

- *Data efficiency:* Transfer learning significantly reduces the need for large, labeled datasets. By leveraging pretrained models, it can adapt to new tasks with smaller amounts of data, making it more suitable for domains with limited data availability.
- *Faster training:* Compared to training a model from scratch, transfer learning typically requires less time and computational resources. Utilizing pre-learned features allows the model to converge faster, accelerating the training process.

Table 9.2 Predominant disease prognosis challenges in Biomedicine 4.0: technology and application perspective.

References	Year	Challenges	Technology	Application	Possible technology contribution
[17]	2021	Data integration and interoperability	AI and big data	Electronic health records (EHRs)	Advanced algorithms for data fusion and seamless integration across all platforms
[18]	2021	Ethical use of AI in diagnosis	AI decision-making processes and explainability	Diagnostic imaging	Development of AI models with transparent
[19]	2021	Cybersecurity and data privacy	Blockchain	Telemedicine	Decentralized and secure data management using blockchain
[20]	2022	Limited access to healthcare data	Cloud computing	Health research databases	Cloud-based systems for secure and efficient sharing of healthcare data
[21]	2022	Real-time disease monitoring	IoT	Remote patient monitoring	IoT devices and sensors for continuous monitoring and early detection of diseases
[22]	2022	Personalized medicine	Genomics	Precision medicine	Advancements in genomic sequencing technology for tailored treatment plans
[23]	2022	Drug discovery and development	Machine learning	Pharmaceutical Research	ML algorithms for drug design and optimization to accelerate development process
[24]	2021	Patient empowerment and adherence	Mobile apps	Mobile health apps	Mobile applications for patient education and tracking treatment adherence
[25]	2022	Health data bias and inclusivity	Natural language processing (NLP)	Public health initiatives	NLP techniques to identify and mitigate biases in health data
[26]	2021	Interdisciplinary collaboration	Virtual reality	Healthcare institutions	VR platforms for Remote collaboration among healthcare professionals

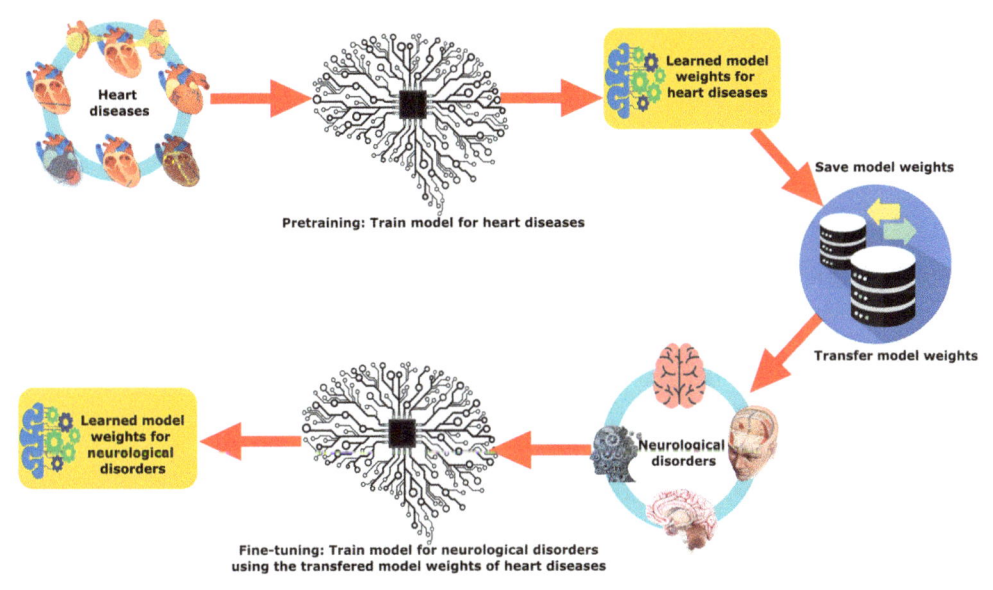

Fig. 9.3 Deploying transfer learning for transferring the model weights from the model that learns heart diseases to the neurological disorder learning model.

- *Improved generalization:* Transfer learning helps improve model generalization by capturing high-level patterns and representations from the source domain. These learned representations can be beneficial for related tasks, resulting in better performance on new and unseen data.
- *Domain adaptation:* In scenarios where the target domain has distinct characteristics from the source domain, transfer learning can facilitate domain adaptation. It enables the model to adapt and generalize well to the new domain, enhancing its applicability in real-world settings.
- *Effective feature extraction:* Transfer learning extracts relevant features from the source domain, even if the features are not explicitly known. This ability to learn discriminative features enables the model to focus on task-specific information, leading to improved predictions.
- *Enhanced performance:* By leveraging knowledge from well-established domains, transfer learning can boost the performance of models on complex and challenging tasks. It leverages prior knowledge effectively, reducing the risk of overfitting and enhancing model accuracy.
- *Versatility and flexibility:* Transfer learning is versatile and applicable across various domains and tasks. It allows models to adapt and perform well on a wide range of problems, making it a valuable technique in diverse fields, including healthcare, computer vision, and natural language processing.

- *Interpretable knowledge transfer:* Transfer learning enables knowledge transfer between tasks, making the model's decision-making more interpretable. The model can leverage insights from one domain to inform its predictions in another domain, providing a clearer understanding of the underlying reasoning.

9.4.3 Eliminating the need to build models from scratch

One of the significant advantages of transfer learning is its ability to eliminate the need to build ML models from scratch. Traditional ML methods typically require starting the training process with randomly initialized parameters and training the model on a specific dataset for the task at hand. This process can be computationally intensive and time-consuming, especially when dealing with large datasets or complex models. However, with transfer learning, we can leverage pretrained models that have been trained on large and diverse datasets for different tasks or domains.

These pretrained models have already learned meaningful and generalizable features from the data, capturing valuable patterns and representations. By using these pretrained models as a starting point, we can save considerable effort and time in the model-building process.

Transfer learning allows us to adapt these pretrained models to new tasks or domains by fine-tuning or retraining them on the target dataset. Fine-tuning involves updating the model's parameters on the new dataset while keeping the learned representations intact. This process is much faster and requires fewer training iterations than training from scratch. The ability to eliminate the need to build models from scratch is particularly advantageous in scenarios with limited labeled data. Transfer learning can bridge the gap by leveraging knowledge from other related tasks or domains, improving performance even with smaller datasets.

Furthermore, transfer learning enhances model performance and generalization. By starting with pretrained models that have learned from vast amounts of data, the model is exposed to rich features and patterns, allowing it to perform better on new and unseen data.

9.5 Enhancing disease prognosis models

This section explores advanced techniques such as transfer learning and ensemble methods to enhance disease prognosis models. From multimodal data integration to ethical considerations, we investigate how these models are revolutionizing healthcare. Our goal is to equip researchers with the tools to improve patient outcomes and transform medical practice.

9.5.1 Enhanced accuracy in prognostic models

In the pursuit of improved healthcare outcomes, enhancing the accuracy of prognostic models has become a crucial objective. This section delves into cutting-edge methodologies, including advanced ML techniques, feature engineering, and data integration, that elevate the predictive power of prognostic models. By harnessing the wealth of medical data and knowledge, we aim to empower clinicians and researchers to make more precise prognostic assessments, enabling early detection, personalized treatment strategies, and, ultimately, better patient care.

In the quest for enhanced accuracy in prognostic models, researchers are exploring novel avenues to integrate diverse data sources, such as genomics, proteomics, imaging, and electronic health records. By fusing these multimodal datasets and leveraging sophisticated feature extraction methods, prognostic models gain a deeper understanding of disease complexities and patient-specific factors. Additionally, advancements in transfer learning enable the model to draw insights from related domains, capitalizing on pretrained knowledge to refine predictions for specific diseases. Ethical considerations remain at the forefront as these models hold significant implications for patient care and treatment decisions. As we embrace these advancements, a key focus is ensuring transparency, fairness, and interpretability to build trust among healthcare professionals and patients. By achieving enhanced accuracy in prognostic models, we pave the way for a more proactive and personalized approach to healthcare, revolutionizing how we diagnose, treat, and manage diseases for improved quality of life.

9.5.2 Superior results than other ML methods

By incorporating learned representations from related tasks or domains, transfer learning can effectively adapt to new prognostic tasks, resulting in higher accuracy and efficiency. Moreover, ensemble methods, where multiple models are combined, have demonstrated exceptional predictive power in disease prognosis. By aggregating the diverse insights of individual models, ensembles provide more robust and reliable predictions, leading to superior results.

Additionally, deep learning, with its ability to automatically learn hierarchical representations from complex data, has shown great promise in disease prognosis. Deep neural networks can capture intricate patterns and relationships within medical data, enabling them to outperform traditional ML methods in many cases.

The continuous exploration and integration of these advanced techniques can revolutionize disease prognosis by providing more precise and personalized predictions. As researchers continue to refine and expand these methods, the healthcare industry can anticipate even superior results in the future, leading to enhanced patient care and better medical decision-making.

9.5.3 Improved treatment outcomes

Enhancing disease prognosis models plays a pivotal role in improving treatment outcomes for patients. By accurately predicting disease progression and identifying high-risk individuals, clinicians can intervene proactively, leading to early detection and timely interventions. These enhanced models also enable personalized treatment strategies, tailoring therapies to individual patient profiles and specific disease characteristics.

With the aid of advanced ML techniques like transfer learning and deep learning, prognostic models can better capture complex relationships within medical data, enabling more precise predictions. This, in turn, empowers healthcare providers to make informed decisions, optimize treatment plans, and allocate resources effectively.

Furthermore, by leveraging multimodal data integration and ensemble methods, prognostic models gain a comprehensive view of patient health, considering diverse factors like genomics, clinical history, imaging, and lifestyle. This comprehensive approach fosters a deeper understanding of diseases and their progression, contributing to improved diagnostic accuracy and treatment efficacy.

The deployment of enhanced prognostic models in clinical practice holds the potential to transform patient care. Through early intervention, personalized treatments, and data-driven decision-making, these models can enhance treatment outcomes, reduce hospitalization rates, and improve patient well-being. As research in this domain continues to advance, we anticipate even greater strides in optimizing healthcare and delivering improved treatment outcomes for individuals around the world.

9.5.4 Reduced healthcare costs

Enhancing disease prognosis models can have a substantial impact on reducing healthcare costs. By accurately predicting disease progression and identifying high-risk patients, healthcare providers can implement preventive measures and early interventions. This proactive approach can potentially prevent costly hospitalizations and emergency treatments, leading to significant cost savings in the long run.

Moreover, by leveraging advanced ML techniques like transfer learning and ensemble methods, prognostic models can optimize resource allocation. Healthcare facilities can efficiently direct their resources toward patients who require immediate attention, while also streamlining care for low-risk individuals. This targeted allocation of resources helps in cost containment and ensures that medical interventions are prioritized where they are most needed.

Personalized treatment strategies, enabled by enhanced prognostic models, can also contribute to cost reduction. By tailoring treatments to individual patient profiles, healthcare providers can avoid unnecessary procedures or medications, minimizing both financial and physical burdens on patients and the healthcare system. Furthermore, improved diagnostic accuracy achieved through multimodal data integration and deep learning can lead to fewer misdiagnoses and unnecessary tests, avoiding redundant expenses and medical errors.

As enhanced disease prognosis models continue to evolve and become more widespread, healthcare systems stand to benefit from reduced costs, better resource utilization, and improved patient outcomes. By harnessing the potential of data-driven prognostic insights, healthcare organizations can take substantial strides toward a more sustainable and cost-effective healthcare landscape.

9.6 Conclusion

The significance of disease prognosis in Biomedicine 4.0 and its role in improving medical diagnosis, treatment, and patient outcomes is highlighted in this chapter. The challenges of limited data and disease complexity are addressed through the application of ML and AI algorithms, with a particular focus on the transformative potential of transfer learning. By eliminating the need to build models from scratch and outperforming traditional ML methods, transfer learning enhances the accuracy and efficiency of disease prognosis models. Through data-driven insights, these sophisticated models empower healthcare professionals with precise prognostic information, leading to improved treatment outcomes and reduced healthcare costs. As we embrace these advancements, personalized medicine and proactive healthcare become attainable goals, shaping a future where patient care is revolutionized and tailored to individual needs.

References

[1] P. Roman-Naranjo, A. Parra-Perez, J. Lopez-Escamez, A systematic review on machine learning approaches in the diagnosis and prognosis of rare genetic diseases, J. Biomed. Inform. (2023) 104429, https://doi.org/10.1016/j.jbi.2023.104429.

[2] M. Liu, J. Zhang, C. Lian, D. Shen, Weakly supervised deep learning for brain disease prognosis using MRI and incomplete clinical scores, IEEE Trans. Cybern. 50 (7) (2019) 3381–3392.

[3] A. Johansson, O.A. Andreassen, S. Brunak, P.W. Franks, H. Hedman, R.J. Loos, B. Meder, E. Mel'en, C.E. Wheelock, B. Jacobsson, Precision medicine in complex diseases—molecular subgrouping for improved prediction and treatment stratification, J. Intern. Med. (2023), https://doi.org/10.1111/joim.13640.

[4] Y.-H. Zhou, K.R. Hess, V.R. Raj, L. Yu, L. Liu, A.W. Yung, M.E. Linskey, Establishment of prognostic models for astrocytic and oligodendroglial brain tumors with standardized quantification of marker gene expression and clinical variables, Biomark. Insights 5 (2010). pp. BMI–S6167.

[5] K.-S. Lee, J.-Y. Jang, Y.-D. Yu, J.S. Heo, H.-S. Han, Y.-S. Yoon, C.M. Kang, H.K. Hwang, S. Kang, Usefulness of artificial intelligence for predicting recurrence following surgery for pancreatic cancer: retrospective cohort study, Int. J. Surg. 93 (2021) 106050, https://doi.org/10.1016/j.ijsu.2021.106050.

[6] F. Gu, S. Hu, B. Tian, T. Ma, Y. Xu, Y. Yang, B. Gu, Intelligent diagnostic system for cryptococcus: switch-controllable nanocatcher and cnn-based artificial intelligence, Chem. Eng. J. 465 (2023) 142674, https://doi.org/10.1016/j.cej.2023.142674.

[7] P.M. Douglass, T. O'Connor, B. Javidi, Automated sickle cell disease identification in human red blood cells using a lensless single random phase encoding biosensor and convolutional neural networks, Opt. Express 30 (20) (2022) 35 965–35 977.

[8] C. McGenity, E. Clarke, C. Jennings, G. Matthews, C. Cartlidge, H. Freduah-Agyemang, D. Stocken, D. Treanor, Diagnostic test accuracy (dta) of artificial intelligence in digital pathology: a systematic review, meta-analysis and quality assessment, arXiv preprint arXiv:2306.07999 (2023).

[9] J. Stojanowski, A. Konieczny, L. Lis, W. Frosztega, P. Brzozowska, A. Ciszewska, K. Rydzyn'ska, M. Sroka, K. Krakowska, T. Golebiowski, et al., The artificial neural network as a diagnostic tool of the risk of clostridioides difficile infection among patients with chronic kidney disease, J. Clin. Med. 12 (14) (2023) 4751, https://doi.org/10.3390/jcm12144751.

[10] M.N. Islam, T.T. Inan, S. Rafi, S.S. Akter, I.H. Sarker, A.N. Islam, A systematic review on the use of ai and ml for fighting the covid-19 pandemic, IEEE Trans. Artif. Intell. 1 (3) (2020) 258–270, https://doi.org/10.1109/TAI.2021.3062771.

[11] O. Ali, W. Abdelbaki, A. Shrestha, E. Elbasi, M.A.A. Alryalat, Y.K. Dwivedi, A systematic literature review of artificial intelligence in the healthcare sector: benefits, challenges, methodologies, and functionalities, J. Innov. Knowl. 8 (1) (2023) 100333, https://doi.org/10.1016/j.jik.2023.100333.

[12] A. Qayyum, J. Qadir, M. Bilal, A. Al-Fuqaha, Secure and robust machine learning for healthcare: a survey, IEEE Rev. Biomed. Eng. 14 (2020) 156–180.

[13] Y. Kumar, A. Koul, R. Singla, M.F. Ijaz, Artificial intelligence in disease diagnosis: a systematic literature review, synthesizing framework and future research agenda, J. Ambient. Intell. Humaniz. Comput. (2022) 1–28.

[14] M. Shehab, L. Abualigah, Q. Shambour, M.A. Abu-Hashem, M.K.Y. Shambour, A.I. Alsalibi, A.H. Gandomi, Machine learning in medical applications: a review of state-of-the-art methods, Comput. Biol. Med. 145 (2022) 105458, https://doi.org/10.1016/j.compbiomed.2022.105458.

[15] M. Zhang, X. Zeng, C. Huang, J. Liu, X. Liu, X. Xie, R. Wang, An AI-based radiomics nomogram for disease prognosis in patients with covid-19 pneumonia using initial CT images and clinical indicators, Int. J. Med. Inform. 154 (2021) 104545, https://doi.org/10.1016/j.ijmedinf.2021.104545.

[16] S. Sankaranarayanan, E. Gunasekaran, G. Rao, et al., A novel survival analysis of machine using fuzzy ensemble convolutional based optimal RNN, Expert Syst. Appl. (2023) 120966, https://doi.org/10.1016/j.eswa.2023.120966.

[17] M. Sreenivasan, A.M. Chacko, Interoperability issues in ehr sytems: research directions, in: Data Analytics in Biomedical Engineering and Healthcare, 2021, pp. 13–28.

[18] K. Lekadir, R. Osuala, C. Gallin, N. Lazrak, K. Kushibar, G. Tsakou, S. Auss'o, L.C. Alberich, K. Marias, M. Tsiknakis, et al., Future-AI: guiding principles and consensus recommendations for trustworthy artificial intelligence in medical imaging, arXiv preprint arXiv:2109.09658 (2021).

[19] B. Zaabar, O. Cheikhrouhou, F. Jamil, M. Ammi, M. Abid, Healthblock: A secure blockchain-based healthcare data management system, Comput. Netw. 200 (2021) 108500, https://doi.org/10.1016/j.comnet.2021.108500.

[20] P. Chinnasamy, P. Deepalakshmi, Hcac-ehr: hybrid cryptographic access control for secure EHR retrieval in healthcare cloud, J. Ambient Intell. Humaniz. Comput. (2022) 1–19.

[21] A. Sujith, G.S. Sajja, V. Mahalakshmi, S. Nuhmani, B. Prasanalakshmi, Systematic review of smart health monitoring using deep learning and artificial intelligence, Neuroscience Informatics 2 (3) (2022) 100028, https://doi.org/10.1016/j.neuri.2021.100028.

[22] M. Sahu, R. Gupta, R.K. Ambasta, P. Kumar, Artificial intelligence and machine learning in precision medicine: a paradigm shift in big data analysis, Prog. Mol. Biol. Transl. Sci. 190 (1) (2022) 57–100, https://doi.org/10.1016/bs.pmbts.2022.03.002.

[23] S. Nag, A.T. Baidya, A. Mandal, A.T. Mathew, B. Das, B. Devi, R. Kumar, Deep learning tools for advancing drug discovery and development, 3 Biotech 12 (5) (2022) 110.

[24] S.S. Volpi, D. Biduski, E.A. Bellei, D. Tefili, L. McCleary, A.L.S. Alves, A.C.B. De Marchi, Using a mobile health app to improve patients' adherence to hypertension treatment: a non-randomized clinical trial, PeerJ 9 (2021) e11491, https://doi.org/10.7717/peerj.11491.

[25] S. Khurshid, C. Reeder, L.X. Harrington, P. Singh, G. Sarma, S.F. Friedman, P. Di Achille, N. Diamant, J.W. Cunningham, A.C. Turner, et al., Cohort design and natural language processing to reduce bias in electronic health records research, NPJ Digit. Med. 5 (1) (2022) 47.

[26] S.Y. Liaw, T. Choo, L.T. Wu, W.S. Lim, H. Choo, S.M. Lim, C. Ringsted, L.F. Wong, S.L. Ooi, T.C. Lau, "Wow, woo, win"-healthcare students' and facilitators' experiences of interprofessional simulation in three-dimensional virtual world: a qualitative evaluation study, Nurse Educ. Today 105 (2021) 105018, https://doi.org/10.1016/j.nedt.2021.105018.

CHAPTER 10

Voice and chatbot: A hybrid framework using XAI for improving mental health

Debmitra Ghosh, Sayani Ghatak, and Hrithik Paul
CSE Department, JIS University, Kolkata, India

10.1 Introduction

Mental health is something that has come to the forefront in the recent decade. More than a billion people from around the world have experienced mental illness at some point in their lives. Mental health includes our social, psychological, and emotional well-being. It affects the way we behave, think, feel, handle stressful situations, relate to others, and make choices. Having mental health issues can degrade some individuals' lives. There can be several factors leading to mental illness, for example, childhood abuse, trauma, social isolation or loneliness, facing discrimination, bereavement (losing someone close to you), severe stress, long-term stress, etc. There can also be a genetic link to mental health; for example, if someone has a parent suffering from schizophrenia, the child is more likely to develop the same mental condition. Traditional treatment for mental illness includes psychotherapy. Psychotherapy is the treatment of mental illness that is provided by a trained medical professional. This treatment involves the professional conducting multiple sessions to explore the thoughts, feelings, and behavior of the individual, trying to find out the underlying cause of the individual's current mental status, thus seeking to improve his/her well-being. Some cases of mental illness require the patient to consume antidepressants, antipsychotics, antianxiety, or such drugs, which, if consumed in a certain amount, are safe. Still, in many cases, it is seen that consumers become addicted to the drug. But due to the recent advances in technology, people tend to spend more time on social networks and over the internet. Thus, what people see and what people respond to are 70%–80% of the time present online. Thus, it is a calculated fact that mental illness nowadays is mostly related to the internet world. Chatbots are becoming very popular these days, where people and businessmen opt to add a service or a bot that will answer some FAQs of the people who visit their website or application. Most or all of these chatbots are made with the help of machine learning (ML) methods to answer every question the customer asks related to the website. Our study aims to use chatbots' power and utility to address mental illness in people worldwide. The chatbot framework works in this way, some questions are given as input or spoken to the chatbot, wherein the data that is given is audio. The algorithm converts the voice input/data into text.

Then various algorithms are applied directly to the text data, like natural language processing (NLP), or first converted to numeric data using LabelEncoder and similar algorithms. After that, the data is used to train various machine learning and deep learning models according to respective use cases to get some predicted results. The chatbots that are developed during the recent advances in NLP are applied to various domains like support systems, voice assistants, and medical sciences. Chatbots, in particular, that are used in medicine to diagnose medical conditions based on the patient's symptoms, have growing use cases and popularity.

Explainable AI (XAI) is a rapidly growing field focused on making the decision-making processes of AI models more understandable to humans. In simple terms, XAI is like a "transparent" model that allows us to see how and why it makes certain decisions. This is in contrast to "black box" models, where the decision-making process is hidden and unclear. One of the main goals of XAI is to make the inner workings of AI models interpretable, so users can understand the logic and steps involved in the model's decisions. However, XAI can do much more than just making AI decisions interpretable. Two of the most popular XAI techniques are Local Interpretable Model-Agnostic Explanations (LIME) and Shapley Additive Explanations (SHAP). LIME helps us understand how a machine learning model makes predictions for individual cases. It works by creating several modified versions of the input data with slight changes and then observing how these changes affect the model's predictions. For example, if the input data is a piece of text, LIME might remove certain words to see how their absence changes the outcome. This helps us see which parts of the input data are most important for the model's decision. LIME can be used with various types of data, including text, images, and tables [1]. SHAP is another widely used XAI method that provides detailed explanations for a model's predictions. It uses a concept from game theory called Shapley values to show how each feature in the data contributes to the final prediction [2]. In other words, if your dataset has multiple features, SHAP can show you how much each feature is influencing the model's decision. This approach is valuable because it offers a clear visual representation of the importance of each feature in the decision-making process [3].

This study includes an XAI analysis of both the mentioned packages. XAI can prove very significant and helpful in the healthcare and medical domains, owing to its increased interpretability. The report, charts, or visual representation generated by the XAI facilitated the medical professionals to get a better and next-level understanding of the conditions of the patient, who is using the chatbot, based on certain symptoms. As our study is concerned, patients will be able to communicate with the chatbot, conveying their feelings, symptoms, and similar information. The model working behind the chatbot will be able to generate appropriate responses concerning the asked questions and thereby predict the current mental status of the patients. Further, the chatbot will be able to provide some instant methods to make the individual feel better. Also, the applied XAI technique will be able to generate certain important and useful representations based on the data the chatbot has received.

The main contribution of this paper is:
- To provide a solution to the field of mental disease prediction.
- To provide treatment to individuals using machine learning methods and XAI.
- The model can take voice and text as input from the patients and analyze the input and provide predictions about the mental status of the patients.
- The XAI goes a step forward and explains the prediction of the model using visual representations.

The rest of the paper is organized as follows: There are several existing state-of-the-art methods available for predicting mental health diseases described in Section 10.3 "Literature survey." In Section 10.2, the problem statement is described. In Section 10.4, we describe the preliminary aspects of our project. The description of datasets is discussed in Section 10.5. Section 10.6 stands for methods that we apply in our project. The next part is the proposed result, which is described in Section 10.7, and lastly, Section 10.8 describes the conclusion and limitations.

10.2 Problem statement

Our study mainly focuses on predicting the mental health status of patients that are communicating with the chatbot using machine learning and deep learning algorithms. The model runs predictions on the data it receives from the patient in voice form or text form. It then gives suitable predictions and then also suggests some diagnostics. With the help of XAI, we get a proper format of report regarding the model's prediction, which accounts for features that positively impacted the decision and the features that harmed the same. This helps to understand the predictions of the model in a better human interpretable fashion.

10.3 Literature survey

The demand for mental health services during the COVID-19 epidemic is reported to have outstripped the supply in this study [1], which provides chances for digital technology solutions to cover this new gap and, in the process, exhibit capacities to improve their efficacy and efficiency. Reconceptualized models and frameworks have been used to overcome the persistent failure of these implementations, and there have been several initiatives to connect dissimilar developers and clinical researchers to provide them with a key for advancing evaluative research. During the epidemic, web-based treatments are being utilized more often, making psychological therapy more accessible and inexpensive. To overcome engagement hurdles, particularly with predictive technologies, it is also claimed that a greater grasp of the consequences and functions of human-computer interaction is necessary. To achieve beneficial and responsible results, explainable artificial intelligence (AI) is being included in the implementation of digital mental health. For real-time screening, tracking, and treatment, investing in digital platforms and related apps holds the potential of being cost-effective for vulnerable groups. To help policymakers adopt digital mental health, it is necessary to effectively integrate decision support tools due to the limits of an evidence-based approach. Effectiveness, fairness, access, and ethics all have complicated problems that need to be solved. It is necessary to build exceptional digital products and services, evidence-informed policies, and the technical know-how to use and sustain these solutions. Digital mental health investments should guarantee their viability and safety. End users should promote the adoption of cutting-edge techniques to urge developers to thoroughly assess their goods and services and make them an investment worth making. In a hybrid model of care, technology-enabled services are most likely to be successful [1]. In this paper [2] a topic on human-computation interaction (HCI) in mental health problems is discussed. This article, How digital devices and AI can be used to identify, predict, and overcome various kinds of mental health problems and suicide attempting disorders, is explained very well. Real-time machine learning algorithms can be used for outdated treatment as well as the identification of various kinds of mental health disorders. Applications based on HCI mapping can assist in effectively identifying, preventing, and acknowledging the inequalities of several mental health disorders and in the digital therapeutic alliance. Chen et al. [3] provide an overview of how machine learning (ML) and AI play vital roles in the era of psychiatry. Combining AI and ML with neuromodulation technologies can be used to improve treatment. Neuroimaging, neuromodulation, and modern mobile technologies with machine learning algorithms are grouped in the psychiatry study. How XAI and neuromodulation correlate with each other to define machine learning prospects in the extraction of multi-media information and multi-media data fusion. In this study [4], four challenges are discussed related to human-AI interactions. The writers of this article deeply research the need for conceptualizing and experimental study about the challenges based on testing limitations, real-life problems, and limitations of AI and ML in human-AI interactions. The paper [5] focuses on psychological health, especially depression. This study uses social media data to predict the mental health status of an individual with the help of machine learning, NLP, and conventional techniques. This study includes state-of-the-earth techniques, features, datasets, and performance metrics. It also proposes a framework for mental health surveillance. The paper [6] focuses on the integration of AI technologies into the mental health domain. It describes a framework for "pragmatic AI-augmentation" that addresses the difficulties that mental health clinicians have to face due to the integration of AI-based clinical practices. It also elaborates on the medical benefits offered by these technologies, the challenges the clinicians may face from these technologies, and some solutions regarding the same. The paper [7] focuses on attention deficit hyperactivity disorder (ADHD). It is a disorder in children where they face difficulty in maintaining focus and completing daily tasks due to impaired executive function, which leads to the downfall of self-image in front of society, family, and themselves. So the study presents a voice bot (conversational agent) intervention that provides support for both the children and their parents in dealing with the disorder. Moret-Tatay et al. [8] use Azure voice bot to screen cognitive impairment of health workers' experience, WAY2AGE. A survey of 30 workers has been done to analyze the results. In the back end, Azure is used to trial surveys. The main limitation of WAY2AGE is coherent problems that are found in older people. They face problems with the transcript of audio to text [9]. ADHD child patients got assistance to perform their daily tasks using a voice bot. The dialogue structure method and token-based economics methods were used for the voice bot. Raspberry Pi is used to develop the voice bot. This voice bot was successfully shown to have an effective result in that most of the patients increased their self-efficacy. Mezzi et al. [10] proposed an efficient tool for mental health detection for Arab-speaking patients. Their proposed system follows bidirectional encoder representations from the transformers (BERT) model and the International Neuropsychiatric Interview (MINI) for intent recognition to diagnose mental health. Datasets are collected from the Military Hospital of Tunis in Tunisia. Excellent performance of the system has been shown with better accuracy in mental health diagnosis for five disorders (depression, social phobia, suicidality, panic disorder, and adjustment disorder). In this review paper [11], an overview of the features of most of the chatbots that have been reviewed that were used in mental health. Seven bibliographic databases were extracted for this work. Study selection and data extraction were followed by two individuals. There were different classifications for each chatbot based on various aspects. Out of several citations, 53 unique works on chatbots have been reviewed. The most common use of chatbots was for therapy, training, and screening. There was also a classification based on types of conversations; some chatbots only used input modality in written language, and some chatbots used a combination of written, spoken, and visual languages. But the majority of chatbots represented visual representations. Ito et al. [12] inaugurated a mental healthcare course using VR devices. It was a self-guided course. The main objective of this course was to reduce stress. In addition, this study added a new version. In the new version, smartphones and chatbots were used to enhance its convenience for use and to maintain motivation for the user to use it daily. Cameron et al. [13] outlined how to design and develop chatbots for mental healthcare that administer self-assessment scales as well as provide well-being and self-help guidance and information. The name of the chatbot was iHelpr. In addition, managing risk and ethical considerations should be included in a chatbot in the healthcare sector. Best practices and proficiencies are used to develop the iHelper chatbot [14]. Outcomes, features, and performance of previously published trials for the prevention and treatment of internet intervention for different kinds of mental disorders are reviewed. The main focus of this work is depression and anxiety disorders. After reviewing 29 reports, 26 trails passed the test cases for finalized trails. The study of Abd-Alrazaq et al. [15] is focused on evaluating how effective and safe chatbots are to improve mental health by analyzing and pooling the results of previous studies. The study is a systematic review carried out from different citations from bibliographical databases like MEDLINE, EMBASE, etc. The study examined a total of 12 studies for the purpose. Certain weak evidence shows that chatbots are effective in the case of depression, stress, anxiety, etc. Also, according to some similar evidence, it is shown that there is no significant effect statistically using chatbots on psychological well-being. Christine [16] discussed how the chatbot is developed, highlighting its participatory, co-design process with the youth, who are considered the primary stakeholder to benefit from this digital tool. Research from the interviews, surveys, etc. helps to develop the chatbot's personality and its character design. The primary focus of the paper is how all the digital tools, such as chatbots, can provide support for the mental health of people in conjunction with the health care team.

Sweeney et al. [17] focused on understanding the attitude of the professionals working in the mental health domain regarding the use of chatbots for supporting mental health and well-being. The results of this survey conducted during this study show that almost half of the participants in the survey agreed about the benefits associated with mental healthcare chatbots, along with a higher perception of their importance. A majority of the participants also agreed that mental healthcare chatbots will be able to help their clients manage their health in a better manner. This study also shows that with the increase in the years of experience, there was a corresponding increase in the belief that healthcare chatbots might help clients better manage their mental health. The study by Shi et al. [18] proposed a transfer learning-based English language learning chatbot that produced output generated by GPT-2, which can be explained by the corresponding ontology graph. Three levels were designed for systematic English learning, which include the phonetics level for speech recognition and correcting pronunciation, semantic levels, and the simulation of free-style conversation by XAI that helps to visualize the connections of the neural network in bionics and explain the output sentence from the language model. The study by Zeng et al. [19] proposed an XAI-based language learning chatbot using ontology and transfer learning methodology. Three levels were designed for systematic English learning, which include the phonetics level for speech recognition and correcting pronunciation, the semantic level for specific domain conversation, and the simulation of free-style conversation. An ontology graph is used to explain the performance of free-style conversation, with the help of XAI, which aids in visualizing the connections of neural networks in bionics and explaining the output sentence from the language model.

10.4 Preliminaries

The main concepts of a number of the components of this research work are briefly discussed, including the RNN model, CNN Model, Integrated Stacked Ensemble Model, and NLP, voice engines.

10.4.1 RNN

recurrent neural network (RNN) is a type of neural network that is commonly used in NLP tasks such as language modeling, machine translation, and chatbot development. RNNs give results of one step and are fed into the current step as input. Traditional neural networks have inputs and outputs that are independent of one another, but there is a need to remember the previous words in situations where it is necessary to anticipate the next word in a sentence. As a result, RNN was developed, which utilized a hidden layer to resolve this problem. The hidden state, which retains some information about a sequence, is the primary and most significant characteristic of RNNs. RNNs have a "memory" that retains all data related to calculations. It executes the same action on all of the input or hidden layers to produce the output, using the same settings for each input. In contrast to other neural networks, this minimizes the complexity of the parameter set. Every piece of knowledge is retained by an RNN over time. Only the ability to remember past inputs makes it helpful for time series prediction.

$$h_i = f(Wh_{i-1} + Ux_i) \tag{10.1}$$

where W and U are matrices containing the weights (parameters) of the network. f is a nonlinear activation function, which can be the hyperbolic tangent function.

10.4.2 CNN

Artificial neural networks are commonly used for tasks such as classifying words, audio, and images. Different types of neural networks are suited to different tasks. For instance, RNNs, particularly long short-term memory networks (LSTMs), are often used for predicting the order of words. On the other hand, convolutional neural networks (CNNs) are typically employed for image classification. In this paper, we will cover the fundamentals of CNNs. A typical neural network consists of three types of layers: input, hidden, and output layers. During the feedforward stage, data is passed through the network, layer by layer, to produce an output. When calculating error, functions like cross-entropy and squared loss are often used. After determining the error, backpropagation is applied to update the network's weights and minimize the loss. Backpropagation is a key process used to improve the model's accuracy over time. One potential application of a CNN in a chatbot is to assist with NLP tasks, such as sentiment analysis or text classification. For example, a CNN could be trained to categorize incoming user messages as positive, negative, or neutral, which could then be used to tailor the bot's responses accordingly.

10.4.3 Integrated stacked ensemble

When using neural networks as submodels, it may be desirable to use a neural network as a meta-learner. Specifically, the sub-networks can be embedded in a larger multi-headed neural network that then learns how to best combine the predictions from each input sub-model. It allows the stacking ensemble to be treated as a single large model. The benefit of this approach is that the outputs of the submodels are provided directly to the meta-learner. Further, it is also possible to update the weights of the submodels in conjunction with the meta-learner model, if this is desirable. This can be achieved using the Keras functional interface for developing models. After the models are loaded as a list, a larger stacking ensemble model can be defined where each of the loaded models is used as a separate input head to the model. This requires that all of the layers in each of the loaded models be marked as not trainable, so the weights cannot be updated when the new larger model is being trained. Keras also requires that each layer has a unique name; therefore, the names of each layer in each of the loaded models will have to be updated to indicate to which ensemble member they belong.

$$f = \sum (w_i * p_{i-1})/w_i \qquad (10.2)$$

Here f is the final prediction, w_i is the weight assigned to the i-th base model, and p_i is the prediction produced by the i-th base model. The weights assigned to each model in the ensemble are typically learned during the training process. One common approach is to use a meta-learning algorithm such as gradient boosting or neural networks to learn the weights that minimize the error of the ensemble on a validation set. In an Integrated Stacked Ensemble, the base models are typically trained on different subsets of the data or with different algorithms, which helps to reduce overfitting and improve the generalization performance of the ensemble.

10.4.4 NLP

This seemingly complex process can be identified as one that allows computers to derive meaning from text inputs. Put simply, NLP is an applied AI program that helps chatbots analyze and understand the natural human language communicated with users. Chatbots can understand the intent of the conversation rather than just use the information to communicate and respond to queries. Business owners are starting to feed their chatbots with actions to "help" them become more humanized and personal in their chats. Chatbots have, and will always, help companies automate tasks, communicate better with their customers, and grow their bottom lines. But the more familiar consumers become with chatbots, the more they expect from them. With personalization being the primary focus, we need to try and "train" the chatbot about the different default responses and how exactly it can make customers' lives easier by doing so. With NLP, the chatbot will be able to streamline more tailored, unique responses, interpret and answer new questions or commands, and improve the user's experience according to their needs.

Here, NLTK is used, which is a Python package that can be used for NLP. A lot of the data that could be analyzed is unstructured data and contains human-readable text. Before one can analyze that data programmatically, one first needs to preprocess it. Three components of NLTK have been used here. Such as "punkt," "wordnet," and "om-1.4." Punkt Sentence Tokenizer: This tokenizer divides a text into a list of sentences by using an unsupervised algorithm to build a model for abbreviation words, collocations, and words that start sentences. It must be trained on a large collection of plaintext in the target language before it can be used. WordNet is a lexical database for the English language that was created by Princeton and is part of the NLTK corpus. One can use WordNet alongside the NLTK module to find the meanings of words, synonyms, antonyms, and more.

10.4.5 Voice engines

A voice engine is a software component for two-way audio communication that is often used in telecommunications systems to mimic a phone conversation. It performs the same function as a speech data pump for audio data. Embedded systems frequently employ the voice engine. With the widespread use of voice-over-internet protocol technology in software DSP systems after 2000, the term gained popularity. Unlike earlier generations of systems, which required specialized, math-optimized digital signal processor chips, speech engines manage the voice processing for an IP Phone system on a normal CPU. Because voice filtering and speech coding involve mathematically sophisticated signal processing, voice engines are highly optimized software subsystems. A voice engine's filter stages and coding components are made to function with a larger telecommunications system and only perform a narrow range of processing, which reduces the memory and CPU demands on the voice engine. A voice engine is created to adhere to certain industry standards for interoperability, unlike software desktop programs that may use plugins to continuously increase flexibility or extensibility.

10.4.6 XAI

Machine learning algorithms' output and outcomes can now be understood and trusted by human users because of a set of procedures and techniques known as explainable artificial intelligence (XAI). An AI model, its anticipated effects, and potential biases are all described in terms of XAI. It contributes to defining model correctness, fairness, transparency, and outcomes in decision-making supported by AI. When putting AI models into production, an organization must first establish trust and confidence. A company can adopt a responsible approach to AI development with the aid of AI explainability.

Humans find it difficult to understand and trace the steps taken by the algorithm as AI develops. The entire mathematical procedure is reduced to a "black box" that is unintelligible and is sometimes referred to as such. The data are used to generate these black box models. Furthermore, nobody, not even the engineers or data scientists who developed the algorithm, is able to comprehend or describe what exactly is going on inside of them, let alone how the AI algorithm came to a particular conclusion. The LIME and SHAP module, which will be briefly discussed and shown in use cases in the methodology sections, has been used for carrying out such activities.

10.5 Dataset description

The used dataset is a JSON file. JSON is an open standard file format and data exchange format that employs text that can be read by humans to store and transport data objects made up of arrays and attribute-value pairs (or other serializable values). It is a typical data format having a wide range of applications in electronic data exchange. The JSON file includes the key, tag, and associated queries and questions. As an illustrative example, "Greetings" is key in a JSON file, and under this key, there will be some patterns of

Table 10.1 Description of dataset.

Key	Queries pattern	Answers pattern
Greetings	["Hey," "Hello," "Hi," "Good Day"]	["Hello," "Hey," "How can I help you?" "What can I do for you?" "hi beautiful," "Hola people"]
Goodbye	["See you," "Thank you"]	["Bye Bye," "You're most welcome," "Thank you," "See you soon my friend"]
bad feeling	["I am feeling bad," "I have a bad feeling," "I am confused and feeling bad"]	["Why are you feeling bad, is something bothering you? you can tell me freely," "If something bothers you"]

questions and replies. Each "key" in a JSON file is designated as the main thing that divides the queries and inquiries. The pattern of questions and replies, or inquiries, comes next. There will be some questions in the "question/queries" area that will aid the bot in remembering the format of questions/queries. The bot will then go to the "answer" section based on the format of the questions/queries. The replies section outlines the kinds of questions the bot will answer and the general format it will use.

Three keys are seen in Table 10.1. With questions and answers, these keys have been the most frequently utilized. The word "Key" is a tag in Table 10.1, and keys like "Greetings," "Goodbye," and "poor emotion" are found under this tag. There are more keys than even in the dataset. There are 20 keys in the dataset. Also, there are patterns for questions and answers under each of the 20 keys. The query pattern aids the bot in determining the nature of the user's questions and requests. Also, the pattern of the response includes information about the types of answers that should be provided in response to user requests. The dataset consists of 2000+ data points along with different keys and different tags. For improved working, even more information has been added. The mental health dataset was created by gathering information from actual doctors. The signs of a patient's mental instability and the kinds of questions he asked have already been gathered. It has also been used in the section on query patterns that were previously discussed. After that, the doctor's solutions and recommendations were gathered and presented in the "answers pattern" section.

10.6 Proposed method

The showcase of methodology is quite important, where it will be shown how the model works, its internal structure, and how the model gives accurate answers to the corresponding users.

Data preparation is required after data collection and dataset construction. An essential phase in the data mining process is data preparation. It describes the processes of preparing data for analysis by cleansing, converting, and integrating it. The purpose of data preprocessing is to enhance the data's quality and suitability for the particular data mining operation. Thus, to that end, preprocessing the data in the JSON dataset file. The dataset is imported first, and after that, remove all the extra letters like "?" and "!". The data is then used and tokenized after that. Tokenization is carried out to operations using the word tokenize. Next, the tag is saved, and word values are in a different variable for pattern matching. The class values for the tag values will thereafter be kept. Next, classes and words are sorted. After sorting, create a lot of words to keep the unique words. Then, both classes are transformed and a collection of words into an integer series. Classes were turned into multidimensional binary arrays in this instance, or category label encoding with class data. After that, the bot's classes and features have been stored as training data. Next, models are built. First, the RNN model is built where the input shape is the length of training data that has got after data preprocessing. It is the input shape of our model.

From Fig. 10.1, shows the structure of the RNN model, where first an input layer is the basic RNN input layer. Then the two hidden layers, or dense layers, are added. And lastly, the output layer has a length of the class. The model is compiled with categorical_crossentropy loss and the "Adam" optimizer function. Among the layers, there are two dropout layers for removing overfitting-related issues. Then the training data is fitted in the model with 300 epochs with batch_size 5. Then a CNN model is built, where the input shape is the length of feature training data and it consists of other layers.

As it is shown in Fig. 10.2, the input shape from training data is used here. Afterward, 2000 filters and an embedded layer were utilized, with the input shape being the length of the feature. Following the use of max pooling and the 3Conv1D layer with 32,32,64 filters each, the 3Conv1D layer is utilized with 12,32,64 filters again. Subsequently, the conv1D layer and the max pooling layer are applied to unit 1 together. There are seven conv1D layers in all. In the end, two dense layers are employed, with the first layer having 128 units and the output layer's final layer having a class length. The model was

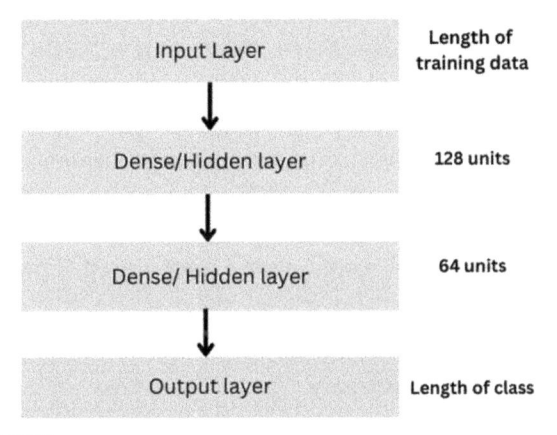

Fig. 10.1 Structure of RNN.

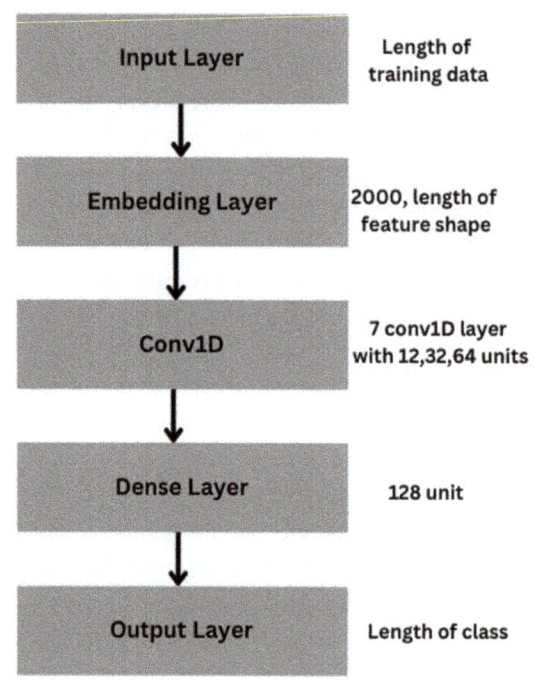

Fig. 10.2 Structure of CNN.

then put together using the "Adam" optimizer with categorical_crossentropy loss. The training data has then been fitted using batch size 5 and the same epoch 300.

From Table 10.2, RNN has better accuracy after 300 epochs with the lowest loss. CNN is also closer to RNN. But this model has given good responses also to the user, but when concatenating is done in these two models, the accuracy becomes highest and performance gives greater and better than the previous.

In Fig. 10.3, build models are loaded with the CNN model and the RNN model. The model is saved with the .h5 extension when it is built. Hierarchical Data Format (HDF) is a set of file formats (HDF4, HDF5, h5) designed to store and organize large amounts of data. Originally developed at the U.S. National Center for Supercomputing Applications, it is supported by The HDF Group, a non-profit corporation whose mission is to ensure the continued development of HDF5 technologies and the continued accessibility of data stored in HDF. After saving, these two models are loaded. Each model is taken as input and layer. After that, a concatenate layer is used. The concatenation layer

Table 10.2 Tabular form of accuracy and loss of RNN and CNN model.

Model	Accuracy	Loss
RNN	0.9788	0.0368
CNN	0.9634	0.0876

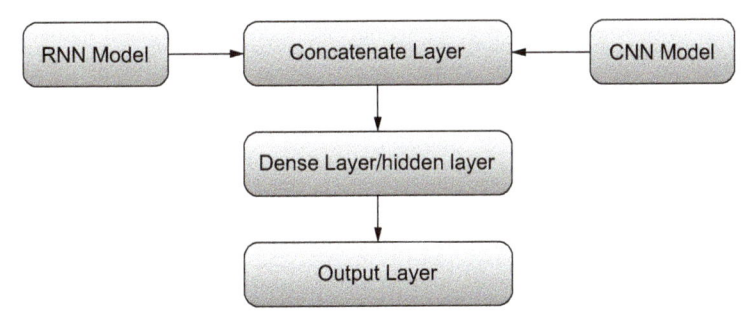

Fig. 10.3 Flow chart of integrated stacked ensemble.

takes inputs and concatenates them along a specified dimension. Then, after concatenation, a hidden layer or dense layer is used with 128 units, and then the output layer is used to specify the output of the model prediction.

Table 10.3 shows model layer comparison, where each layer is vital for building the model. And also, Stacked Ensemble has all the layers that have been used in CNN, RNN, and Stacked Ensemble. After building the model, fit the training data into a stacked model. Then, got the highest accuracy of 0.9898 and a loss of 0.043, which makes the model better.

Table 10.4, shows that while the accuracy between RNN and CNN is slightly closer, their differences in loss are far greater. Yet, among the three models, the accuracy of the stacked model is the highest. The stacking model, which provides superior accuracy and performance, was created using this implemented model. And it also increases performance, and users get more accurate and well-written answers. Even training the stacked model takes fewer epochs. In 200 epochs, it gives better accuracy than RNN and CNN with minimum loss.

Table 10.5 shows that the stacked model takes fewer epochs and iterations to reach the highest accuracy, which is 0.9898. Where RNN and CNN both take 300 epochs to get the highest accuracy, which decreases the execution time and training time.

Table 10.3 Comparison of layers of different models.

Model	Dense layer	Dropout	Conv1D	Concatenate	Embedding layer
CNN	3 Dense layer	5 Dropout (0.2)	7 Conv1D layer	—	1 Embedding layer (len (features))
RNN	3 Dense layer	2 Dropout layer(0.2)	—	—	—
Stacked ensemble	2 Dense layer	1 Dropout layer(0.2)	—	1 Concatenate layer (RNN and CNN)	—

Table 10.4 Accuracy and loss comparison between three different models.

Model	Accuracy	Loss
RNN	0.9788	0.0368
CNN	0.9634	0.0876
Stacked model	0.9898	0.043

Table 10.5 Comparison of various epochs with various models.

Model	Epochs
RNN	300
CNN	300
Stacked model	200

The line graph in Fig. 10.4 demonstrates that each model's accuracy rises at a particular epoch iteration stage. The accuracy of all three of them is 0 for the 0 epoch before increasing with each succeeding epoch. The accuracy of the stacked model overtook the other two after 50 epochs. And in a 200 epoch, it becomes maximal and constant, which implies that after the 200 epoch, the accuracy does not fluctuate and delivers stable accuracy up to the 300 epoch. For this reason, it is important to gather and highlight the accuracy data that occurs at 200 epochs first. But in the case of the other two models, the accuracy difference with stacked is high. So, up to 300 epochs, the accuracy differences become low, and getting the highest point where the difference is low means CNN and RNN got their highest accuracy, and the difference with the highest accuracy is also low.

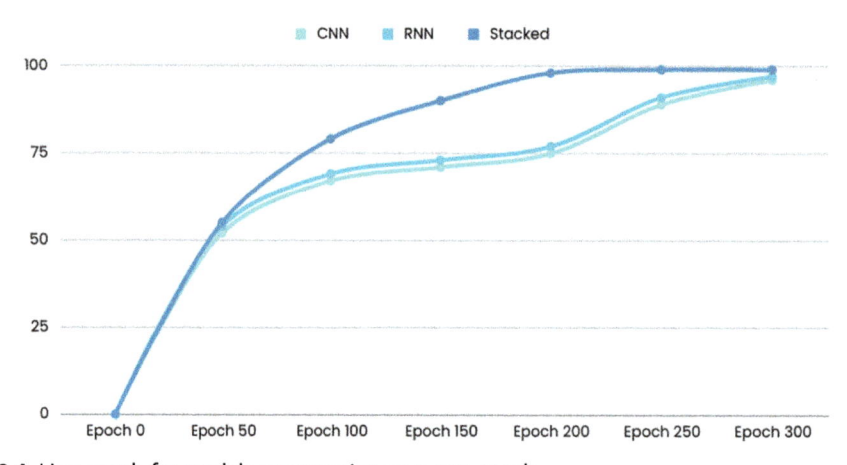

Fig. 10.4 Line graph for models accuracy increase per epoch.

So, for better performance and better results, then choose the stacked model. Then our model is used to predict user queries, and the model gives closer predictions and solutions to the user's problems. Voice engines are set so users can ask the bot in voice mode also. For voice engines, Google API is used. The Google API has been invoked using the pyttsx3 module, which helps in voice recognition. And the tts engine is also used, which means text-to-speech, where the user will get their solution in voice mode also. The model is known as "switch mode."

From Fig. 10.5 it has been shown the voice mode and text mode are both contained in "switch mode." Here, if the user wants to use anyone mode at the time during their conversation, they can simply use the switch mode to change the mode. The "switch mode" helps the user to interchange between text mode to speech mode or speech mode to text mode. It makes communication easy and builds a strong interconnection relationship between the user and the bot. After training and prediction, the stacked model is set for XAI. LIME and SHAP are used for XAI. LIME is the acronym for Local Interpretable Model-Agnostic Explanations and is a technique that approximates any black box machine learning model with a local, interpretable model to explain each prediction. In the case of SHAP, it is a mathematical method to explain the predictions of machine learning models. It is based on the concepts of game theory and can be used to explain the predictions of any machine learning model by calculating the contribution of each feature to the prediction. After training the model, LIME and SHAP are used for the model interpretable. Where LIME gives tabular results and SHAP gives a graphic illustration. Then the model is interpretable.

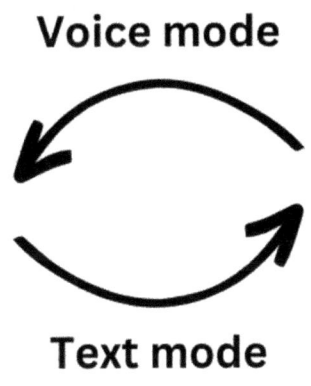

Fig. 10.5 Switch mode concept.

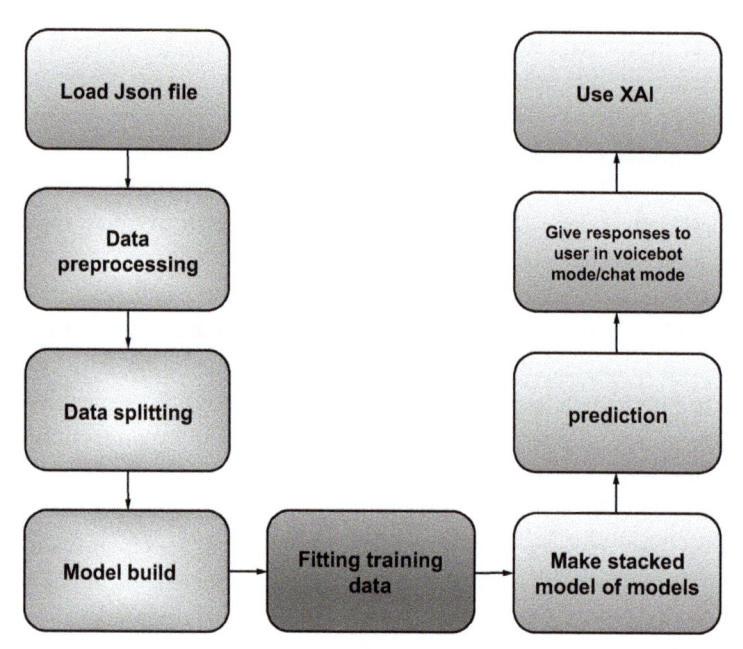

Fig. 10.6 Proposed workflow.

In Fig. 10.6, the suggested work is observed as an architecture or chart from the above figure. Where our dataset is loaded initially. A JSON file is loaded because the dataset is in JSON format. Following that, the data is processed. Links have been cleared after the symbols underwent data preparation. After that, the data was divided into classes and features. After dividing it and constructing the suggested models, such as RNN and CNN, using a few hyperparameters. Next, the training set is fitted with classes and features. After the model has been trained, two models are taken and combined to create a stacked model. The stacked model is fitted after building it. Finally, using test data, the stacking model is anticipated or provided to a user for feedback. The bot then responds by applying prediction analysis to the model. The bot has two modes: chat and voice. The user can switch from chat mode to voice mode and vice versa. XAI is added to establish confidence after all of this prediction analysis. The XAI makes the model interoperable and helps users understand the black box model.

10.7 Result and analysis

Results and analysis is a crucial area where the various experimental findings, model performance, and XAI findings are displayed. From this, it is possible to determine whether the suggested work fits the existing problem statement and resolves the user's key problems or not.

The below Algorithm 1 pseudocode shows how the model has been built, training, prediction, and giving XAI results through different steps. It shows all internal works and how each step gives a major role from data preprocessing to XAI.

ALGORITHM 1 Pseudocode of the proposed BOT system.

Step 1: Make a JSON file along with tags, patterns, and responses. Here, tags will represent the group, patterns represent the question or query format of the user and the response represents how the bot will respond.

Step 2: load json file, intents=json.loads(open('intents.json').read().

Step 3: First task to ignore unnecessary letters, ignore_letters= ['?','!']

Step 4: Store each word of patterns and tags, and lemmatize them. words=[lemmatizer. lemmatize("word") for a word in words if the word is not in ignore_letters].

Step 5: Sort the words to not repeat the same word in the model and make it unique, words=sorted(set(words))

Step 6: Open the files in binary mode and make a dump file for it,
    pickle.dump(words, open('words.pk1', 'wb'))
    pickle.dump(words, open('class.pk1',' wb'))

Step 7: Add all words and patterns after lemmatizing to training list training=[], empty list
    word_patterns=[lemmatizer. l emmatize("word. lower"()) for a word in word_patterns], for lemmatizing Loop: word in word list -:(will take each element from words word list)
    bag.append(1) if the word in word_patterns or if it is not in word_patterns, bag append the value of "0"
    output_Row=list of output empty, list(output_empty)
    output_Row of classes.index of documents =1
    training. append(list of bag and output_Row)

Step 8: shuffle all words in the training list, random.shuffle(training)

Step 9: Then store training list one part to train_x which will our feature part and another part to train_y which is our class part

Step 10: Then build individual model

Step 11: For RNN model, use sequential model, RNN=Sequential()

Step 12: add 3 hidden layers,2 dropout Model.add(Dense_layer)x3
    Model.add(Dropout_layer)x2

Step 13: Then compile the model and train it. Model. Compile (categorical loss), Model. Train (train_x and train_y)

Step 14: Then For the CNN model, the same Sequential model has been used, CNN=Sequential()

Step 15: 7 CNN layer, 5 Dropout layer added.
    Model.add(CNN_layer)x7
    Model.add(Dropout)x5

Step 16: Compile the model, Model.compile(categorical_loss)

Step 17: Train the model, CNN.train(train_x and train_y)

(Continued)

> **ALGORITHM 1 Pseudocode of the proposed BOT system—cont'd**
>
> **Step 18**: After building and training two models, the two of them have been loaded into a list, list=[RNN, CNN]
> **Step 19**: Then list has passed to Stacked architecture function, define_stacked(list)
> **Step 20**: in the function, stack=input_of_models(list1), list1= for loop RNN to CNN
> **Step 21**: Concatenate them stack=concatenate(list1)
> **Step 22**: add two hidden layers, stack.add(Dense_layer)x2
> **Step 23**: compile the model and stack.compile(categorical_loss)
> **Step 24**: here features value become 2 tensors as our input and model both concatenate, x=train_x for loop stack.input.first_layer to stack. input.last_layer
> **Step 25**: train the model and stack.train(x,train_y)
> **Step 26**: prediction, stack.predict(user's query)
> **Step 27**: for giving the predictive response, switch mode has enabled
> If switch mode==" text". Then text mode is invoked and stacked.predict(user's query) in chat mode . otherwise
> then voice mode invoked,Then tts engine has been invoked and the user gets a reply on voice mode
> **Step 28:** now Send the user's query value to Lime, SHAP for XAI
> **Step 29**: For Lime, Lime tabular has been used explainer=Lime.tabular(user's query, features, and classes)
> **Step 30**: Lime.show_as_notebook(stack .predict)
> **Step 31**: For SHAP, kernel explainer has been used, shap_explainer=kernel_explainer(stack . predict, user's query).
> **Step 32**: shap.summary_plot(here the kernel values come and other features) for showing the summary plot XAI.

10.7.1 Experimental setup

Experimental setup is quite important for any work. It tells in which environment the system has been working and its research work has been done. In the case of this research work, the experimental setup is below:-

- Processor: Core i3, Intel
- Processor type/architecture: x86_64
- CPU cores: 2
- SSD: 128GB
- Ram: 12GB
- OS:- Elementary os
- A Linux distribution based on Ubuntu LTS is called elementary OS. With a pay-what-you-want business model, it positions itself as a "thoughtful, competent, and ethical"

alternative to Windows and macOS. The desktop environment, the operating system, and related software are created and maintained by Elementary.
- Version: "6.1 Jólnir"
- VERSION_CODENAME=jolnir
- Version of the kernel: 5.15.0-67-generic
- Text-editor: VScode
- Programming language: Python
- Version: 3.8.10
- Extension of files: .ipynb, .json, .h5
- Here .ipynb extension indicates python jupyter file extension. .json JSON file extension is used in our dataset. .h5 is used for model extension.

10.7.2 Time complexity analysis

As we know, each proposed work has a time range to complete its execution. And each algorithm takes a time to run. So, in our proposed work, it has a certain amount of time taken to execute. Opening a website and making a connection with each user takes $O(1)$ notation time. Whereas for predicting a certain query through voice or text mode, the proposed algorithm takes $O(n)$ notation where n stands for the number of lines in the query.

The three models that have been used in our work, have been taken three different distinct times to train.

Table 10.6 shows the training time comparison between the proposed methods. Here, each time has been indicated as the amount of time it has taken to train a certain model. The CNN model takes a large amount of time as the number of neurons and layers is more. Then comes the RNN model, which takes a medium range of time to train. And in the end, the stacked model gives more accurate results in fewer epochs, which have been discussed before in Table 10.5, giving less amount of time in training.

10.7.3 Optimizer analysis

Optimizers are techniques or approaches that are used to minimize an error function (loss function) or to maximize production efficiency. Optimizers are mathematical functions that are affected by the model's learnable parameters, such as weights and biases.

Table 10.6 Training time/execution time comparison.

Model	Time (s)
CNN model	88.89 s
RNN model	13.58 s
Stacked model	11.32 s

Table 10.7 Optimizer comparison.

Optimizer function	Accuracy	Loss
Adam	0.9898	0.043
Rmsprop	0.9643	0.0689
Adagrad	0.2679	2.4714
Adadelta	0.1250	2.5979
SGD	0.9464	0.5389

Optimizers assist in determining how to modify the weights and learning rate of a neural network to minimize losses.

Table 10.7 shows the optimizer comparison between optimizers that have been used in our proposed model. After doing research with those optimizers, the results have been shown in the tabular format where two columns exist, "Accuracy" and "Loss." Here, it is observed that adagrad and adadelta both have the lowest accuracy and highest loss, which makes our model performance low. On the other hand, there are SGD, RMSpropo, and Adam. And among those optimizers, it has been observed that SGD has the highest low among the three optimizers. In the end, the comparison goes between "Adam" and "RMSprop," where both have better accuracy and loss, but among them, "Adam" has the highest accuracy with the minimum loss, which is best for the proposed model's performance. So, for our proposed study and work, the "Adam" optimizer has been chosen to build and train the proposed model. And it gives better performance and more accurate prediction of the user's query.

10.7.4 Result

This XAI bot is intelligent enough to help users get rid of their problems. At the same time, this bot can produce predicted output in text as well as voice format. Like this bot, users can also give input in the voice as well as text format. Some snapshots of the bot are given below in Fig. 10.7A and B.

In Fig. 10.7A, a user is giving input that the user is feeling low at that time. This XAI bot is updated enough for giving solutions that work well. XAI is always ready for giving better solutions to the user for his/her problems. Here, this conversational agent will give a better solution than other things. When one cannot express their mental pressure to others, then this bot will help them to come out of their mental disorder. Fig. 10.7B is explaining how this bot is also giving output for any health-related problem. Fever is a common problem in humans. Sometimes, fever indicates a serious issue for people. This bot is specifically made by doctors' consultants. Only doctors can identify what the correct reason is for fever or other diseases. So this bot is made with their advice.

Fig. 10.8 shows that the bot is replying formally and decently. It works like a human who will help one in a bad time.

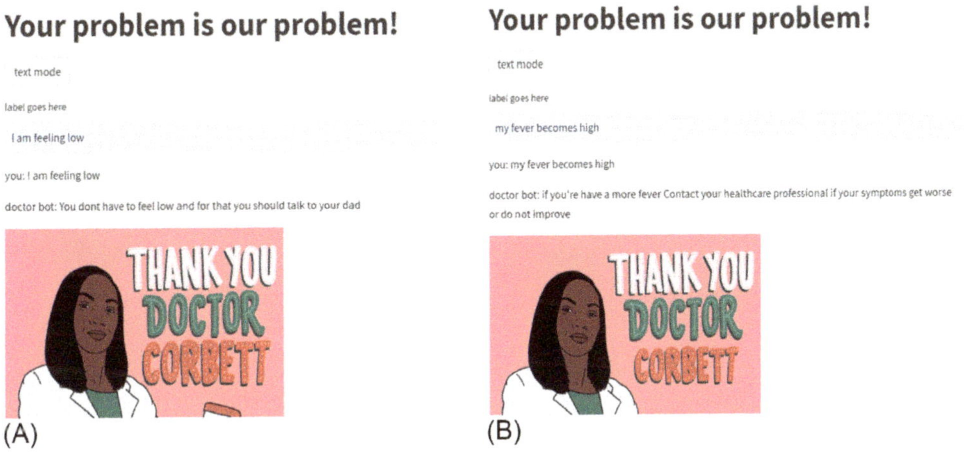

Fig. 10.7 (A): Feeling low problem and its solution. (B): Increasing fever problem and its solution.

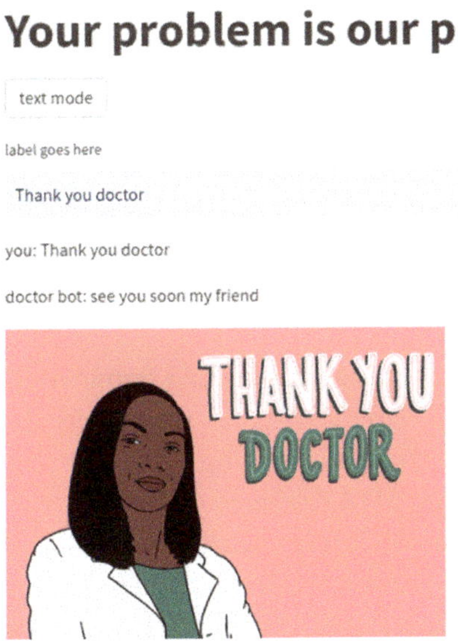

Fig. 10.8 Responding to greetings.

LIME, or Local Interpretable Agnostic Explanation, is an XAI framework that is used to explain the black box structure of machine learning models, which helps in the interpretability of the models. These interpretations are in the form of visual representations that help to get a better insight into the factors affecting the prediction of the model, or, in rather simple terms, it helps to gain an understanding of what the contributions of the features of a dataset are in the prediction of the model that is made

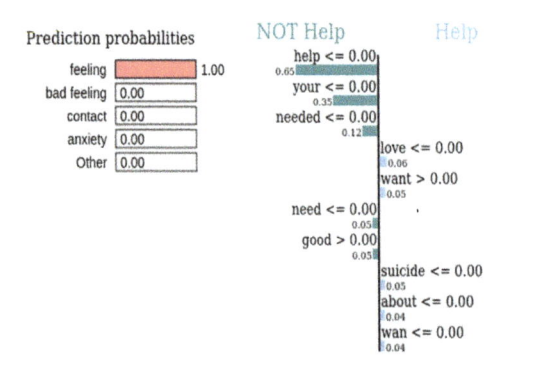

Fig. 10.9 LIME Tabular Explainer showing an explanation of a prediction.

upon the data. It can also explain the prediction for a particular data point in the whole dataset.

Fig. 10.9 shows the prediction of a particular data point out of the whole dataset. In the prediction, there are prediction probabilities, where the feeling of the individual is mentioned after the prediction is performed. The structure in the middle of the image helps us to understand what are the features that contributed to the classes "NOT Help" and "Help." For example, from the same image, the features "help," "your," "needed," etc. contribute to the prediction of the class "NOT Help." Whereas, the features "love," "want," "Suicide," etc. contribute to the prediction of the class "Help." The feature value lists all the features that are considered in the prediction, along with the contribution values.

Shapley Additive Explanation, or SHAP, is a famous XAI framework that provides model-agnostic local explainability for a variety of types of datasets. It is a thoracic approach that explains the output of any machine learning model. It connects optimal credit allocation with the local explanation. SHAP is based on Shapley values (a concept popularly used in game theory). By definition, Shapley values are the mean marginal contribution of each feature value across all possible values in the feature space. In simple terms, if there are 10 features in the dataset, then SHAP gives some visual representation of the contributions of each of the features to the prediction of the model in a given problem.

The SHAP summary plot defines the global interpretation of the feature and their contributions to the prediction of each class. In the figure, the feature "about" is having the largest impact on the prediction of that class. Also from the feature "about," all the classes like love, suicide, give up, etc., have their impact on the prediction. Similar is the case for other features of the dataset, Fig. 10.10.

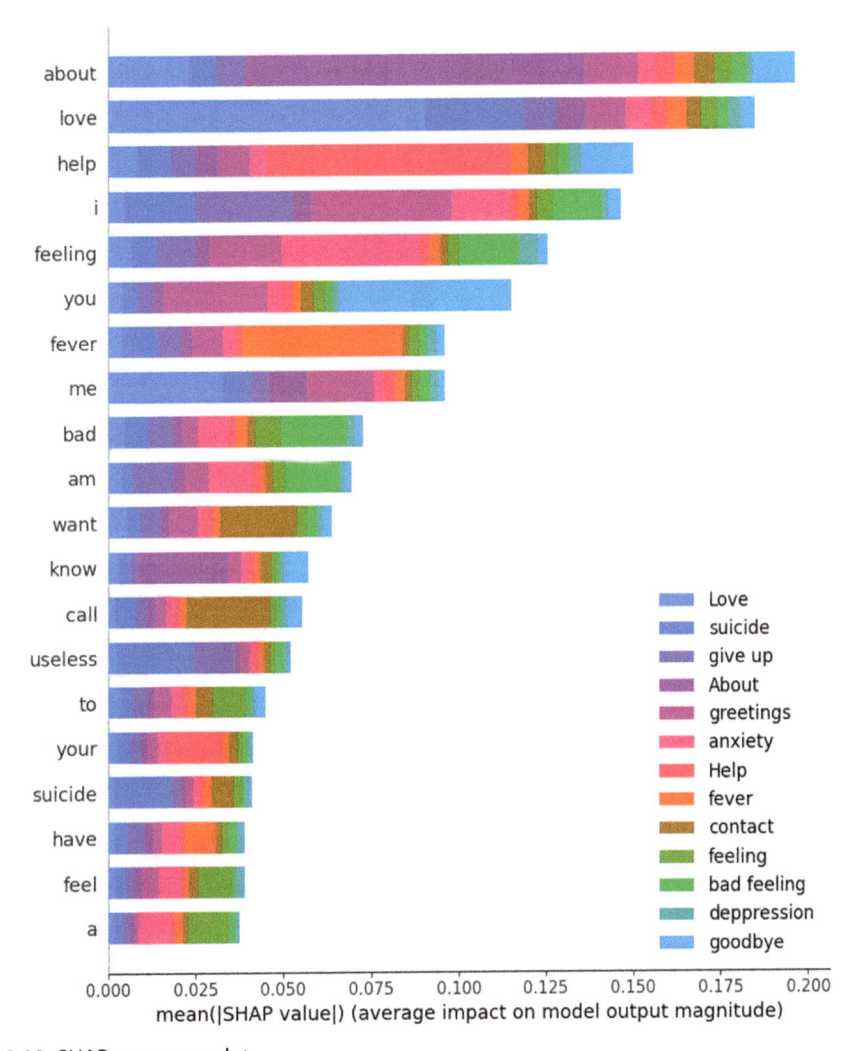

Fig. 10.10 SHAP summary plot.

10.7.5 Comparison

Table 10.8 is the comparison of our study and some related works in the same domain. The study by Shi et al. [18] proposed a transfer learning-based English language learning chatbot that produced output generated by GPT-2, which can be explained by the corresponding ontology graph. Three levels were designed for systematic English learning, which include the phonetics level for speech recognition and correcting pronunciation, semantic levels, and the simulation of free-style conversation by XAI that helps to

Table 10.8 A comparison study with our proposed model with and three existing models.

	Our proposed model	Shi et al. [18]	Ali et al. [15]	Malhotra et al. [5]
User model	Stack ensemble learning	Transfer learning	None	Conventional machine learning and NLP techniques
Interface	Dual interface	Dual interface	No interface	No interface
Use of XAI	Yes	Yes	No	No
Use of social media data	No	No	Yes	Yes

visualize the connections of the neural network in bionics and explain the output sentence from the language model. The main focus of this work is depression and anxiety disorders. After reviewing 29 reports, 26 trails passed the test cases for finalized trails. This study also does not involve the usage of social media data. The study of Abd-Alrazaq et al. [15] is focused on evaluating how effective and safe chatbots are to improve mental health by analyzing and pooling the results of previous studies. The study is a systematic review carried out from different citations from bibliographical databases like MEDLINE, EMBASE, etc. The study examined a total of 12 studies for the purpose. Certain weak evidence shows that chatbots are effective in the case of depression, stress, anxiety, etc. Also, according to some similar evidence, it is shown that there is no significant effect statistically using chatbots on psychological well-being. As this is a systematic review, it does not involve the usage of any models, interfaces, or datasets. The paper [5] focuses on psychological health, especially depression. This study uses social media data to predict the mental health status of an individual with the help of machine learning, NLP, and conventional techniques. This study includes state-of-the-earth techniques, features, datasets, and performance metrics. It also proposes a framework for mental health surveillance. This study used conventional machine learning and NLP techniques, and there was no use of XAI. The dataset used was social media data. No interface was built for the study or the model.

10.7.6 Benefits

- **Instant response:** This chatbot is very fast to respond to users. After putting input, users get output within a few milliseconds. In addition, the chatbot tries to maintain average time complexity for every type of input from the users.
- **24/7 Service time:** This proposed chatbot works at all times. There is no break time for this intelligent bot. Users can use it at all times without any delay. Due to its 24/7 service time, it can be used in any emergency medical system.

- **Correct information:** The chatbot is always ready to produce correct information for users. With the average response time, the conversational agent always tries to generate output with a high rate of accuracy.
- **User friendly:** First of all, the chatbot does not reveal the personal information of any mental patients. So, this bot gives a comfort zone to the users. At the same time, the use of it is very easy. Everyone can use it without any confusion. In addition, users can give input in the form of verbal as well as in language.

10.8 Limitation and conclusion

The system or the bot has some limitations, which can be solved in the future. Limitations of mental healthcare are stress and time pressures: difficulties managing assignments, prioritizing tasks, and meeting deadlines as a result of time pressures and multiple tasks. Having a problem with multitasking. It is difficult for them to get along with others, fit in, contribute to group work, and read social cues when interacting with others. Across the globe, many people who require mental health care are unable to access high-quality services. There is a treatment gap in mental health because of stigma, human resource shortages, fragmented service delivery models, and a lack of research capacity for implementation and policy change. There are three most common diagnoses when it comes to anxiety disorders, depression, and post-traumatic stress disorder. In addition to seeing, hearing, and moving, communication, cognition, and self-care are all considered functional limitations. This mental health care bot will help to resolve this problem easily. In the case of voice mode, if the voice is not clear or leads to too much noise, it may deal with the wrong speech-to-text conversion, which can lead to the wrong prediction of the bot. On the other hand, the system is unable to take input as a picture from the user. There are a few limitations with the system or the bot that can be resolved in the future. When using voice mode, if the speech-to-text conversion is not clear or has too much noise, the bot may make the wrong prediction based on the speech-to-text conversion. In contrast, the system cannot accept input from a user in the form of a picture. The study uses various kinds of algorithms to build an XAI-based voice and chatbot. RNN, CNN, and integrated stack ensemble are used in this study. Among these applied algorithms, stack ensemble provides better accuracy with 98.98% and a loss of 0.043. In this work, a conversational agent is used to deal with mental health disorders in the healthcare world. All kinds of solutions for different kinds of mental health problems are available to this powerful bot. Not only in the primary stage, but the bot is also responsible enough to handle the critical stage of any disease. This study is related to mental health disease, but this work can be used in other healthcare sections also, like cancer, HIV, heart disease, etc. More features can be added in the future to get better accuracy with better output also. Day by day, new algorithms are coming into the market. We can apply more new technology to enhance the performance of this work. In the future, we plan to recommend perfect medicines as per the inputs of users' common health problems through this bot with high-level accuracy.

Declaration of data availability

The authors declare that the data that support the findings of this study are not openly available due to reasons of sensitivity and are available from the corresponding author upon reasonable request.

Declaration of conflicts of interest statement

The authors whose names are listed in the paper have NO affiliations with or involvement in any organization or entity with any financial interest (such as honoraria; educational grants; participation in speakers' bureaus; membership, employment, consultancies, stock ownership, or other equity interest; and expert testimony or patent-licensing arrangements) or non-financial interest (such as personal or professional relationships, affiliations, knowledge, or beliefs) in the subject matter or materials discussed in this manuscript.

References

[1] L. Balcombe, D. De Leo, Digital mental health challenges and the horizon ahead for solutions, JMIR Ment. Health 8 (3) (2021) e26811.
[2] L. Balcombe, D. De Leo, Human-computer interaction in digital mental health, in: Informatics, vol. 9, No. 1, MDPI, 2022, p. 14.
[3] Z.S. Chen, I.R. Galatzer-Levy, B. Bigio, C. Nasca, Y. Zhang, Modern views of machine learning for precision psychiatry, Patterns 3 (11) (2022) 100602.
[4] B. Abedin, C. Meske, I. Junglas, F. Rabhi, H.R. Motahari-Nezhad, Designing and managing human-AI interactions, Inf. Syst. Front. 24 (3) (2022) 691–697.
[5] A. Malhotra, R. Jindal, Deep learning techniques for suicide and depression detection from online social media: a scoping review, Appl. Soft Comput. (2022) 109713.
[6] K.C. Kellogg, S. Sadeh-Sharvit, Pragmatic AI-augmentation in mental healthcare: key technologies, potential benefits, and real-world challenges and solutions for frontline clinicians, Front. Psychiatry 13 (2022) 990370.
[7] D.E. Park, Y.J. Shin, E. Park, I.A. Choi, W.Y. Song, J. Kim, Designing a voice-bot to promote better mental health: UX design for digital therapeutics on ADHD patients, in: Extended Abstracts of the 2020 Chi Conference on Human Factors in Computing Systems, 2020, pp. 1–8.
[8] C. Moret-Tatay, H.M. Radawski, C. Guariglia, Health professionals' experience using an azure voice-bot to examine cognitive impairment (WAY2AGE), in: Healthcare, vol. 10, No. 5, MDPI, 2022, April, p. 783.
[9] D.E. Park, J. Lee, J. Han, J. Kim, Y.J. Shin, A preliminary study of Voicebot to assist ADHD children in performing daily tasks, in: International Journal of Human–Computer Interaction, 2023, pp. 1–14.
[10] R. Mezzi, A. Yahyaoui, M.W. Krir, W. Boulila, A. Koubaa, Mental health intent recognition for Arabic-speaking patients using the Mini international neuropsychiatric interview (MINI) and BERT model, Sensors 22 (3) (2022) 846.
[11] A.A. Abd-Alrazaq, M. Alajlani, A.A. Alalwan, B.M. Bewick, P. Gardner, M. Househ, An overview of the features of chatbots in mental health: a scoping review, Int. J. Med. Inform. 132 (2019) 103978.
[12] T. Kamita, T. Ito, A. Matsumoto, T. Munakata, T. Inoue, A chatbot system for mental healthcare based on SAT counseling method, in: Mobile Information Systems, 2019. 2019.
[13] G. Cameron, D. Cameron, G. Megaw, R.R. Bond, M. Mulvenna, S. O'Neill, M. McTear, Best practices for designing chatbots in mental healthcare–a case study on iHelpr, in: British HCI Conference 2018, BCS Learning & Development Ltd., 2018.
[14] K.M. Griffiths, L. Farrer, H. Christensen, The efficacy of internet interventions for depression and anxiety disorders: a review of randomised controlled trials, Med. J. Aust. 192 (2010) S4–S11.

[15] A.A. Abd-Alrazaq, A. Rababeh, M. Alajlani, B.M. Bewick, M. Househ, Effectiveness and safety of using chatbots to improve mental health: systematic review and meta-analysis, J. Med. Internet Res. 22 (7) (2020) e16021.
[16] C. Grové, Co-developing a mental health and wellbeing chatbot with and for young people, Front. Psychiatry 11 (2021) 606041.
[17] C. Sweeney, C. Potts, E. Ennis, R. Bond, M.D. Mulvenna, M.F. Mctear, Can chatbots help support a person's mental health? Perceptions and views from mental healthcare professionals and experts, ACM Trans. Comput. Healthc. 2 (3) (2021) 1–15.
[18] N. Shi, Q. Zeng, R. Lee, The Design and Implementation of Language Learning Chatbot with XAI using Ontology and Transfer Learning, arXiv preprint arXiv, 2020, p. 13984.
[19] N. Shi, Q. Zeng, R. Lee, Xai language tutor–a Xai-based language learning Chatbot using ontology and transfer learning techniques, IJNLC 9 (2020).

Further Reading

A.A. Abd-Alrazaq, M. Alajlani, N. Ali, K. Denecke, B.M. Bewick, M. Househ, Perceptions and opinions of patients about mental health chatbots: scoping review, J. Med. Internet Res. 23 (1) (2021) e17828.
P. Amiri, E. Karahanna, Chatbot use cases in the Covid-19 public health response, J. Am. Med. Inform. Assoc. 29 (5) (2022) 1000–1010.
R.H. Aswathy, AGRIMART: An E-platform for agro products with voice based Chat Bot, in: 2022 Second International Conference on Advanced Technologies in Intelligent Control, Environment, Computing & Communication Engineering (ICATIECE), IEEE, 2022, December, pp. 1–5.
S. Athikkal, J. Jenq, Voice Chatbot for Hospitality, 2022. arXiv preprint arXiv:2208.10926.
T.W. Bickmore, S. Ólafsson, T.K. O'Leary, Mitigating patient and consumer safety risks when using conversational assistants for medical information: exploratory mixed methods experiment, J. Med. Internet Res. 23 (11) (2021) e30704.
C. Bradley, D. Wu, H. Tang, I. Singh, K. Wydant, B. Capps, B. Srivastava, et al., Explainable Artificial Intelligence (XAI) User Interface Design for Solving a Rubik's Cube, in: HCI International 2022–Late Breaking Posters: 24th International Conference on Human-Computer Interaction, HCII 2022, Virtual Event, June 26–July 1, 2022, Proceedings, Part II, Springer Nature Switzerland, Cham, 2022, pp. 605–612.
S. Chakraborty, H. Paul, S. Ghatak, S.K. Pandey, A. Kumar, K.U. Singh, M.A. Shah, An AI-based medical Chatbot model for infectious disease prediction, IEEE Access 10 (2022) 128469–128483.
M. Gao, X. Liu, A. Xu, R. Akkiraju, Chat-XAI: a new chatbot to explain artificial intelligence, in: Intelligent Systems and Applications: Proceedings of the 2021 Intelligent Systems Conference (IntelliSys) Volume 3, Springer International Publishing, 2022, pp. 125–134.
S. Hepenstal, L. Zhang, N. Kodagoda, B.L.W. Wong, Developing conversational agents for use in criminal investigations, ACM Trans. Interact. Intell. Syst. 11 (3–4) (2021) 1–35.
M. Kuźba, Conversational Explanations of Machine Learning Models using Chatbots.
G.H. Sai, M.M. Nair, V. Vani, INTELLIBOT-Intelligent voice assisted Chatbot with sentiment analysis, COVID dashboard and offensive text detection, in: Cyber Warfare, Security and Space Research: First International Conference, SpacSec 2021, Jaipur, India, December 9–10, 2021, Revised Selected Papers, Springer International Publishing, Cham, 2022, pp. 311–323.
A. Shafeeg, I. Shazhaev, D. Mihaylov, A. Tularov, I. Shazhaev, Voice assistant integrated with chat GPT, indones. J. Electrical Eng. Comput. Sci. 12 (1) (2023).
C.T. Wolf, K.E. Ringland, Designing accessible, explainable AI (XAI) experiences, ACM SIGACCESS Accessibility and Computing 125 (2020) 1.
T. Yue, D. Au, C.C. Au, K.Y. Iu, Democratizing Financial Knowledge with ChatGPT by OpenAI: Unleashing the Power of Technology, Available at SSRN, 2023, p. 4346152.

CHAPTER 11

Wearable sensors: The pathway to applications of on-body electronics

Viktorija Makarovaite and Robert Horne
School of Engineering, University of Kent, Canterbury, United Kingdom

This chapter explores on-body electronics and the transformative pathway leading to diverse applications in the radio frequency (RF) domain. Wearable sensors, designed for low power, epidermal adherence, and conformal mounting, serve as the cornerstone of this exploration. Delving into the intricate design aspects, we discuss the essential considerations vital for the development of these devices.

The majority of wearable RFID sensor publications are related to healthcare information systems such as object telemetry, logistics, and environmental sensing. These have been reviewed for chipless RFID sensors in Ref. [1]; however, here we will review chipped RFID systems. There are a number of challenges such technologies must overcome before full implementation including reliability, energy consumption, and scalability as described in Ref. [2]. To address some of these challenges, Amato et al [3] described an S-band (3.6 GHz) epidermal RFID loop design to increase transfer data speed and to reduce design complexity and [4] suggested that 5G antenna designs such as a single dipole at 5.8 GHz or a 23-element array of dipoles at 60 GHz can produce similar read ranges to UHF RFID epidermal tags but with smaller less-intrusive designs. Some such arrays have been described in Ref. [4] and Hughes et al. [5]. Hughes showed that on-body application of a 5G S-band array could produce a 6 m read range in passive mode. Utilizing RFID tags as sensor nodes within a wireless sensor network has also been explored [6]. However, there are still many concerns about implementing RFID technology as wearable sensors of which scalability and reliability remain on top [7,8].

Altogether these allow us to understand how electromagnetic fields can be measured by antennas for wearable applications. To delve further into the topic of wearable sensors, Section 1 will cover the background of RF design and considerations. Section 2 will cover the fundamentals of sensor fabrication at low volume levels focusing on the understanding of materials. Section 3 will detail the scaling up of printed sensors and electronics suitable for mass market production using techniques such as flexographic printing to achieve roll-to-roll mass manufacturing. Finally, Section 4 will conclude this chapter.

11.1 RFID wearables: Design consideration

At the core of this exploration lies the interaction between the human body and electric and magnetic fields, a complex dynamic deciphered through fundamental electromagnetic equations such as Coulomb's law, Ohm's Law, and Maxwell's equations. Distinctions between permittivity, conductivity, and permeability emerge as key elements, with a particular focus on simplifying considerations based on the human body's weak magnetic properties [9]. Assuming a permeability of 1 ($\mu r = 1$) for human tissue simplifies considerations, making permittivity and conductivity the primary focus for most RF wearable device applications.

Similarly, understanding "lossiness" in materials is crucial in wearable sensors. Perfect dielectrics (lossless materials with no free charges ($\sigma = 0$)) do not absorb power or generate heat from electromagnetic waves, making them excellent electrical insulators. Common materials such as plastics and glass are nearly lossless, with human skin and fat tissue exhibiting similar properties. For improved sensor development in human body applications, refer to [10] for dielectric properties of various human tissues.

This section will delve into RFID wearable sensors and devices, emphasizing their diverse applications in healthcare. These wearables are preferred for their easy installation compared to tethered sensors, attributed to their compact form factors, facilitating high-density deployment at reduced costs by eliminating excess wiring on components. Notably, RFID sensors excel over optical counterparts by enabling measurements without the necessity for transparent packaging. Among the most prevalent categories of wireless RFID sensors are thickness shear mode [11], magnetic acoustic resonance [12], and resonant inductor-capacitor-resistor (LCR) transducers (Fig. 11.1). The majority of these sensors possess the capability for either passive or active sensing, detecting physical, chemical, and biological changes in their specified targets. These methodologies provide cost-effective solutions for fully wireless on-body healthcare applications.

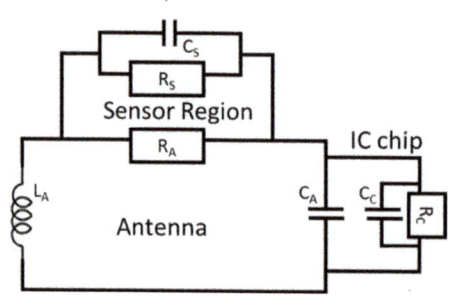

Fig. 11.1 General RFID sensor configuration consisting of an antenna, sensor area, and IC impedance matching network.

11.1.1 RFID basic principles of design

The LCR circuit RFID tag stands out as the most promising and cost-effective approach for medical applications. It excels in ultrahigh-frequency (UHF) applications, enabling long-distance detection—outperforming other common sensor methods—and offering easier adjustment of dielectric solutions to influence impedance [13]. LCR's advantages include compatibility with standard IC chips, enhancing the robustness and repeatability of sensor operation, especially when producing multiple copies of the device [13]. In a basic RFID sensor, the LCR circuit is formed by the sensing antenna and integrated circuit (IC) chip's inductance, resistance, and capacitance [14]. In UHF scenarios, a resonant RFID tag antenna receives an RF signal from the RFID reader, leading to voltage build-up on the antenna terminals. This activation of the chip allows for signal transmission back to the RFID reader, incorporating backscatter signal modulation over several meters [15].

The electrical field produced by an RFID sensor is susceptible to ambient environmental influences. This susceptibility creates an opportunity to sense the external environment [13,16]. The external environment can range from a sample of food, liquid, gas, or human body within the tag electrode's electric field. In these cases, the impedance presented to the tag transponder (IC) relies on changes in capacitance and resistance within the sensing region or entire tag [13,17]. In RF applications, understanding the real and imaginary impedance components in calculations can improve the sensor's accuracy and precision. Calculation of additional spectral parameters, such as the "real" impedance magnitude, frequency position, and resonant and antiresonant frequencies of "imaginary" impedance, further contributes to improving sensor accuracy [13]. Resonant frequency occurs when the circuit becomes purely resistive with an imaginary portion of impedance (Z) at zero. This resonance can be determined using the resonant frequency formula (11.1):

$$f_0 = \frac{1}{2\pi\sqrt{LC}} \quad (11.1)$$

with capacitance (C) and inductance (L) of the circuit included.

11.1.2 Human tissue considerations for tag design

When developing any wearable sensor, the body dielectrics should always be accounted for in the antenna and transponder chip impedance matching. Makarovaite et al. [18] described that in their wearable sensor approach, they utilized a "shunting" method previously described in Ref. [19] to reduce the near-body effects such as capacitive loading caused by the lossy properties of human tissue. If left unaccounted for, the near-body effects will reduce read ranges as gain drops causing large frequency shifts. This is why designing a wearable RFID antenna sensor without testing on the body or only simulating in the air is a poor approach; these readings and measurements will not account for the antenna attenuation due to human tissue or the degradation of the radiation efficiency or radiation pattern fragmentation [20,21]. This will be further discussed in the following section. Therefore, the only reason to use "air" measurements in wearable RFID sensors is as a calibration check to make sure that the antenna has not been detuned or damaged before reuse. In all other situations, it is imperative to design and tune the tag while attached to a body (or any other lossy material) as described in Ref. [19]. The only exceptions should be for systems that are shielded from the capacitive loading of human tissue such as designs with backings or designs that utilize this capacitive loading as a method for sensing.

Shunt scaling for resistance approach

Adjusting the real part of impedance in antenna design proves challenging without altering the antenna geometry. Nevertheless, this can be achieved by employing a shunt scaling approach [19]. When reactance (X_p) is shunted (placed in parallel) with the antenna impedance (Z_A), the following relationship holds:

$$Z_A = \frac{R_C \cdot X_p^2}{R_C^2 + (X_C + X_p)^2} + j\frac{X_p \cdot [R_C^2 + X_C \cdot (X_C + X_p)]}{(R_C^2 + [X_C + X_p]^2)}$$

The source impedance (Z_C) comprises real (R_C) and imaginary (X_C) components. Calculating X_p requires the use of an alpha scalar ($\alpha = R_A/R_C$) [19]. This alpha scalar can take either a capacitive or inductive form even with a negative reactance:

$$X_p = \mp \frac{\sqrt{\alpha}}{1 \pm \sqrt{\alpha}} \cdot X_C$$

Capacitance exhibits a frequency dependence that is linear and, therefore, is better suited for UHF applications.

However, using traditional methods, such as inductive path reduction, to limit ohmic losses is not often done for epidermal designs. Changing the geometry of an antenna design can adjust input reactance but is unlikely to cause a large change in input resistance as often there are space constraints due to intended tag placement. However, shunt scaling [19] and electric density centralization [22] can overcome these issues. These two approaches are based on loop-matching networks (reviewed in Ref. [23]) for impedance matching. The shunt scaling approach directly adjusts the tag resistance (real part of impedance) with a parallel placement of an extra component, whereas electric density centralization instead alters the antenna design geometry to limit the lossy material proximity effect. As shunt scaling improves impedance matching between transponder IC and epidermal tag by incorporating an extra component (capacitor or inductor) in an existing design, it reduces the need to change tag geometry. This often can be a necessity for reducing epidermal tag size while improving impedance matching (and often radiation efficiency). The human body's proximity effect can destroy an antenna's radiation efficiency severely limiting the read range. Therefore, both of these more novel approaches can improve epidermal tag function and help overcome the capacitive loading of human tissue.

Electric density centralization
Centralizing electric density involves shifting it away from the borders of a tag design to isolate it from a lossy substrate, as recommended for on-body tag design to minimize tag thickness [22]. This insulation strategy eliminates the need for a ground plane as a shield against the proximity effect of the lossy substrate, allowing for thinner, more flexible, and comfortable epidermal tags. Adjusting tag geometry to centralize electric density toward the tag center, which is frequency-independent, is a crucial step. Simulations should be employed to visualize electric density changes in epidermal designs, enhancing tag decoupling from the skin and ultimately increasing antenna robustness and radiation efficiency.

Due to this effect of the body on antenna attenuation, it is difficult to design any epidermal RFID sensor that can have read ranges above 3 m while on the body without the utilization of a power source. This issue can be even further complicated as tissue dielectric properties change with antenna placement on the human body not just from one volunteer to the next but also on different body locations of the same person [24]. This is because the human body has varying levels of fat-to-muscle ratios throughout and muscle is more conductive with a higher permittivity than fat, causing it to have a greater effect on antenna tuning and impedance matching [10,25,26]. Human skin dielectric properties have been known to change even due to sun exposure [27]. Understanding human body dielectric variability is key for epidermal sensor design as tissue conductivity alters antenna efficiency while permittivity affects resonant frequency [20].

11.1.3 Ultra-lower power live streaming through UHF RFID

To effectively utilize the ultra-low power data transmission capabilities of Ultrahigh-Frequency Radio Frequency Identification (UHF RFID), it is imperative to adapt conventional methodologies to accommodate the streaming of live data. Standard RFID communication predominantly involves static data transmission for identification purposes, such as tracking merchandise. This process typically tolerates low data rates, around 8–16 bytes of data. However, the foundational principles of RFID technology do permit dynamic data transfer at rates sufficient for biological measurement streaming. Biological data streaming, for instance, includes body-centric information like acceleration (60–200 Hz, 3 axis, 8–10 bit per axis) or cardiac data such as photoplethysmogram

(PPG) or electrocardiogram (ECG) at approximately 250 Hz with 8–10-bit resolution. In contrast to popular fitness devices in the consumer market that transmit data using low-power Bluetooth, UHF RFID offers a more efficient solution in terms of power consumption for reliable data transmission.

Typically, RFID systems access EEPROM memory, a static type with a limited lifespan (100,000 read/write cycles) and moderate latency (20–50 ms). While adequate for static data or infrequently changing applications, this medium is less suitable for data altering several hundred times per second. Alternatively, some UHF RFID chips incorporate a smaller volatile memory segment within RAM registers. This segment, although losing data upon power-off, offers significantly lower latency and greater endurance (approximately 10,000,000,000 read/write cycles). However, this RAM-based memory is constrained by limited space, with devices typically having only 16 bytes available in this area.

For dynamic data handling, an RFID transponder alone is insufficient. A Microcontroller Unit (MCU) is essential for scheduling data capture, processing sensor data, and transmitting it to the RFID chip seamlessly. A crucial function of the MCU is to prevent data clashes, which occur when the RFID reader and the MCU simultaneously attempt communication with the RFID chip, potentially leading to data corruption and validation challenges.

11.2 RFID wearable sensor fabrication and applications

Wearable device challenges encompass comprehending operational frequencies, considering the impact of surrounding biological tissues, addressing antenna design and miniaturization issues, ensuring compliance with international safety guidelines, and implementing suitable fabrication processes that tolerate epidermal antenna stretching [28]. We present here a few attempts to address these problems.

11.2.1 Wearable sensor stretchability

To overcome some of the expected antenna stretching issues, we looked at the effect on conductive ink (Voltera Flex 2 Ink) printing and temperature (Table 11.1). The recommended setting for this ink is at 160°C for 30 min, the wearable polymeric backing we use cannot withstand 135°C. Therefore, understanding the adjustments needed for wearable conductive ink printing is necessary. The initial test comprises 15 samples, featuring straight 15 mm-long tracks illustrated in Fig. 11.2A. Each sample is printed with varying widths on FR-4 substrates and subjected to different temperatures and durations of baking. The objective was to identify the temperature and duration that yield the track with the lowest resistance (Ω).

Since the resistance measured from the tracks sintered at 120°C and 130°C was comparable, the flexible conductor was sintered at 120°C to mitigate the risk of damaging the polymer dermal backing. Given that the curing temperatures are lower than

Table 11.1 Average resistance(Ω) for tracks bake in different temperatures and time.

		Track width utilized to measure average resistance (Ω)				
Temperature (°C)	Time (min)	0.25 mm	0.35 mm	0.45 mm	0.55 mm	0.65 mm
90	40	0.678	0.453	0.373	0.283	0.218
	50	0.688	0.473	0.380	0.285	0.228
	60	0.535	0.383	0.295	0.230	0.190
100	40	0.780	0.455	0.323	0.258	0.198
	50	0.333	0.215	0.168	0.143	0.120
	60	0.253	0.258	0.200	0.160	0.133
120	30	0.333	0.220	0.173	0.135	0.110
	40	0.300	0.185	0.143	0.113	0.093
	50	0.370	0.225	0.178	0.145	0.128
130	30	0.240	0.180	0.133	0.110	0.095
	40	0.337	0.247	0.168	0.150	0.128
	50	0.348	0.175	0.138	0.108	0.088
140	30	0.323	0.205	0.168	0.125	0.105
	40	0.368	0.243	0.190	0.133	0.108
	50	0.300	0.193	0.148	0.113	0.095

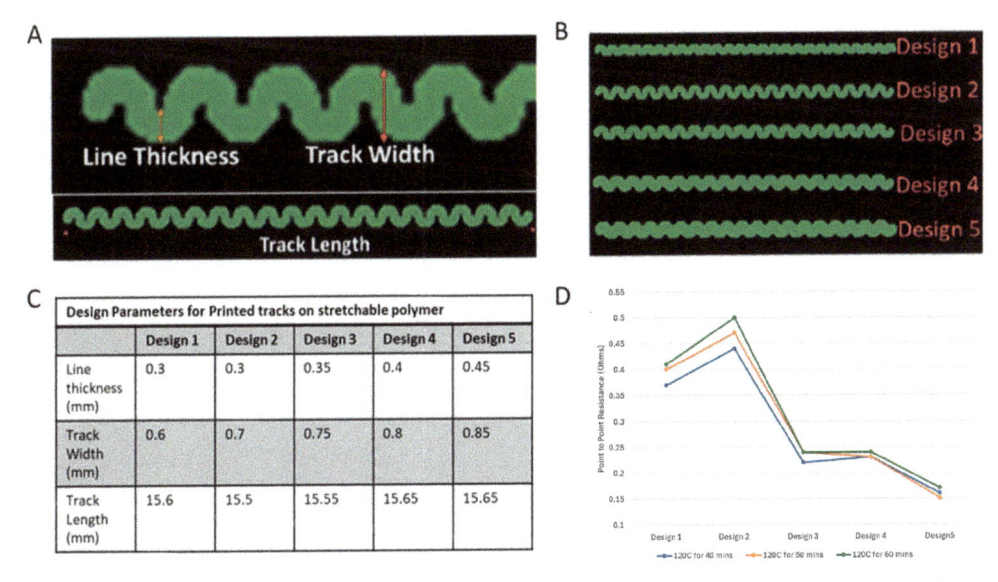

Fig. 11.2 Average values of conductive ink tracks sintered at 120°C for Different Times on Polymer Dermal Backing. (A) The characteristics adjusted between stretchable track designs. (B) The designs utilized during the experiment. (C) The dimension details for each design utilized in the experiment. (D) The average resistance for each design at 40, 50, or 60 min of sintering.

recommended, the curing time for the conductor was extended to 40 and 50 min. We then were able to test both the strength and resistivity of the conductive ink when printed on stretchable dermal polymer (Fig. 11.2). The lowest resistance was when the designs were sintered at 60°C; however, the overall difference was about 0.1Ω. Therefore, to prevent dermal polymer damage, 40 min at 120°C was utilized.

Finally, all the printed designs needed to be tested for stretchability and strength when placed on human skin. Design 5 had the least breaks after stretching, many of the breaks appeared where the vertical and horizontal tracks portions met, therefore it was decided to thicken these areas when utilizing for on-body applications (Fig. 11.3). However, breaks still appeared, so the serpentine design had to be adjusted with the addition of an arc.

These new designs, unlike previous designs, could be printed without breaks and withstand stretchability (Fig. 11.4). However, they could not withstand continued wear throughout the day. Therefore, further adjustment is needed to improve the longevity of a printed wearable and stretchable circuit.

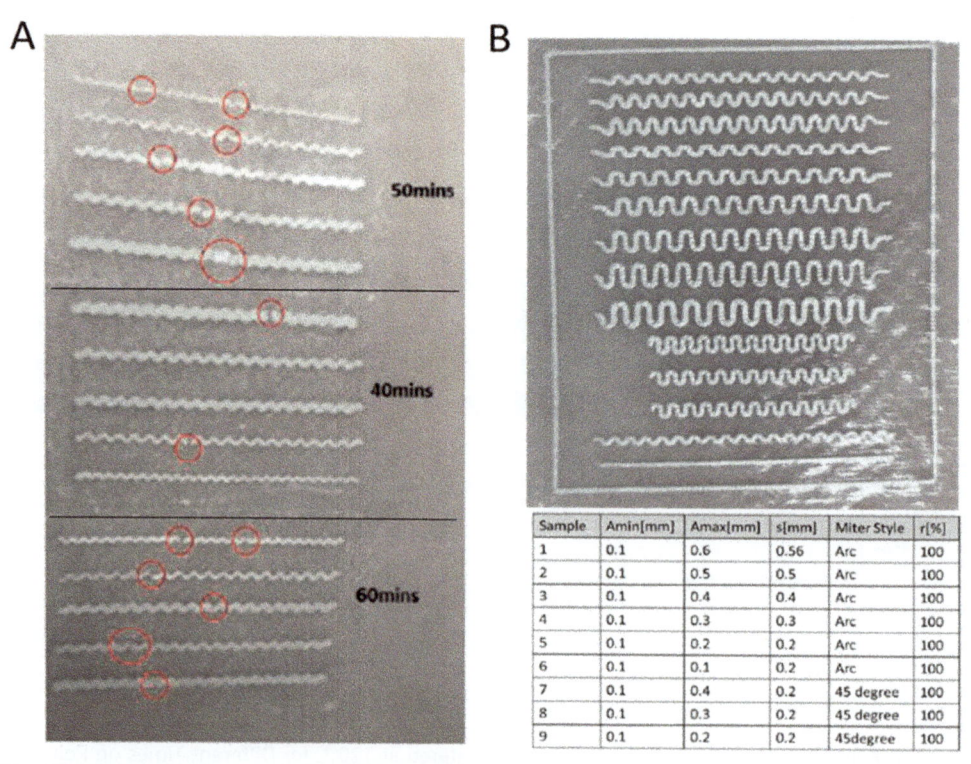

Fig. 11.3 Printed designs and adjusted printed designs to improve stretchability and wear resistance. (A) Printed tracks at varying sintering temperatures after a stretch was applied. (B) Readjusted serpentine designs to improve design thickness and stretchability.

Wearable sensors 215

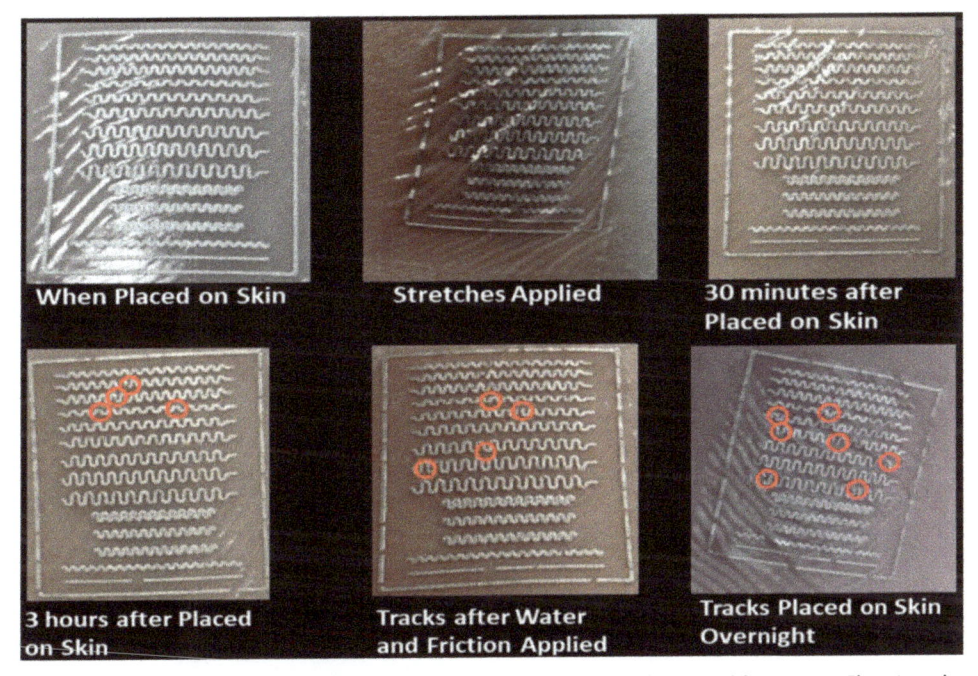

Fig. 11.4 Printed design testing for tolerance to epidermal stretching and longevity. Showing that there are no longer any breaks after printing till after 3 h when a stretch was applied.

This was followed by including protective layers over the expected break points from previous experiments. A functional design was able to be printed, stretched, and worn for over 24 h without any breaks (Fig. 11.5), suggesting that to improve printed wearable design longevity, a protective layer is necessary.

This allowed the lifespan of the device to extend to multiple days of normal everyday wear (Fig. 11.6). To design wearable devices with printed circuits, a protective layer is necessary to improve stretchability and wearability. The following testing circuit was fully functional even after 5 days of continuous wear.

11.2.2 Wearable sensors and variable human tissue dielectrics

In an attempt to address the problem of variable tissue dielectrics, Makarovaite et al described how a single wearable epidermal sensor could be utilized by a range of individuals with various dielectric skin properties with minimal loss to sensor read range (Fig. 11.7) [29]. It was suggested that decoupling the sensor from the skin for individuals with high muscle content (permittivity above 30) could negate the need for multiple sensor geometry adjustments [29]. This approach was continued in the smart PIVC (peripheral intravenous catheter) moisture sensor.

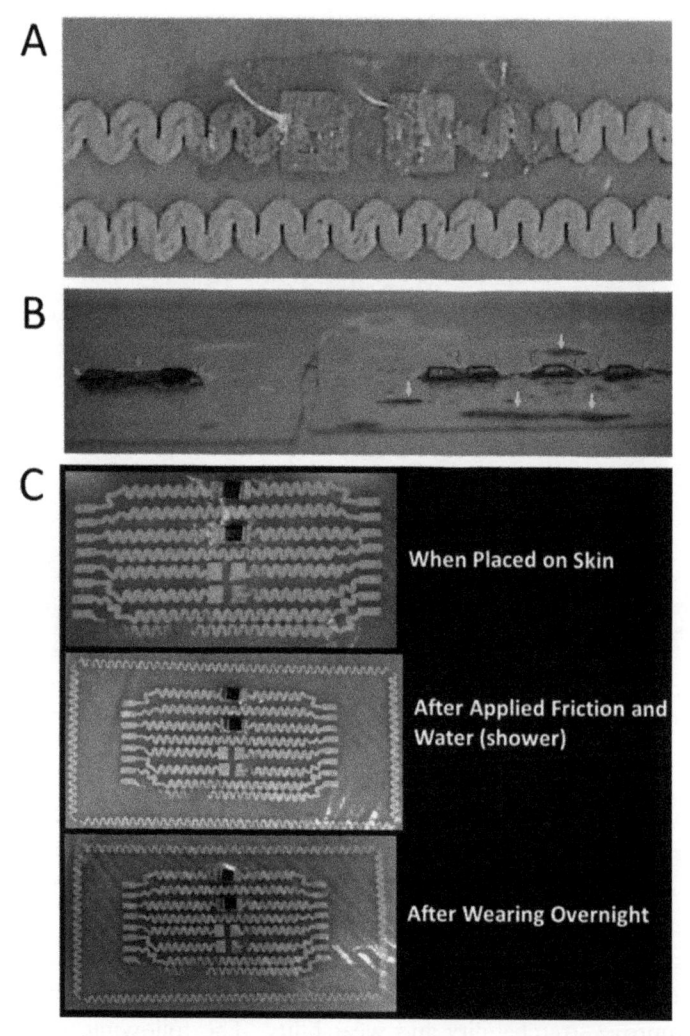

Fig. 11.5 Protection of printed wearable circuits. (A) Example of polymer layer addition to protect printed circuit. (B) Cut cross-section of printed circuit where the tracks are visually present under the protective polymer layer. (C) Stretch and wear test of 24 h.

The utilization of a PIVC is required for treatment in approximately 90% of hospitalized patients. However, the substantial range of failure rates, ranging from 36% to 63%, poses significant risks to patient safety and has notable financial implications [30]. This can lead to skin necrosis, catheter-associated bloodstream infections, disruption of medical treatments, venous depletion, and extended hospitalization periods and often necessitate PIVC removal [30]. Therefore, the understanding and detection of these PIVC failures can improve patient outcomes. In a recent study, PIVC-related adverse events (PIVCAE) accounted for 52.3 out of 100 PIVC insertions [31]. Specifically, out of these total events,

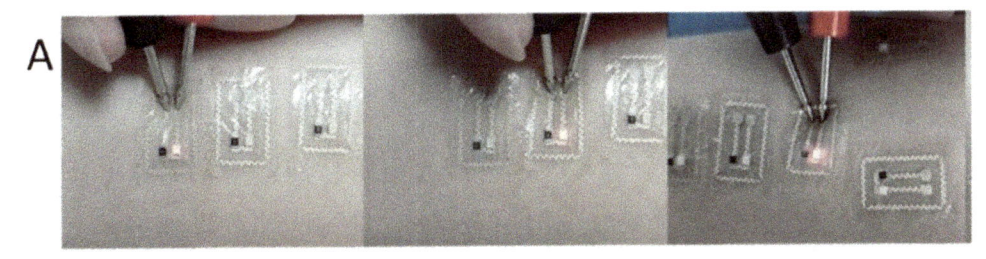

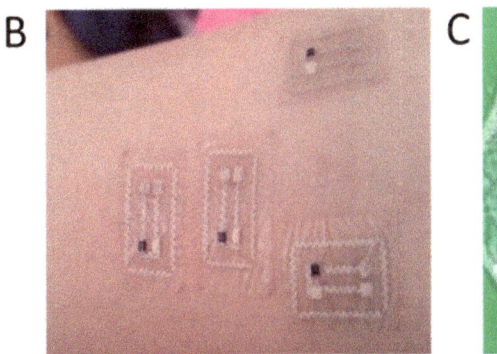

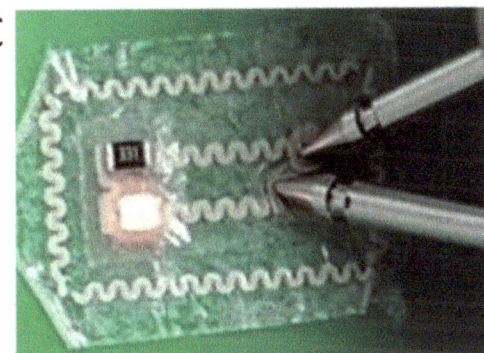

Fig. 11.6 Polymer Protected circuit with functional LED tested for stretchability and longevity on skin. (A) LED functionality of design replicates once placed on skin. (B) Designs after 5 days of continuous wear. (C) Tested of LED function once the circuits were removed after 5 days of continuous wear, showing full functionality of device.

"liquid/blood escape" accounted for 13.1 out of 100 PIVCAEs [31]. Here, we present a UHF RFID-based passive dressing design that can detect PIVC leakage with a diameter of less than 3 cm (Fig. 11.7).

Using the CST Microwave Studio software [32], an arm phantom was simulated, and the SPEAG Dak-3.5 probe system [33] was employed to obtain the dielectric properties of volunteer forearms, which could be utilized in creating appropriate body models. To incorporate moisture leakage sensing functionality into the skin tag [18] and enhance the sensitivity of the IC, the design was tailored to accommodate the Higgs-4 IC chip (with a matching impedance of 23Ω -j120 (915 MHz)) [34]. Testing (with a PIVC-insertion mimic) was carried out on seven volunteers (Table 11.2) with both saline and food-grade porcine blood.

Switching to a more sensitive IC allowed for the adjustment of the substrate material (between the skin and tag) to cotton gauze (dielectric constant near 2.2) [35] with a thickness of 0.2 mm (915 MHz) or 0.1 mm (865 MHz) for optimal matching, while maintaining the overall antenna design (Fig. 11.2A). Increasing volunteer numbers was necessary to assess a broader range of tissue dielectric properties (Table 11.2) and evaluate tag functionality. Moisture sensing using DI water and cotton gauze was conducted on the forearm, following the setup shown in Fig. 11.7B. Introduction of an IV line involved

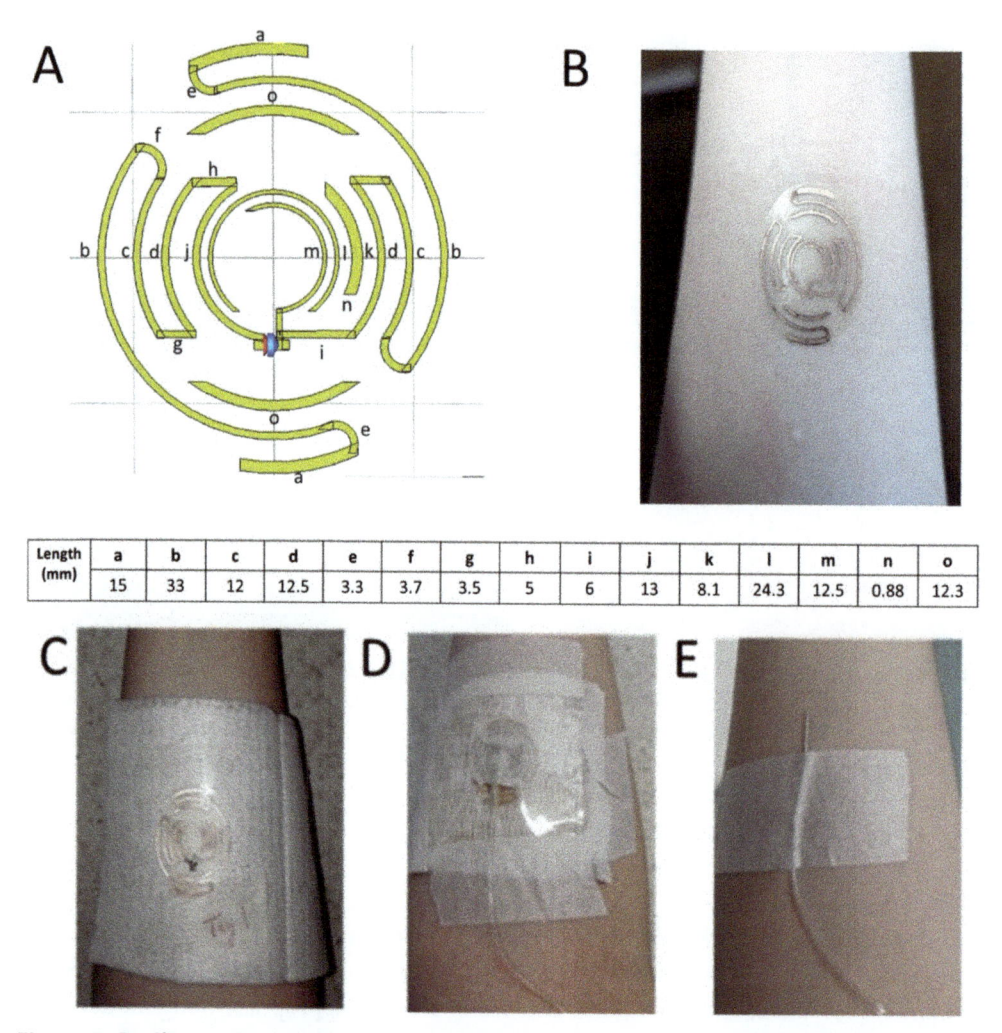

Length (mm)	a	b	c	d	e	f	g	h	i	j	k	l	m	n	o
	15	33	12	12.5	3.3	3.7	3.5	5	6	13	8.1	24.3	12.5	0.88	12.3

Fig. 11.7 On-Skin UHF matched RFID antenna design utilizing a Higgs-4 IC. (A) Dimensions (mm); (B) On-skin copper etched tag with a polyurethane layer; (C) Same on-skin copper etched design but with a cotton gauze layer; (D) 18-gauge equivalent and 16mm length "needle" with the needle inserted through tag design center and attached with medical tape mimicking a saline IV line; (E) View of saline IV line and "needle" with medical tape only.

switching to a medical-grade saline solution (0.9% sodium chloride) (Fig. 11.7D). A 16mm length steel wire (equivalent to an 18-gauge needle) simulated an IV line inserted through the open center of the sensor to detect leaks and assess the impact of the IV line and steel metal "needle" (Fig. 11.7D and E). Lastly, to understand the moisture-sensing ability of the tag design on human body fluids, porcine blood was utilized as an analog.

Table 11.2 Tissue dielectric properties for moisture sensing collected on volunteer forearms.

	\multicolumn{6}{c}{SPEAG probe measured dielectric properties}
	Relative permittivity, ε' (294.25 K)		Conductivity, σ (S/m)		Tan (δ)	
Volunteer	915 MHz	865 MHz	915 MHz	865 MHz	915 MHz	865 MHz
#1	20.3	22.2	0.18	0.22	0.19	0.20
#2	31.4	26.2	0.42	0.30	0.28	0.23
#3	36.6	37.4	0.56	0.57	0.32	0.32
#4	27.7	25.8	0.30	0.26	0.23	0.21
#5	34.0	34.4	0.42	0.43	0.26	0.26
#6	31.8	31.9	0.43	0.43	0.28	0.28
#7	22.0	24.2	0.27	0.27	0.21	0.22

In the US UHF frequency band (902 to 928 MHz), all volunteers using a dry tag of 0.2 mm thickness achieved a minimum 1 m read range (Fig. 11.8). For the EU UHF frequency (865 to 868 MHz), the gauze layer needed reduction to a thickness of 0.1 mm. Despite the thinner gauze layer, the tag maintained a minimum 0.5 m read distance for all volunteers. It is important to note that the EU-adjusted tag exhibited increased variability in read range across all volunteers. Volunteers 7 and 5 were selected to investigate the impact of increased moisture levels, representing the maximum and minimum tag read distances (865 MHz and 915 MHz), as depicted in Fig. 11.9. Volunteer 7 exhibited the optimal read range for both EU and US frequency bands. This tag demonstrates a minimum read range of 0.5 m (up to 1.5 m) and a detection threshold ranging from 10 µL to 30 µL at 865 MHz and from 20 µL to 50 µL at 915 MHz. Comparable results were observed with food-grade porcine blood (Fig. 11.9C). Additionally, this design maintains functionality even when embedded within gauze at a proximity of approximately 5 cm (Fig. 11.9D), making it an ideal smart dressing solution for medical environments. These findings indicate practical read ranges for individuals with varying body types.

These sensors have a common feature: they identify environmental changes in close proximity to the RFID tag by detecting alterations in tag impedance or phase. The capacity to sense is ultimately dictated by the fabrication methods and materials employed.

11.3 Wearable sensor mass fabrication

Previously, in this chapter, we have mentioned the difficulty of improving stretchability, wearability, and conductive ink resistivity; however, there are other significant challenges associated with the mass printing of electronic sensors. Addressing these challenges requires understanding operational frequencies, considering the impact of surrounding tissues, designing effective antennas, ensuring miniaturization, complying with safety

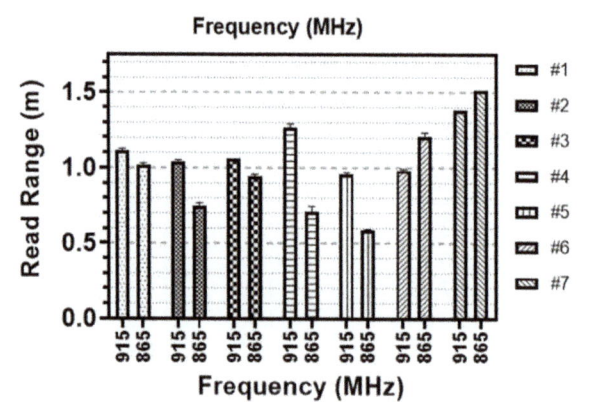

Fig. 11.8 Moisture tag measured read ranges for seven volunteers, highlighting differences between 865 and 915 MHz measurements in the case of a dry tag application. The measured data comprises three replicates, each demonstrating consistent results with no noticeable variation.

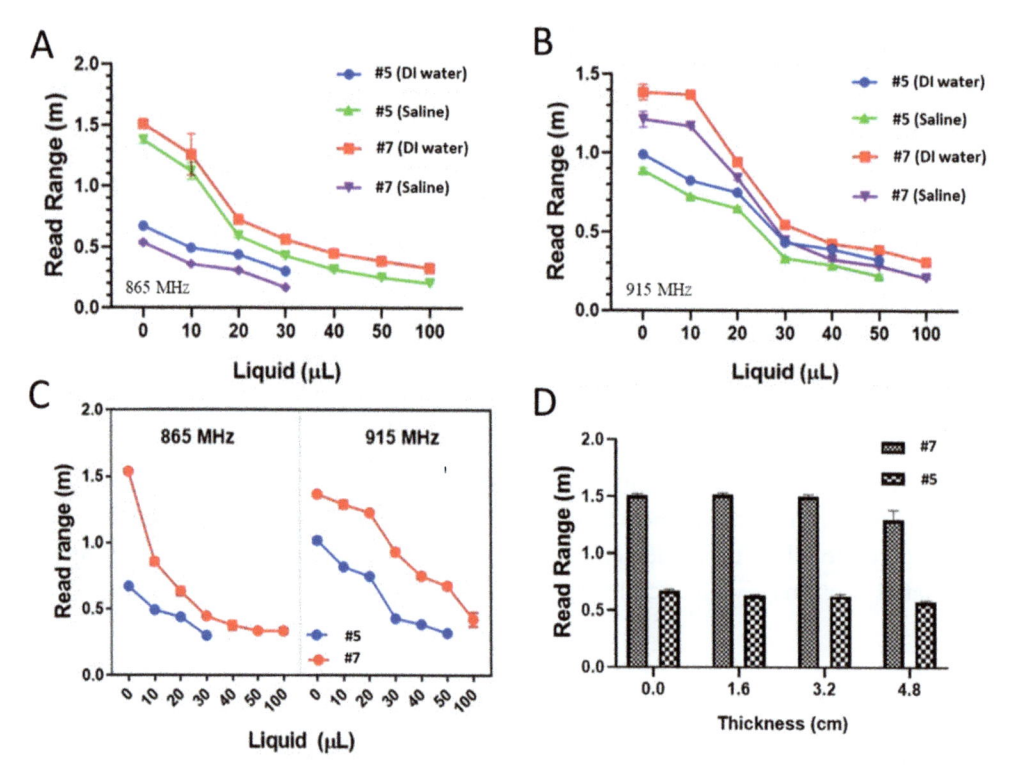

Fig. 11.9 Functionality of the moisture sensing tag with varying fluid amounts on volunteers with maximum (#7) and minimum (#5) read responses (see Table 11.2 for tissue dielectric values). (A) DI water and Saline response for both (A) 0.1 mm (865 MHz) and (B) 0.2 mm (915 MHz) cotton gauze tag backing and where (C) utilised porcine blood at both frequencies. (D) Measured effect on read range when tag covered by varying thickness (0–4.8 cm) of gauze. After allowing all samples to air dry and rereading them, there was no deviation from the original 0 μL dry readings for both volunteers or frequency bands of interest. Data represents three replicates with no noticeable variation.

guidelines [36], and implementing fabrication processes, including tolerance for epidermal antenna stretching. Inkjet printing [37] stands out as a common method for RFID tag fabrication, but it comes with certain limitations [36,38–40], such as printing resolution, robustness, printed layer thickness, and conductivity consistency. These limitations arise because inkjet printing is an additive fabrication method that involves depositing conductive nanoparticles (with silver nanoparticles having a conductivity above 10^7 S/m) through an inkjet printer nozzle, and its printing resolution depends on the chosen printer. A variety of conductive inks have been reviewed in Ref. [41].

In RFID tag areas where increased current density is necessary, an additional conductive ink can be applied, a method referred to as drop-on-demand (DOD) printing. To achieve a consistent printed layer, multilayer printing is often employed, typically assisted by sintering to eliminate excess ink solvent and improve layer conductivity. Multilayer inkjet printing has even been utilized for producing passive components [42,43]. While multilayer printing offers benefits such as enhanced read range, guaranteed continuity of the conductive path, and accommodation of surface-mounted elements like transistors, capacitors, inductors, and resistors [44], it also presents drawbacks, including heightened costs and an increased risk of manufacturing defects, often due to printer nozzle clogging.

Other methods of sensor fabrication include screen printing, flexible wires, conductive thread, gravure printing, and etching. Screen printing involves the use of conductive inks similar to inkjet printing. However, instead of depositing ink drop by drop, the ink is pressed through a mesh onto a substrate, excluding the areas blocked by the stencil [45]. In a study by Ref. [46], screen printing techniques were employed on fabric to create wearable RFID antennas for use with implantable sensors (ranging from Bluetooth to 5G designs) and with a single sensor integrated into clothing (915 MHz design).

Over the last decade, flexographic printing has garnered significant attention for its ability to economically and eco-friendly manufacture advanced electronics. This process, particularly advantageous for creating conductive traces, is now recognized as a viable option for low-cost electronics production on paper substrates, with some studies noting improved antenna performance with water-based inks [47]. The process's precision is highlighted by optimization methods that focus on high-resolution conductive lines, utilizing statistical and engineering techniques like gray relational analysis in conjunction with the Taguchi method [48].

The flexographic printing process's adaptability is further underscored by the control it allows over ink delivery. This is achieved through careful selection of the anilox roll, which enables highly variable film thicknesses, essential for tailoring electrical properties. Using specialized Ag nanoparticle inks, researchers have successfully printed conductive traces with impressive electrical resistivity and mechanical precision, demonstrating the process's ability to meet stringent electrical requirements [49,50]. Moreover, the technique has been effectively applied in the roll-to-roll manufacturing of transparent conductive films and transistor devices, achieving significant advancements like conductive circuits with low resistivity and transistors with efficient power switch ratios [51].

Flexography's integration capabilities are also notable, allowing for the combination of printing with various additional processes in a single pass operation, which brings significant economies of scale. With the capability to operate at high speeds and reliably print on diverse substrates, flexographic printing stands out for its speed and reliability, catering to the growing demand for versatile and rapid production methods in the electronics industry. Within Figs. 11.10 and 11.11, we can see a board built using a flexographic process with a pick-and-place selection of components added post sintering. The flexographic process has allowed for an effective stack up of 15-μm silver traces to enable additive tracking routing, through the creation of mixed material bridging.

To summarize, this section discusses the challenges in mass printing electronic sensors, focusing on RFID tags and wearable electronics. It highlights issues like stretchability, wearability, and conductive ink resistivity. The section delves into various printing methods:

- Inkjet printing: A common method for RFID tag fabrication, inkjet printing faces limitations such as resolution, robustness, and consistency in layer thickness and

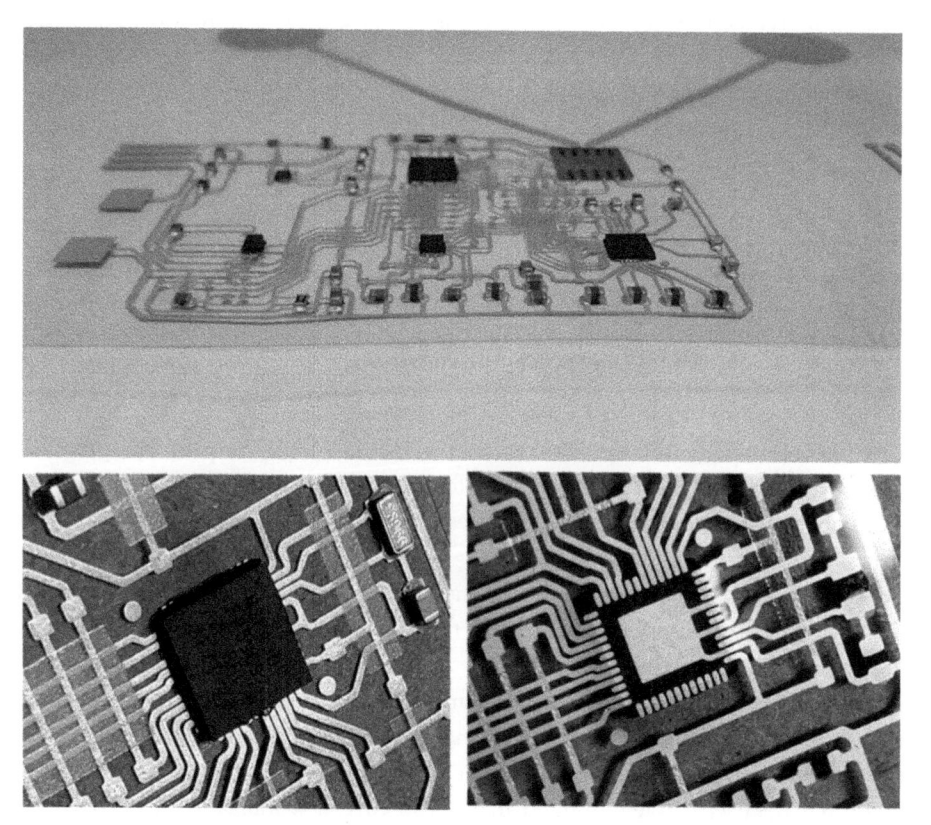

Fig. 11.10 Flexographic printed echocardiogram device with multilayer stack up.

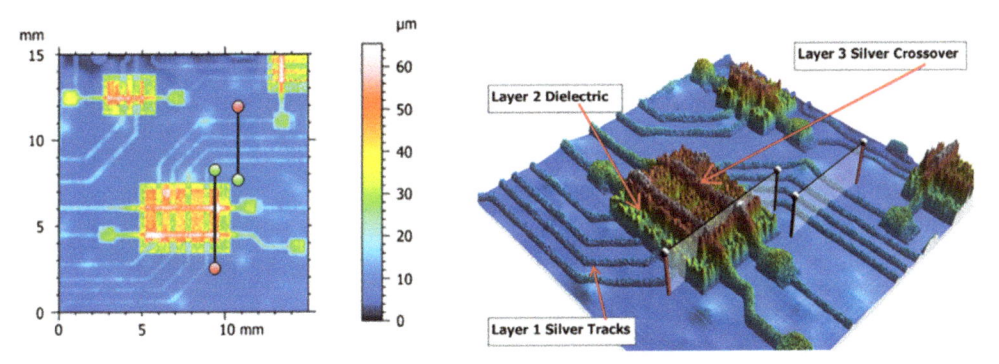

Fig. 11.11 Imaging of flexographic print with layer height mapping.

conductivity. Conductive nanoparticles, particularly silver, are used, and multilayer printing with sintering improves layer conductivity. However, this method can be costly and prone to manufacturing defects.
- Drop-on-demand (DOD) printing: This method involves applying additional conductive ink in areas of high current density, often used in tandem with multilayer printing.
- Screen printing: This technique differs from inkjet printing by pressing ink through a mesh, useful for creating wearable RFID antennas on fabric.
- Flexographic printing: This method is gaining attention for its eco-friendly and cost-effective production of advanced electronics. It is suitable for creating conductive traces on paper substrates and is known for its high-resolution capabilities. Flexography is adaptable, allowing control over ink delivery and film thickness, essential for electrical properties. It has been used in manufacturing transparent conductive films and transistor devices, showcasing its efficiency in integrated printing processes.

Overall, the section emphasizes the importance of understanding operational frequencies, tissue impact, antenna design, miniaturization, safety compliance, and fabrication tolerances. It recognizes the potential of each printing method while acknowledging their respective limitations and advancements.

11.4 Conclusion

In conclusion, this chapter highlights the transformative potential of low-power, epidermal-adherent, and conformally mounted wearable sensors, actively enhancing human experiences. From understanding the fundamental principles of UHF RFID to diverse applications in healthcare, these sensors serve as a cornerstone in integrating technology with the human body. Through the integration of RFID UHF-based wearable sensors and printed electronics via methods such as Inkjet Printing, Drop-on-Demand, and Flexographic Printing, we can approach more complex sensing applications while maintaining compatibility with human tissue. Highlighting the transformative potential of both RFID UHF-based technology and flexible, stretchable printed sensors in wearable applications is crucial for understanding the limitations and improvements still needed in the RF field.

References

[1] A.J. Healey, P. Fathi, N.C. Karmakar, RFID sensors in medical applications, IEEE J. Radio Freq. Identif. 4 (3) (2020) 212–221, https://doi.org/10.1109/JRFID.2020.2997708.
[2] H. Landaluce, et al., A review of IoT sensing applications and challenges using RFID and wireless sensor networks, Sensors 20,9 (2020) 2495, https://doi.org/10.3390/s20092495.
[3] F. Amato, A.D. Carlofelice, C. Occhiuzzi, P. Tognolatti, G. Marrocco, S-band testbed for 5G epidermal RFIDs, in: 2020 XXXIIIrd General Assembly and Scientific Symposium of the International Union of Radio Science, 2020, pp. 1–3, https://doi.org/10.23919/URSIGASS49373.2020.9232255.
[4] F. Amato, S. Amendola, G. Marrocco, Upper-bound performances of RFID epidermal sensor networks at 5G frequencies, in: 2019 IEEE 16th International Conference on Wearable and Implantable Body Sensor Networks (BSN), 2019, pp. 1–4, https://doi.org/10.1109/BSN.2019.8771071.
[5] J.D. Hughes, C. Occhiuzzi, J. Batchelor, G. Marrocco, Miniaturized grid array antenna for body-centric RFID communications in 5G S-band, in: 2020 50th European Microwave Conference (EuMC), 2021, pp. 796–799, https://doi.org/10.23919/EuMC48046.2021.9338030.
[6] L. Catarinucci, R. Colella, L. Tarricone, A cost-effective UHF RFID tag for transmission of generic sensor data in wireless sensor networks, IEEE Trans. Microw. Theory Techn. 57 (5) (2009) 1291–1296, https://doi.org/10.1109/TMTT.2009.2017296.
[7] M. Haddara, A. Staaby, RFID applications and adoptions in healthcare: a review on patient safety, Procedia Comput. Sci. 138 (2018) 80–88.
[8] P.J. Hawrylak, J. Hale, Data privacy issues with RFID in healthcare, in: A. Gkoulalas-Divanis, G. Loukides (Eds.), Medical Data Privacy Handbook, Springer, Cham, 2015. https://doi.org/10.1007/978-3-319-23633-9_21.
[9] D. Cohen, Phys. Today 28 (8) (1975) 34, https://doi.org/10.1063/1.3069110.
[10] C. Gabriel, Dielectric properties, in: IT'IS Foundation, 1996. itis.swiss/virtual-population/tissue-properties/database/dielectric-properties/.
[11] A. Saitoh, T. Nomura, Wireless Sensor System Using Surface Acoustic Wave Devices, 2009. ICCAS-SICE. 2009.
[12] R. Muthupillai, et al., Low frequency acoustic shear wave imaging in tissue-like media using magnetic resonance, in: 1995 IEEE Ultrasonics Symposium. Proceedings. An International Symposium, 1995.
[13] R.A. Potyrailo, et al., Battery-free radio frequency identification (RFID) sensors for food quality and safety, J. Agric. Food Chem. 60 (35) (2012) 8535–8543.
[14] J.-G. Guan, Y.-Q. Miao, Q.-J. Zhang, Impedimetric biosensors, J. Biosci. Bioeng. 97 (4) (2004) 219–226.
[15] P.V. Nikitin, et al., Sensitivity and impedance measurements of UHF RFID chips, IEEE Trans. Microw. Theory Techn. 57 (5) (2009) 1297–1302.
[16] J.S. Daniels, N. Pourmand, Label-free impedance biosensors: opportunities and challenges, Electroanalysis 19 (12) (2007) 1239–1257.
[17] R.A. Potyrailo, et al., Selective quantitation of vapors and their mixtures using individual passive multivariable RFID sensors, in: 2010 IEEE International Conference on RFID (IEEE RFID 2010), 2010.
[18] V. Makarovaite, A.J.R. Hillier, S.J. Holder, C.W. Gourlay, J.C. Batchelor, Passive wireless UHF RFID antenna label for sensing dielectric properties of aqueous and organic liquids, IEEE Sensors J. 19 (11) (2019) 4299–4307, https://doi.org/10.1109/JSEN.2019.2896481.
[19] S. Zuffanelli, P. Aguilà, G. Zamora, F. Paredes, F. Martín, J. Bonache, An impedance matching method for optical disc-based UHF-RFID tags, in: Proc. IEEE Int. Conf. RFID (IEEE RFID), 2014, pp. 15–22.

[20] D.O. Oyeka, J.C. Batchelor, A.M. Ziai, Effect of skin dielectric properties on the read range of epidermal ultra-high frequency radio-frequency identification tags, Healthc. Technol. Lett. 4 (2) (2017) 78–81.
[21] M.E. Daniel Marques, P. Pannier, Broadband UHF RFID tag antenna for bio-monitoring, Prog. Electromagn. Res. B. 67 (2016) 31–44.
[22] G.A. Casula, et al., Energy-based considerations for ungrounded wearable UHF antenna design, IEEE Sensors J. 17 (3) (2017) 687–694.
[23] G. Marrocco, The art of UHF RFID antenna design: impedance-matching and sizereduction techniques, IEEE Antennas Propag. Mag. 50 (1) (2008) 66–79.
[24] D. Oyeka, J.C. Batchelor, M.A. Ziai, J.S.R. Wheeler, S. Yeates, Tag diversity of inkjet printed body-worn radio frequency identification integrated medical sticking plasters for wireless monitoring, IET Healthc. Technol. Lett. Vol. 3 (4) (2016) 257–262.
[25] T. Sunaga, et al., Measurement of the electrical properties of human skin and the variation among subjects with certain skin conditions, Phys. Med. Biol. 47 (1) (2002) N11–N15.
[26] M. Kanesan, D.V. Thiel, S.G.O. Keefe, The effect of lossy dielectric objects on a UHF RFID meander line antenna, in: Proceedings of the 2012 IEEE International Symposium on Antennas and Propagation, 2012.
[27] P. Heydari, A. Heydari, H.I. Maibach, Sunlight exposure and skin thickness measurements as a function of age: Risk factors for melanoma, in: M.A. Farage, K.W. Miller, H.I. Maibach (Eds.), Textbook of Aging Skin, Springer, Berlin, Heidelberg, 2010, https://doi.org/10.1007/978-3-540-89656-2_60.
[28] S.G. Kirtania, A.W. Elger, M.R. Hasan, A. Wisniewska, K. Sekhar, T. Karacolak, P.K. Sekhar, Flexible antennas: a review, Micromachines 11 (9) (2020) 847, https://doi.org/10.3390/mi11090847. PMID: 32933077; PMCID: PMC7570180.
[29] V. Makarovaite, C. Gourlay, A.J.R. Hillier, J.C. Batchelor, S.J. Holder, Adjustable passive RFID skin mounted sticker, in: 2019 IEEE 16th International Conference on Wearable and Implantable Body Sensor Networks (BSN), Chicago, IL, USA, 2019, pp. 1–4, https://doi.org/10.1109/BSN.2019.8771069.
[30] A. Bahl, et al., Early recognition of peripheral intravenous catheter failure using serial ultrasonographic assessments, PLoS One 16 (6) (2021) e0253243, https://doi.org/10.1371/journal.pone.0253243.
[31] K. Miliani, et al., CATHEVAL Study Group, Peripheral venous catheter-related adverse events: evaluation from a multicentre epidemiological study in France (the CATHEVAL Project), PLoS One 12 (1) (2017) e0168637, https://doi.org/10.1371/journal.pone.0168637.
[32] Dassault Systemes, CST- Computer Simulation Technology, Available at www.cst.com, accessed: March 06, 2023. [Online].
[33] SPEAG, DAK - Dielectric Assessment Kit Product Line. Available at speag.swiss/products/dak/dielectric-measurements, accessed: April 10, 2023. [Online].
[34] Higgs 4 RFID IC, Alien Technology, www.alientechnology.com/products/ic/higgs-4/, accessed: April 10, 2023. [Online].
[35] S. Sankaralingam, B. Gupta, Determination of dielectric constant of fabric materials and their use as substrates for design and development of antennas for wearable applications, IEEE Trans. Instrum. Meas. 59 (12) (2010) 3122–3131.
[36] A. Kiourti, RFID antennas for body-area applications: from wearables to implants, in: IEEE Antennas and Propagation Magazine, vol. 60, no. 5, 2018, pp. 14–25, https://doi.org/10.1109/MAP.2018.2859167.
[37] C.L. Baumbauer, M.G. Anderson, J. Ting, et al., Printed, flexible, compact UHF-RFID sensor tags enabled by hybrid electronics, Sci. Rep. 10 (2020) 16543, https://doi.org/10.1038/s41598-020-73471-9.
[38] S. Amendola, A. Palombi, L. Rousseau, G. Lissorgues, G. Marrocco, Manufacturing technologies for UHF RFID epidermal antennas, in: 2016 46th European Microwave Conference (EuMC), 2016, pp. 914–917, https://doi.org/10.1109/EuMC.2016.7824493.
[39] D.O. Oyeka, J.C. Batchelor, V. Sanchez-Romaguera, S.G. Yeates, R.E. Saunders, Effect of conductive area trimming on the read range of inkjet printed epidermal RFID tags, in: 2015 9th European Conference on Antennas and Propagation (EuCAP), 2015, pp. 1–4.

[40] S. Amendola, A. Palombi, G. Marrocco, Inkjet printing of epidermal RFID antennas by self-sintering conductive ink, IEEE Trans. Microw. Theory Techn. 66 (3) (2018) 1561–1569, https://doi.org/10.1109/TMTT.2017.2767594.

[41] Y. Khan, A. Thielens, S. Muin, J. Ting, C. Baumbauer, A.C. Arias, A new frontier of printed electronics: flexible hybrid electronics, Adv. Mater. 32 (2020) 1905279, https://doi.org/10.1002/adma.201905279.

[42] C. Mariotti, F. Alimenti, L. Roselli, M.M. Tentzeris, High-performance RF devices and components on flexible cellulose substrate by vertically integrated additive manufacturing technologies, IEEE Trans. Microw. Theory Techn. 65 (1) (2017) 62–71.

[43] J. Horn, P. Vasireddy, I. Mahbub, R. Hossain, A.B. Kaul, Simulation and fabrication of inkjet-printed mm-sized capacitors for wearable temperature sensing applications, in: 2020 IEEE Texas Symposium on Wireless and Microwave Circuits and Systems (WMCS), 2020, pp. 1–6, https://doi.org/10.1109/WMCS49442.2020.9172399.

[44] J.G.D. Hester, J. Kimionis, M.M. Tentzeris, Printed motes for IoT wireless networks: state of the art challenges and outlooks, IEEE Trans. Microw. Theory Techn. 65 (5) (2017) 1819–1830.

[45] G.G. Xiao, Z. Zhang, S. Lang, Y. Tao, Screen printing RF antennas, in: 2016 17th International Symposium on Antenna Technology and Applied Electromagnetics (ANTEM), 2016, pp. 1–2, https://doi.org/10.1109/ANTEM.2016.7550245.

[46] U. Hasni, M.E. Piper, J. Lundquist, E. Topsakal, Screen-printed fabric antennas for wearable applications, IEEE Open J. Antennas Propag. 2 (2021) 591–598, https://doi.org/10.1109/OJAP.2021.3070919.

[47] R. Kattumenu, M. Rebros, M. Joyce, A.E. Hrehorov, P.D. Fleming, Evaluation of flexographically printed conductive traces on paper substrates for RFID applications, Tech. Assoc. Graph. Arts J. 5 (2008).

[48] H.A.D. Nguyen, C. Lee, K.-H. Shin, Approach to optimizing printed conductive lines in high-resolution roll-to-roll gravure printing, Robot. Comput. Integr. Manuf. 46 (2017) 122–129. ISSN 0736-5845.

[49] M. Joyce, L. Pal, R. Hicks, et al., Custom tailoring of conductive ink/substrate properties for increased thin film deposition of poly(dimethylsiloxane) films, J. Mater. Sci. Mater. Electron. 29 (2018) 10461–10470.

[50] R. Kattumenu, M. Rebros, M. Joyce, P.D. Fleming, G. Neelgund, Effect of substrate properties on conductive traces printed with silver-based flexographic ink, Nord. Pulp Pap. Res. J. 24 (2009) 101–106.

[51] Y. Wang, Y. Huang, Y.-Z. Li, C. Pan, S.-y. Cheng, Q. Liang, Z.-Q. Xu, H.-J. Chen, Z.-s. Feng, A facile process combined with roll-to-roll flexographic printing and electroless deposition to fabricate RFID tag antenna on paper substrates, Compos. B Eng. 224 (2021) 109194 (ISSN 1359-8368).

Index

Note: Page numbers followed by *f* indicate figures and *t* indicate tables.

A

Abdominal interventions, continuum robots in, 8
Actigraphy, 113
Active interaction control, 48–49
Actuators and batteries challenges, 80
Additive manufacturing (AM) techniques, 1, 5–6, 17–18, 20–21
Advanced signal processing techniques, 2–3
Alzheimer's disease (AD) prediction from MRI, 135–136
   accuracy, 144
   brain MRI samples, 138*f*
   convolutional neural network (CNN), 141–142
   data augmentation, 140–141
   data set description, 137–140
   evaluation metrics, 144–145
   F1 score, 145
   machine learning models, 141–143
   precision, 144–145
   recall, 145
   Residual Network (ResNet-50), 143
   support, 145
   Visual Geometry Group (VGG-16) model, 142–143
Anechoic chamber, 89, 89–90*f*
Ankle–foot orthosis (AFO) design, 65–66, 69, 70*f*
   actuators and batteries challenges, 80
   articulated, 69
   biomechanics of biological ankle and foot, 67–68
   ergonomics challenges, 80
   future directions, 81–82
   human–robot interaction (HRI) challenges, 78–79
   materials and safety challenges, 80
   orthoses design for lower limb, 69–74
   orthotic manufacturing, advances in, 74–78
   sensors and controllers challenges, 79
   structural design challenges, 79
   technical challenges, 78–80
Area difference (ArD) index, 101
Artifact removal, techniques for, 99–100
Artificial intelligence (AI), 1–4, 25*f*, 168–171
   efficient analysis of medical data, 169–170
   forecasting disease outcomes, 170–171
Artificial organs, 9–10
Assistive devices for motor rehabilitation, 56
Attention deficit hyperactivity disorder (ADHD), 181–184
Automation, technological advancements in, 20–27
   diagnosis of diseases, equipment for, 24–26
   implantable devices, 20–23
   treatment of diseases, equipment for, 26–27
   wearable devices, 23–24
Automation in biomedical devices, 16–20
   definition and scope, 16–17
   diagnosis of diseases, equipment for, 19–20
   emergence of, 17–20
   implantable devices, 16–17*f*, 17–18
   technological advancements, 20–27
   treatment of diseases, equipment for, 20
   wearable devices, 16*f*, 18
Azure voice bot, 181–184

B

Backpropagation (BP) neural network algorithm, 51, 51*f*
Bed-embedded sensors, 118
Bidirectional encoder representations from the transformers (BERT) model, 181–184
Big data analytics, 22
Biomedical devices
   automation in. (*see* Automation in biomedical devices)
   background, 15
   case studies and applications, 27
   connectivity across platforms, 34
   cyber security and cyber-attacks ethical considerations, 34–35
   drawbacks and challenges, 30–35
   initial cost and initial investment, 32
   internet, 33
   medical device regulations, compliance with, 30
   objective, 15
   regulatory and safety considerations, 27–30
   sensor's failure/device malfunction, 33–34

Biomedical devices (Continued)
  software failure, 34
  specialized training and workforce adaptation, 32–33
  standardization and validation, 30
  technical failures and malfunctions, 33–34
Biomedical engineering, computational intelligence in, 3–4
Biomedical field, robots types in, 43f
Biomedical robotics. *See also* Soft robotics; Surgical robotics, mathematics in
  in healthcare field, 42f
  mathematical concept used in, 44f, 50–52
Biomedicine 4.0, transfer learning in, 165–166
  AI/ML in disease prognosis, 168–171
  disease complexity and variability, 167–168
  disease prognosis, challenges in, 166–168
  disease prognosis, transfer learning for, 171–174
  disease prognosis in, 166, 166f
  disease prognosis models, enhancing, 174–177
  lack of standardization in prognostic models, 168
  limited data availability, 167
Bladder pathologies, continuum robots in, 8
Body sensor network (BSN), 121
Brain disorders, 3–4
Brain-machine interfaces (BMIs), 56–57
Brain MRI samples, 138f
Brain surgery, continuum robots in, 7

C

Capek, Karel, 41–42
Cardiac surgery, continuum robots in, continuum robots in, 7
Central Drug Standards Control Organization (CDSCO), 28–30
Centroid Difference, 101
Chatbots, 179–181, 186
China Food and Drug Administration (CFDA), 28–30
Clinical notes, 29t
Clinical sleep assessments, hierarchy of, 112
Closed-loop control systems, 57–58
Cloud computing, 170
Computational intelligence, 2–4
Computational intelligence in biomedical engineering, 3–4
Computed tomography (CT), 76, 85
Computed torque control (CTC), 48
Computer-aided design (CAD), 74–78

Computer-aided engineering (CAE) tool, 74–76
Computer-aided manufacturing (CAM) processes, 77
Computerized numerical control (CNC), 74
Computerized tomography (CT), 29t, 41–42
Conformity "Europe" enne (CE) marking, 28–30
Connectivity across platforms, 34
Contact-based sensor technologies, 118
Contactless sensor technologies, 117
Continuum robots, 7–8
Continuum soft robots, 7
Convolutional neural network (CNN), 1–2, 52–53, 141–142, 142f, 146–150, 146t, 147f, 148t, 149f, 170, 185, 189–191, 190t
  -based approach, 154
  structure of, 190f
Coriolis effect, 49
COVID-19 epidemic, 181–184
Craig–Scott orthosis, 71
Cyber-attacks, 34
Cyber physical system (CPS), 15, 22–25, 25f
  cyber CPS, 21
Cyber security and cyber-attacks ethical considerations, 34–35

D

Data privacy, 119
Da Vinci Surgical System, 29t
Decision-level fusion, 122
Deep learning (DL), 1–4
Diagnosis of disease
  biomedical devices for, 18, 22–23
  case studies equipment for, 29t
  equipment for, 19–20, 24–26
  mathematics in medical robotics for, 57–58
Digital Light Processing, 17–18
Dijkstra's algorithm, 53–54
Disease complexity, 167
Disease prognosis, 166
  in Biomedicine 4.0, 166, 166f
  challenges in, 166–168
  disease complexity and variability, 167–168
  lack of standardization in prognostic models, 168
  limited data availability, 167
Disease variability, 167
Driven gait orthosis (DGO), 74
Drop-on-demand (DOD) printing, 223
Dynamic risk assessment, 171

E

EcoFlex range of soft elastomers, 5–6
Electrocardiogram (ECG), 29t, 211–212
Electroencephalography (EEG), 3–4, 56–57, 153–155, 155–156f
Electromyograms (EMG), 155
Electron Beam Melting, 17–18
Electronic KAFO, 73, 73f
Ella model, 99
ESNet method, 158–159
E-textile-based wearable sensor, 28t
EU-funded I-SUPPORT project, 10
European Union (EU), 28–30
Exoskeleton devices, 65–66
Exosuits, 8, 9f
Explainable AI (XAI), 180, 187
  convolutional neural network (CNN), 185, 190f
  dataset description, 187–188
  integrated stacked ensemble, 185–186, 191f
  limitation and conclusion, 203–204
  literature survey, 181–184
  Natural Language Processing (NLP), 186
  problem statement, 181
  proposed method, 188–194, 194f
  recurrent neural network (RNN), 184–185, 188–189, 189f
  results and analysis, 194–203, 199f
    benefits, 202–203
    comparison, 201–202, 202t
    experimental setup, 196–197
    optimizer analysis, 197–198, 198t
    time complexity analysis, 197, 197t
  voice engines, 187

F

False negatives (FN), 144
False positives (FP), 144
Feature-level fusion strategies, 122
Fivefold cross-validation results, 160–161
Flexographic printing process, 221, 222–223f, 223
Food and Drug Administration (FDA), 28–30
Foot movements, 67, 68f
Force control in robotics, 48–50
4D printing, 5–6
Friction Stir Additive Manufacturing, 17–18
Fully connected (FC) layer, 159
Functional near-infrared spectroscopy (fNIRS), 154
Fused deposition modeling (FDM), 17–18, 77

G

Gait cycle, 67–68, 68f
General practitioner (GP), 87
Global Harmonization Task Force (GHTF), 30
Glucometer, 28t
GOST Standard in Russia, 28–30
Graphics processing units (GPUs), 170

H

Healthcare industry, 4
"Help" class, 200
Hemorrhagic brain strokes, detecting, 87–101
Hemorrhagic stroke, 85–86
Hierarchical data format (HDF), 190–191
Hierarchical sensor information fusion, 121–122
Hip-and ankle linked orthosis (HALO), 72
Hip–knee–ankle–foot orthosis (HKAFO), 72
Human body biomechanics, 67, 67f
Human–computer interaction (HCI), 181–184
Human head phantom, description of, 95–96
Humanoid robots, 3
Human–robot interaction (HRI), 3, 78–79
Human sleep behavior, 109–110
  abnormalities in, 110
Human sleep posture sensing technologies, 117–120
  contact-based sensor technologies, 118
  contactless sensor technologies, 117
  sensor technology debate, 118–120
Human walking, 67–68
Huygens principle (HP), 88, 92–95, 93f
Huygens's Principle, 93–94
Hybrid force-motion control (HFC), 49
Hydraulic reciprocating gait hip–knee–ankle foot orthosis (HRGO), 73

I

Impedance control, 49–50
Implantable devices, 16–17f, 17–18, 20–23
  case studies on, 28t
  classification of, 17f
Implanted pacemaker, 28t
In-bed postural activity, temporal analysis of, 125–126
Incomplete spinal cord injury (ISCI), 69
Independent component analysis (ICA) decomposition, 155
Industry 4.0, 27, 30–35
Inertial measurement unit (IMU), 118

Initial cost and initial investment, 32
Inkjet printing, 222
Integrated stacked ensemble, flowchart of, 185–186, 191f
International Classification of Sleep Disorders, 110
Internet, 33
Internet of Medical Things (IoMT), 1, 18, 22–26
  wearable devices used via, 19f
Internet of Things (IoT), 1, 3–4, 34
  connection of wearable devices using, 24f
Ischemic stroke, 85–86

J
JSON file, 187–188, 194

K
Keras functional interface, 185–186
Knee–ankle–foot orthosis (KAFO), 66, 69–73, 71f
  electronic, 73f

L
LabelEncoder, 179–180
Lagrange's dynamics, 45
Laminated Object Manufacturing, 17–18
Laparoscopic surgery (FLS), 153–154
Leave-one-subject-out (LOSO) evaluation, 3–4, 154, 159, 160–162f, 161–162
Linear regression-based classification methods, 125
Local Interpretable Model-Agnostic Explanation (LIME), 180, 193, 199–200, 200f
LokoMat, 66
Longitudinal patient data analysis, 170
LOPES, 66
Lower limb, orthoses design for, 69–74
  ankle–foot orthoses (AFOs)ss, 69
  hip–knee–ankle–foot orthosis (HKAFO), 72
  knee–ankle–foot orthosis (KAFO), 69–72, 71f, 73f
  mobility-enhancing orthotic systems, advancements in, 72–74
Lower limb orthotic devices, 66

M
Machine learning (ML), 1–2, 179–184
  integration in sleep medicine, 2
Machine learning in disease prognosis, 168–171
  efficient analysis of medical data, 169–170
  forecasting disease outcomes, 170–171
Machine learning brain activation topography
  background, 153–154
  data collection, 155
  data preprocessing, 155–157
  fivefold cross-validation results, 160–161
  leave-one-subject-out cross-validation results, 161–162
  topography-preserving 3D-CNN, 157–159
Machine learning models, 141–143
  convolutional neural network (CNN), 141–142
  Residual Network (ResNet-50), 143
  Visual Geometry Group (VGG-16) model, 142–143
Magnetic resonance imaging (MRI), 85, 136
Magneto-inertial measurement unit (M-IMU), 118
Magneto-inertial sensors, 121
Materials and safety challenges, 80
Mathematical concept used in biomedical robotics, 44f
Mathematics in biomedical robotics, 50–52
Mathematics in medical robotics, 57–58
Mathematics in rehabilitation robotics, 55–57
  assistive devices for motor rehabilitation, 56
  neural interfaces and brain-machine interactions, 56–57
  quantitative assessment and personalized therapy, 57
Mathematics in surgical robotics, 52–55
  image processing and analysis, 52–53
  robotic-assisted MIS, 54–55
  surgical navigation and path planning, 53–54
Medical Device Directive (MDD), 28–30
Medical devices
  classification of, as per FDA, 29f
  regulations/guidelines, 30, 31t
MEMS technology, 119
Mental healthcare, robots in, 3–4
Mental illness, chatbots to address, 179–180
Microcontroller Unit (MCU), 212
Microstrip antenna design, description of, 97–99
Microwave cerebral imaging trial product, advancement of, 89–92
Microwave imaging (MWI), 85–89, 95, 105
Microwave tomography (MT), 86
Mild demented (MD) images, 136
Millimeter wave (mmWave) technologies, 117
Minimally invasive surgery (MIS), 42–44
  robotic-assisted, 54–55
Minimally Invasive Surgery, 29t

Ministry of Health and Family Welfare in India, 28–30
Mobility-enhancing orthotic systems, advancements in, 72–74
Moderate demented (MoD) images, 136
Monitoring of patients' health, mathematics in medical robotics for, 57–58
Motion control in robotics, 45–48
Motor rehabilitation, assistive devices for, 56
Movement behavior, 111
Multibackbone robots, 7
Multibistatic antennas, integrating, 87–101
Multibistatic frequency-domain measurements, 85–86
   experimental validation, 101–104
   human head phantom, description of, 95–96
   Huygens principle (HP), 92–95, 93f
   microstrip antenna design, description of, 97–99
   microwave cerebral imaging trial product, advancement of, 89–92
   multibistatic antennas, integrating, 87–101
   phantom models, imaging with, 104
   signal preprocessing techniques, description of, 99–101
   simulated imaging, 101–104
Multiinput multioutput system (MIMO) nonlinear robotic system, 48
Multijet/Polyjet 3D printing, 17–18
Musculoskeletal conditions, 109
Musculoskeletal system, 110–112

N

National Sleep Foundation, 109–110
Natural Language Processing (NLP), 186
Neural interfaces, 56–57
New England Regional Spinal Cord Injury Center (NERSCIC) KAFO, 71
NLTK, 186
Nondemented (ND) images, 136
"NOT Help" class, 200

O

Obstructive sleep apnoea (OSA), 123
Omnidirectional walker (ODW), 56
On-body electronics, 207–208, 214
Operational space control, 45–46
Operator 4.0, 32
Optical motion capture systems, 76

Optimizers, 197–198, 198t
Orthoses design for lower limb, 69–74
   ankle–foot orthoses (AFOs), 69, 70f
   hip–knee–ankle–foot orthosis (HKAFO), 72
   knee–ankle–foot orthosis (KAFO), 69–72, 71f, 73f
   mobility-enhancing orthotic systems, advancements in, 72–74
Orthotic and exoskeleton devices, 66
Orthotic manufacturing, advances in, 74–78
   rapid prototyping technologies (RPT), 77–78
   3D anatomical data acquisition technologies, 76–77
Orthotic Research and Locomotor Assessment Unit (ORLAU) Parawalker, 72
Otolaryngology, continuum robots in, 7

P

Passive interaction control, 48–49
PDMS, 5–6
Peripheral intravenous catheter (PIVC) moisture sensor, 215–217
Peripheral intravenous catheter-related adverse events (PIVCAE), 216–217
Personalized therapy, 57
Personalized treatment strategies, 176
Phantom models, imaging with, 104
Pharmaceuticals Medical Devices Agency (PMDA), 28–30
Photoplethysmogram (PPG), 211–212
Physical therapy, 114
Physiotherapy, 114
Pneumatic active gait orthosis (PAGO), 73
Polyshape Construction, 101
Polysomnography, 112–113
Posterior leaf spring AFO, 69
Powered gait orthosis (PGO), 74
Premarket approval (PMA), 28–30
Prevention of diseases, biomedical devices for, 18
Prostate/bladder pathologies, continuum robots in, 8
Printed designs, 214, 214–215f
Printed wearable circuits, protection of, 215, 216f
Proportional derivative (PD) control, 46–48
   control scheme, 47f
Proportion-integral-derivative (PID) control, 46–48, 51, 51f
   control scheme, 47f

Prosthetic hand, 28t
Prosthetics, 9
Provocative postures, 125
Psychotherapy, 179–180

Q

Quantitative assessment, 57
Quantitative image analysis metrics, 100–101

R

Radio frequency identification (RFID) wearable sensors, 117, 208–212, 208f
   basic principles of design, 209
   fabrication and applications, 212–219
   human tissue considerations for tag design, 209–211
   ultra-lower power live streaming through UHF RFID, 211–212
Rapidly exploring random trees (RRT), 53–54, 77–78
Rapid prototyping technology (RPT) approach, 74–76, 78
Raspberry Pi, 181–184
Reciprocating gait orthoses (RGOs), 72
Recurrent neural network (RNN), 184–185, 188–191, 190t
   structure of, 189f
Regulatory and safety considerations, 27–30
   medical device regulations, compliance with, 30
   standardization and validation, 30
Rehabilitation
   robot-assisted, 3
   soft robotic application for, 11f
Rehabilitation robotics, mathematics in, 55–57
   assistive devices for motor rehabilitation, 56
   neural interfaces and brain-machine interactions, 56–57
   quantitative assessment and personalized therapy, 57
Residual Network (ResNet-50) model, 136, 143, 144f, 146–150, 146t, 147f, 148t, 149f
Robot-assisted rehabilitation, 3
Robotic surgery, 27f
Robots types in biomedical field, 43f
Roszdravnadzor in Russia, 28–30
Rotation Subtraction (RS) Artifact Removal Method, 100
Rule-based classification approaches, 125

S

Scaffolds for medical implants, 28t
Screen printing, 223
Selective Compliant Assembly Robot Arm (SCARA), 50–51
Selective Laser Melting (SLM), 17–18
Selective laser sintering (SLS) system, 17–18, 77
Sensor data, 126
Sensor data classification pipeline, 120–121
   data preprocessing, 120
   feature extraction, 120–121
   model deployment, 121
   model evaluation, 121
   model selection, 121
   model training, 121
Sensors and controllers challenges, 79
Sensor technology debate, 118–120
Sensor's failure/device malfunction, 33–34
Series elastic actuators (SEAs), 79
Shapley Additive Explanation (SHAP), 180, 193, 200, 201f
Signal preprocessing techniques, description of, 99–101
   artifact removal, techniques for, 99–100
   quantitative image analysis metrics, 100–101
   Rotation Subtraction (RS) Artifact Removal Method, 100
Signal-to-clutter ratio (S/C), 101
Signal-to-Noise Ratio, 101
Simulated imaging, 101–104
Single input, single output (SISD) system, 46
Sleep, 109
Sleep analysis, 2
Sleep assessment methods, 112
Sleep disorders
   clinical assessment of, 112–113
   management and treatment practices for, 113–114
   and musculoskeletal conditions, 110–111, 111f
Sleep medicine, machine learning integration in, 2
Sleep posture analysis, 109, 112
   clinical needs and challenges in, 115–116
   contact-based sensor technologies, 118
   contactless sensor technologies, 117
   health complications, 109–116
   human sleep posture sensing technologies, 117–120

in-bed postural activity, temporal analysis of, 125–126
musculoskeletal system, 110–112
sensor technology debate, 118–120
sleep disorders, 112–114
wearable sensor-based, 120–122
wearable sensors, monitoring sleep postures using, 122–125
Small-scale continuum robots, 8
Smart diagnostics, 19–20
Smartphones, 28t, 118
Smartwatches, 28t
Softmax activation, 159
Soft robotics, 4–6. *See also* Biomedical robotics; Surgical robotics, mathematics in
abdominal interventions, 8
application for rehab, 11f
artificial organs, 9–10
assistive technologies, 10
brain surgery, 7
cardiac surgery, 7
exosuits, 8, 9f
for a fruit-picking application, 6f
limitations in, 11
otolaryngology, 7
prosthetics, 9
surgical applications, 6–8
urology, 8
vascular surgery, 8
Software as Medical Devices (SaMD), 1
Software failure, 34
Solid-ankle AFO, 69
Spinal cord injuries (SCI), 72–74
Stable state sleep behavior, 111
Stacked Ensemble, 191
Standard four sleep postures, 122–125
State-of-the-art myoelectric hand prosthetic technology, 9
Steerable soft robotic catheters, 8
Stereolithography (SLA), 17–18, 77–78
Stiffness control, 49
Stroke, detection of, 89–92
Structural Similarity Index Metric, 101
Subcutaneous sensor, 28t
Support, 145
Surgical robotics, mathematics in, 52–55. *See also* Biomedical robotics; Soft robotics
image processing and analysis, 52–53

robotic-assisted MIS, 54–55
surgical navigation and path planning, 53–54
Survival analysis, 170
Switch mode, 193, 193f

T

Tag design, human tissue considerations for, 209–211
Technical failures and malfunctions, 33–34
connectivity across platforms, 34
internet, 33
sensor's failure/device malfunction, 33–34
software failure, 34
Temporal attentive pooling (TAP) layer, 159
Therapeutic Goods Administration in Australia, 28–30
Therapeutic Products Division of Health Canada, 28–30
Thoracolumbosacral orthosis (TLSO), 72
3D anatomical data acquisition technologies, 76–77
3D printed medicine, 28t
3D printing (3DP), 1, 78
3D scanning technologies, 76
Time series analysis, 170
Tissues, biomedical devices interacting with, 17–18, 20–22
TMR-MRS system, 54–55, 54f
Topography-preserving 3D-convolutional neural network (CNN), 157–159
Total artificial hearts (TAH), 10
Traditional surgical robots, 7
Training and workforce adaptation, 32–33
Transfer learning (TL), 2, 142, 174
Transfer learning for disease prognosis, 171–174. *See also* Biomedicine 4.0, transfer learning in
advantages over traditional ML methods, 171–174
eliminating the need to build models from scratch, 174
understanding, 171
Treatment of diseases
biomedical devices for, 18, 22–23
case studies equipment for, 29t
equipment for, 20, 26–27
True negatives (TN), 144
True positives (TP), 144

U

Ultrahigh-Frequency Radio Frequency Identification (UHF RFID)
  ultra-lower power live streaming through, 211–212
  ultra-lower power live streaming through, 211–212
Ultrawideband (UWB) frequency-domain measurements, 91
United States (US), 28–30
Urology, continuum robots in, 8

V

Vascular surgery, continuum robots in, 8
Vector network analyzer (VNA), 86, 98
Ventricle assist devices (VADs), 10
Very mild demented (VMD) images, 136
VGG-16 model. *See* Visual Geometry Group (VGG-16) model
Videosomnography, 113
Vision sensors, 117
Visual Geometry Group (VGG-16) model, 136, 142–143, 143f, 146–150, 146t, 147f, 148t, 149f
Voice bot, 181–184
Voice engines, 187

W

Wearable biosensors coupled with imaging and motion sensors, 28t
Wearable devices, 16f, 18, 23–24
  case studies on, 17f
  connection of, using IoT, 24f
  used via IoMT, 19f
Wearable sensor-based sleep posture analysis, algorithmic trends in, 120–122
  hierarchical sensor information fusion, 121–122
  sensor data classification pipeline, 120–121
Wearable sensors, 4, 118
  in-bed postural activity using, 125–126
  mass fabrication, 219–223
  radio frequency identification (RFID) wearables, 208–212
  stretchability, 212–215
  and variable human tissue dielectrics, 215–219
Weight-bearing control (WBC) orthosis, 74
Wideband (WB) antennas function, 88
WiFi-based sleep posture sensing, 117
Wireless sensors, 117

Milton Keynes UK
Ingram Content Group UK Ltd.
UKHW050230091224
451733UK00028B/11